SOVIET NIGHTINGALES

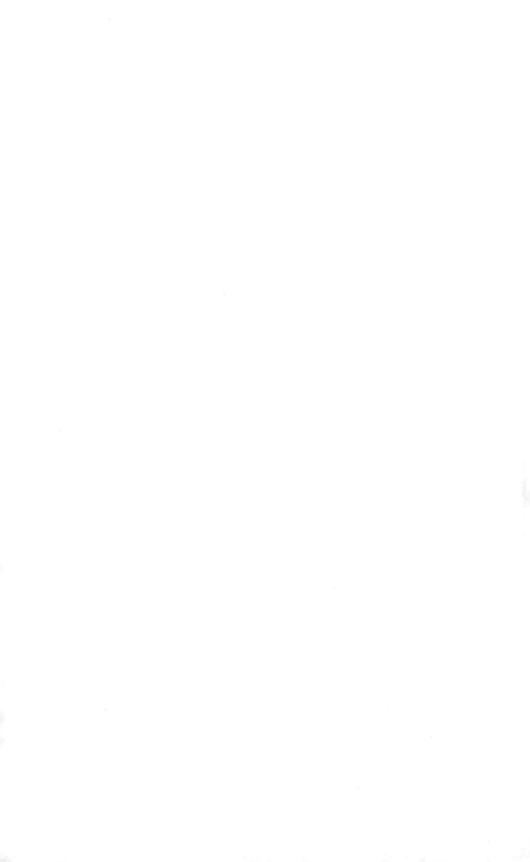

SOVIET NIGHTINGALES

CARE UNDER COMMUNISM

SUSAN GRANT

CORNELL UNIVERSITY PRESS
Ithaca and London

Thanks to generous funding from Liverpool John Moores University, the e-book editions of this book are available as open access volumes through the Cornell Open initiative.

First published 2022 by Cornell University Press

Library of Congress Cataloging-in-Publication Data

Names: Grant, Susan, 1982– author.
Title: Soviet nightingales : care under communism / Susan Grant.
Description: Ithaca [New York] : Cornell University Press, 2022. | Includes bibliographical references and index.
Identifiers: LCCN 2021045769 (print) | LCCN 2021045770 (ebook) | ISBN 9781501763564 (hardcover) | ISBN 9781501762598 (paperback) | ISBN 9781501762604 (pdf) | ISBN 9781501762611 (epub)
Subjects: LCSH: Social medicine—Soviet Union. | Nurses—Soviet Union—History. | Nurses—Soviet Union—Social conditions. | Nursing ethics—Soviet Union. | Medical ethics—Soviet Union.
Classification: LCC RA418.3.S65 G73 2022 (print) | LCC RA418.3.S65 (ebook) | DDC 362.10947—dc23
LC record available at https://lccn.loc.gov/2021045769
LC ebook record available at https://lccn.loc.gov/20210 45770

To Shane,
and in memory of my grandmother, Margaret Grant

CONTENTS

ACKNOWLEDGMENTS

This book has been ten years in the making, and I am grateful to many organizations and people. *Soviet Nightingales* would not have been possible without the generous funding provided by the Irish Research Council / Marie Curie CARA Postdoctoral Mobility Fellowship; the Alice Fisher Society Fellowship Award from the Barbara Bates Center for the Study of the History of Nursing, University of Pennsylvania; University College Dublin (UCD) Seed Funding; a Wellcome Trust Small Grant for a workshop at UCD in 2014; and Liverpool John Moores University (LJMU) Quality Related (QR) research funding.

I could not have asked for two more inspirational and generous mentors in Judith Devlin at University College Dublin and Susan Gross Solomon at the University of Toronto. Their influence has been immense and is written all over this book. The University of Toronto was a stimulating and friendly home, and I thank Seth Bernstein, Mayhill Fowler, Zbigniew Wojnowski, Jennifer Polk, Alison Smith, Peter Solomon, Sioban Nelson, Tracy McDonald, Jana Oldman, Angela Byrne, Lynne Viola, Janet Hyer, and colleagues at the Munk School of Global Affairs for making my time there so enjoyable and productive. At the Barbara Bates Center for the Study of the History of Nursing, University of Pennsylvania, I am particularly grateful for the guidance of Julie Fairman. While in Philadelphia, I also had the immense pleasure of working in the American Friends Service Committee (AFSC) archives and benefited from the help of the wonderful Don Davis.

I am indebted to a number of archive and library staff whose help, guidance, and good humor made working away from home a pleasure. I learned much from my visits to several medical museums, including the Museum for the History of the Sisters of Mercy Communities in Moscow. In St. Petersburg, the Russian Nurses Association, and in particular Valentina Sarkisova and Natalia Serebrennikova, welcomed and helped me in spite of their busy schedules. Yanina Karpenkina provided research assistance. Katherine Stephan, Cath Dishman, and Maria Follett from the LJMU library helped make this book Open Access. Participating in conferences and workshops has been crucial to shaping this research. I am grateful to colleagues for invitations to present papers about nursing and some of the themes in *Soviet Nightingales*.

A number of colleagues and friends have made a mark on this book through various conversations, and some generously read and commented on chapter drafts, as well as pointing me in the direction of research material and sharing sources (and some have done all of this!). In no particular order they include Seth Bernstein, Benjamin Zajicek, Donald Filtzer, Susan Gross Solomon, Johanna Conterio, James Ryan, Dan Healey, Christopher Burton, Melanie Ilic, Elena Kozlovtseva, William A. Glaser, Botakoz Kassymbekova, Mikhail Poddubnyi, Jonathan Waterlow, Sioban Nelson, Elena Zdravomyslova, Gleb Albert, Tony Heywood, Alissa Klots, Chris Read, Frances Bernstein, Claire Shaw, Anne Marie Rafferty, Maria Kunkite, James Crossland, Tom Beaumont, Anna Hajkova, Judith Devlin, Laura Kelly, Mark Jones, Isaac McKean Scarborough, Jaime Lapeyre, and William Glaser. There are so many people whom I met along the way that I might not mention here but to whom I am grateful. Any errors or omissions are naturally my responsibility.

LJMU provided a stimulating and convivial environment in which to finish this book, and I thank my colleagues there, especially Joe Yates, Alex Miles, David Clampin, Tom Beaumont, Gillian O'Brien, Nick White, Olivia Saunders, James Crossland, Lucinda Matthews-Jones, Andrea Livesley, Chris Vaughan, Lucy Dunlop, Matthew Hill, Alison Francis, Janice Johnston and Steve Lawlor. My thanks to friends and colleagues in Dublin, including Niamh Wycherley, Laura Kelly, Maria Falina, Suzanne Darcy, Catherine Cox, and Mercedes Penalba-Sotorrio. Special thanks to James Ryan, Angela Byrne, and Seth Bernstein for making international work so enjoyable.

In Moscow Olga Kleshaeva pulled me away from work to enjoy walks, Sunday afternoon cycles, and pleasant cultural outings around the city. Svetlana Maximenko, who put a roof over my head during my first trip to Moscow in 2005, continues to look out for me. Svet's late mother, Olga Nikolaevna; her daughter, Lera; son Kolya, and partner, Vasily, became my Russian family.

At Cornell University Press I had the great pleasure of working with Roger Haydon before his retirement and later Emily Andrews, Bethany Wasik and Allegra Martschenko. I am also grateful to Cornell's production team and especially Susan Specter. I also thank Kristen Bettcher for overseeing the copyediting process and Susan Certo for indexing. Cornell's peer reviewers provided me with constructive and insightful feedback that greatly enhanced the manuscript. I am also very grateful to the production team at Cornell.

My grandmother, Margaret Grant (1918–2008), trained as a nurse in London in the late 1930s, and my childhood bedtime stories were replete with stories about nursing. She always wanted me to follow her career choice, and even though I chose a different path, she evidently exerted an influence. I thank Thomas, Nora, Richard, and Aoife Grant; Carmel Fraher; and the late Richard Fraher for their love and support. And to Shane—thank you.

Some ideas and material that appear in the book were published elsewhere, and I acknowledge these in the appropriate chapters. Separately, I note the following: Susan Grant, "Creating Cadres of Soviet Nurses, 1936–1941," in *Russian and Soviet Health Care from an International Perspective: Comparing Professions, Practice and Gender, 1880–1960*, edited by Susan Grant (London: Palgrave Macmillan, 2017), 57–75, reproduced with permission of Palgrave Macmillan; Susan Grant, "Nurses in the Soviet Union: Explorations of Gender in State and Society," in *The Palgrave Handbook of Women and Gender in Twentieth-Century Russia and the Soviet Union*, edited by Melanie Ilic (London: Palgrave Macmillan, 2018), 249–265, reproduced with permission of Palgrave Macmillan.

ABBREVIATIONS AND GLOSSARY

AFSC	American Friends Service Committee
akusherka	midwife
BGSO	Be Prepared for Sanitary Defense
Cheka	All-Russian Extraordinary Commission for Combating Counterrevolution and Sabotage
Commissariat	Ministry or Department
delo (d.)	Folder in an opis′
Donprofobr	Don Department of Professional Education
Donzdravotdel	Don Health Department
Gubzdravotdel	Provincial Health Department
feldsher (m) / feldsheritsa (f)	medical worker less qualified than a doctor and usually stationed in rural areas
fond (f.)	archive holding/collection
GAGS	State Archive of Sochi
GARF	State Archive of the Russian Federation
GATO	State Archive of Tambov Oblast
Glavprofobr	Main Committee for Professional-Technical Education

Gosplan	State Planning Agency
GSO	Get Ready for Sanitary Defense
GTO	Get Ready for Labor and Defense
gubernia	territorial unit in Russia (until 1929)
HPSSS	Harvard Project on the Soviet Social System Online
ICN	International Council of Nurses
list (l.)	page (followed by "ob" [*oborot'*] means text is on the reverse side of the page)
LSF	Library of the Society of Friends / Quakers in Britain
Narkomzdrav	People's Commissariat of Health
NEP	New Economic Policy
NKVD	People's Commissariat of Internal Affairs
OMM	Department for the Protection of Mothers and Infants
opis' (op.)	a fond subgroup
Osoaviakhim	Society for the Assistance of Defense, Aircraft, and Chemical Construction
OTE	Department of Technical Use
Rabfak(i)	school(s) for workers
RAC	Rockefeller Archive Center
RGASPI	Russian State Archive of Socio-Political History

RGASPI-M	Russian State Archive of Socio-Political History (Communist Youth League)
RGVA	Russian State Military Archive
ROKK	Russian Society of the Red Cross
RSFSR	Russian Soviet Federated Socialist Republic
sanitarka (s) / *sanitarki* (pl)	orderly
sidelka (s) / *sidelki* (pl)	aide or nurse who "sits" with a patient
SOKK and KP USSR	All-Union Society of the Red Cross and Red Crescent USSR (or SOKK; the Soviet Red Cross as a synonym)
Sovnarkom	Council of People's Commissars
Svodka	secret police report
tekhnikum	medical college
TsDAVO	Central State Archive of the Supreme Organs of Government and Administration of Ukraine
Tsentrokrest	Central Committee of the Russian Society of the Red Cross
TsGAIPD SPb	Central State Archive of Historico-Political Records of St. Petersburg
TsGAM	Central State Archive of the City of Moscow
TsGAMO	Central State Archive of Moscow Oblast
TsGASPb	Central State Archive of St. Petersburg
TsNIAGI	Central Scientific-Research Midwifery-Gynecological Institute

VDNKh	Exhibition of Achievements of the National Economy
Vsemedikosantrud/ Medsantrud	All-Russian Medical-Sanitary Work/ Medical Sanitary Work (Trade Union for Medical Workers)
VTsSPS	All-Union Central Council of Trade Unions
VUZ	Institute of Higher Education
WHO	World Health Organization

Note on Translation and Transliteration

I have followed the Library of Congress system for Russian transliteration. Whenever possible I try to use the more common form (for example, Lunacharsky instead of Lunacharskii or gubernia instead of guberniia), or I have dropped the soft sign for frequently used Russian words (for example, feldsher instead of *fel'dsher*). In keeping with the source material, I transliterate from Russian when referring to cities, towns, and individuals located in the USSR (for example, Kiev instead of Kyiv).

Unless otherwise noted, all translation from Russian to English is my own. I am responsible for any errors or omissions.

SOVIET NIGHTINGALES

Introduction

In 1922 an interesting exchange took place in Moscow's Botkin hospital concerning a "delicate and even shy" patient who had just had a bullet extracted from his neck and was recovering in ward no. 44.[1] The patient wanted to know all about his nurse, the other patients, and the medical personnel. He even asked the nurse why she looked so "bad" and questioned the professor tending to him about why this nurse was "working day and night, without rest." He noticed the physical toll nursing work took on people. Finally, he wanted to know how he could thank this nurse who had been taking care of him. The inquisitive patient was none other than the leader of the world communist revolution, Vladimir I. Lenin. Within a few days the nurse who had tirelessly taken care of Lenin received a resort pass to the Crimea, issued by Commissar of Health Nikolai Semashko on the direct instruction of her thoughtful patient.[2] The busy leader, it seemed, cared about nurses. The account was in a 1980 book on Lenin and Soviet public health, and the moral of the story was that the Soviet state cared about its nurses.

Lenin's nurse—Ekaterina Alekseevna Nechkina—was later featured in the journal *Nurse*. By the time her story appeared in a 1948 issue of the publication, Nechkina had already accumulated some thirty-seven years' work experience. Born into a working-class family, she had the right class credentials, but life was far from easy. Orphaned at just fifteen years old, Nechkina moved from the provinces to Moscow to be under the guardianship of her uncle, a doctor in the Staro-Ekaterinskaia (Old Catherine) hospital. She joined the Sisters of Mercy school attached to the Aleksandrovskaia nursing community and graduated in 1911.[3] After that she entered the Soldatenkovskaia hospital's surgical department (later the Botkin hospital), where she remained for fifteen years. A "thoughtful, dedicated" worker, she was promoted from ward nurse to senior nurse in 1916. As testament to her high standing, she had the "great honor" of caring for Vladimir Ilyich Lenin in April 1922. In the mid-1920s the hospital appointed her head nurse of its new surgical building.[4]

Nechkina was valued as a "highly cultured" worker who had good relations with her patients. She possessed the typical attributes of other Soviet workers—she constantly "worked on herself" to improve her education and was an example to others.[5] We do not know what exactly happened to Nechkina during the revolution, but like so many other nurses who had trained prior to the revolution she continued her hospital work. Her sound working-class background no doubt helped in shielding her from dismissal or arrest. The fact that she had trained in a tsarist nursing community did not negatively affect her career; if anything, she was valued more because of the training and discipline she acquired before the revolution.

Cold War histories tell us that a totalitarian system cowed and repressed Soviet citizens. And while that is true to an extent—the Soviet Union was an illiberal society, after all—people, nurses included, found ways of existing and sometimes thriving in this world. When the Bolsheviks initially set about constructing a socialist society and a New Soviet Person, they were venturing forth into the unknown. They were torn between the old and the new: How would vast numbers of people, predominantly peasants, accustomed to the "old" tsarist ways, help the Bolsheviks build a shiny new world based on Marxist-Leninist principles? They desperately needed healthcare workers to address the public health crisis, but oftentimes these nurses were from the "old" imperial world. If there were nurses and other medical workers who disagreed with the Bolshevik system, they nonetheless continued to work within that system.

Although we might associate the Stalinist years with terror, violence, and repression, and assume that people tolerated these conditions out of fear, we overlook the fact that alternative narratives ran alongside the hunt for enemies. The historian Karl Schlögel's tome on the year 1937 shows us that Soviet citizens continued to go to work, parks, theaters, and concerts and basically got on with their lives as the terror unfolded.[6] The state, while unleashing mechanisms of terror, reminded Soviet citizens that the authorities were constructing metro stations and stadiums and creating a cultured way of life for them. People were told that Stalin and the Soviet government cared about them and that nurses and other medical workers would provide them with the best possible care. But state promises to the people depended on caregivers meeting these expectations. As I show in *Soviet Nightingales*, that was not always the case. The Bolsheviks were too slow to convey sufficient prestige and respect on nursing, and it suffered as a result. Lack of funding and organization undermined standards of nursing care and left medical workers in the hopeless position of working for low salaries in terrible conditions. This situation worsened after the war and only began to improve in the 1950s and 1960s.

For Soviet citizens, good care was, forgive the pun, a game of Russian roulette. The ideological nature of the Soviet system placed nurses in an unusual position. As representatives of the new, socialist order, nurses in the Soviet Union had the vitally important task of caring for future communists. They had to be more than competent: they had to be politically loyal, ideologically literate, and, at varying times, maternal. Yet, nurses inhabited a unique place in Soviet society: as part of a caring profession with roots in charity and the aristocracy, they sat somewhat uncomfortably in the revolutionary world of the Bolsheviks. This book addresses that discomfort by exploring the habitat of Soviet nurses and their colleagues. How did nurses regard the new socialist society? Was it everything they feared or hoped?

At the heart of this book, I show that nurses were crucial symbols of the new Soviet state. The whole ethos and nature of nursing, as the socialist state eventually came to realize, was paramount to the socialist ideological mission. *Soviet Nightingales* analyzes the Bolshevik effort to define the "Soviet" nurse and organize a new system of socialist care for the masses. The process of molding the Soviet nurse was challenging, and I examine the immense educational and organizational tasks that confronted the state as it attempted to identify the kind of nurse that most suited the country's medical, material, and moral needs. Telling the story of nursing necessarily engages with Soviet politics, culture, and society, as well as nursing literature. Nursing ebbed and flowed with the social and political currents, the daily lives of medical professionals and patients shaped by the revolution, the Great Terror, war, "thaw," and glasnost (openness). I analyze living and working conditions, nurse-patient relations, international contact, and education to piece together a holistic picture of the Soviet nurse. Nurses in the Soviet Union have hitherto received insufficient scholarly attention: their history is little known, yet it tells us much about Soviet society.[7]

Defining Soviet Medical Workers

This book deals with a broad typology of medical personnel. Physicians, surgeons, and other medical specialists sat atop the Russian and Soviet healthcare pyramid. The next tier comprised "middle" (*srednyi*) medical workers, a long list of personnel that included, among others, nurses, midwives, feldshers (paramedics), feldsheritsas (female feldshers), dentists, pharmacists, and laboratory workers. Pilloried and praised, the new Bolshevik authorities loathed the feldshers for their lack of scientific background, and they endeavored to completely eliminate this stratum of medical worker.[8] Finally, "junior" (*mladshii*) medical personnel occupied the lowest tier, and included among them were orderlies, *sidelki*, and nannies. The *sidelka*—literally, someone who "sits," such as a nursing aide or caregiver—was a curious figure in Russian and Soviet history. But the *sidelki* often horrified Soviet healthcare authorities, as they were usually uneducated and did not meet the lofty ideals of the revolution and its "New Soviet Person." Although the nurse is the main protagonist of this story, the wider cast of medical workers play important roles too.

The function of middle and junior medical workers was largely seen as facilitating the work of the doctor, and these were not considered particularly prestigious positions. None of the medical professions were especially well remunerated. When researching this book, I quickly realized that a history of Soviet nursing would also have to be a history of a broad spectrum of medical workers. To tell the story of Soviet nursing is also to tell the story of middle and junior medical workers who often shared the same grievances, hardship, suffering, and rewards. And it proved almost impossible to separate them, for two reasons: (1) they were usually lumped together in the source material, and (2) they worked together and interacted every day—care in a socialist society was a team effort. Doctors drift in and out of the book for this same reason: they provided care alongside nurses and orderlies and worked in similar conditions.

The Soviet case is set apart from other international histories of healthcare because the Soviet Union was a worker state: the Bolsheviks quickly set about putting in place structures and policies allowing its citizens to access education so that they could become important contributors to the new socialist society through their labor. It was not uncommon for doctors and nurses in the Soviet Union to have entered the medical profession at the lowest rung as orderlies or middle medical workers and then worked their way up through the healthcare hierarchy and Soviet society.[9] But their journeys reflected the turbulence and uncertainty of a state in flux or in crisis. In the early revolutionary years the state performed a kind of juggling act between the "old" and "new" way of life when it came to establishing a class-based society. Healthcare is a prime example. Nurses, in the form of Sisters of Mercy, and especially feldshers, bore the brunt of campaigns to rid socialist society of its prerevolutionary past. These were not the typical "proletarian" figures deemed worthy of representing the new Soviet state.

Uncertainty about the role and even existence of certain forms of medical worker led to ambiguities in how people perceived nurses and even doctors. In contrast to other countries with a clearly defined system based on the doctor and nurse, the Russian and later Soviet system struggled to work out the best way of delivering care through its three-level system, in place for much of the Soviet period. In this system the orderly and junior medical workers often spent a great deal of time with patients. The Soviet state was built on Marxist-Leninist ideology that strongly influenced healthcare. A prophylactic orientation shaped medical work in theory and in practice. As Soviet healthcare officials examined public health and current social needs, including looking abroad to see how other healthcare systems fared, middle and junior medical workers saw their role and function change over time. Healthcare was subject to seemingly constant review and modification as part of the socialist experiment. New types of nurses in the 1920s tackled mother and child health, military training notched up many hours on nursing curricula in the late 1930s, and attestation arrived in the late Soviet period. Consequently, one of the basic issues for nurses lay in understanding their professional territory. While textbooks outlined their role and function, in practice personnel shortages and labor turnover could result in nurses taking on the work of orderlies. For this reason, issues around workload and salaries receive a good deal of attention in this book.

There are many parallels between the Soviet and contemporary international experience of nursing, none more so than the nursing crisis we so often read about today. Shortages of qualified nurses have led to greater demands for healthcare assistants. In Soviet parlance, these would be "junior" medical workers. Their role was to relieve nurses of their housekeeping work so they could focus on patient care. Much of the discussion in the book centers on debates about these kinds of responsibilities. And such debates continue. In the United Kingdom the Royal College of Nursing (RCN) recommends a skill-mix ratio of 65 percent registered nurses to 35 percent healthcare assistants.[10] The RCN recognizes that healthcare assistants can support registered nurses and assume some of the administrative and housekeeping work to allow nurses to spend more time with patients, but it acknowledges that this "has not been widely enacted upon."[11] In the Soviet Union a skill-mix ratio was already in place, albeit as a necessary consequence of the absence of trained nurses.

The struggle of Soviet medical authorities to increase the quantity of nurses is a problem now faced in many countries, especially in the United Kingdom, where, for the first time in ten years, more nurses left the profession in 2017 than joined the register.[12] Similar conversations about safe staffing levels are taking place in the United States. Even though increasing the number of registered nurses can yield a cost saving of about $3 billion, hospitals in the United States are "feeling pressure to reduce labor costs by eliminating or understaffing registered nurse positions."[13] These problems characterize nursing in Canada, Australia, France, Germany, and many other countries.[14] In the Russian Federation there was a shortage of 130,000 nurses in 2019, while that same year there was a shortage of 137,000 junior medical workers, compared to 2018.[15] In 2019 Russian junior medical worker positions were subject to drastic cuts in hospitals and clinics and their jobs recategorized to "janitors."[16] The reduction in the number of junior medical personnel led to increased workloads for nurses. International nurse staffing standards and conditions for medical workers are still below optimum levels some eighty to ninety years after debates on the same issue in the Soviet Union.

Professional Autonomy, Gender, and Medicine

For nurses the lines between "the duty to care for others and the right to control their own activities in the name of caring" are often blurred.[17] For Soviet nurses the duty to care usually took precedence. Altruism characterized the profession, while autonomy took a backseat.[18] That said, while Soviet nurses may not have had many rights to control their own activities on a macro level, in the micro context of a hospital department they might have had more opportunities for professional autonomy.[19] *Soviet Nightingales* shows that nurses working in a range of healthcare institutions had quite different experiences depending on relationships with head doctors and colleagues and on local politics. And although Soviet nurses did not have a specific nursing union or association with easily identifiable nursing leaders to advance their cause, they nonetheless spoke out when they felt that their rights were infringed on.

As Soviet nurses navigated their professional course, they did so within a healthcare system that suffered from lack of funding, the struggle to modernize, an informal economy, and other shortcomings. Toiling in a vastly bureaucratic system, and often having to do physically and emotionally exhausting work, nurses and middle medical workers were frequently let down by the Soviet system. As the "faces" of healthcare, they saw their situation sometimes worsen because they acted as a buffer between the system and its patients. In an ideological and political context where "cadres" decided everything, nurses and other middle medical workers were often at the receiving end of much criticism. Many of the book's chapters assess the changing positions and fortunes of these workers.

The Russian and Soviet healthcare system overwhelmingly consisted of women workers. Unlike in Western countries, this feminization did not apply just to nursing and auxiliary support: in the Soviet Union large numbers of doctors were women. For that reason, the Soviet case is interesting because many of the developments around gender dynamics arising from increasing numbers of women in medicine were already present in the Soviet Union.[20] Consequently, workplace relations in Soviet healthcare were not strictly delineated along traditional male / doctor or female / nurse lines. Still, men often held senior positions within a medical setting.[21] Male doctors both supported and looked down on nurses, for various reasons explored in *Soviet Nightingales*. In some cases strained professional relationships with male doctors eroded nurses' self-esteem.[22] The relationship between women doctors and female nurses is less clear, although nurses sometimes characterized relationships with senior nurses or women doctors as being supportive. The complexities of the Soviet social and political context, combined with a dearth of source material, make it difficult to draw neat conclusions about complex workplace dynamics and gender relations among healthcare professionals.

Emotions, Identity, and Professionalization

Soviet Nightingales is laden with emotion. This relates to the language of care and the physical act of caring and how both play out in medical and political contexts. "Care" and "compassion" are terms we frequently encounter in the Soviet literature on nursing. Compassion is a feeling but also an action that involves helping others.[23] In the Soviet context mercy and compassion were part of a nurse's tool kit: these were fundamental to providing a high standard of care. In Russian there are two words for care: *zabota* (care, as in concern) and *ukhod* (the act of caring for someone).[24] We see both terms in the sources. Often *zabota* refers to the general delivery of care and can seem more abstract than the personal or individual *ukhod*. Whichever term is used, "care" is seen as intrinsic to nursing. But when nursing shifts from caring to administrative work, we move away from the realm of emotion and feeling and into a world that raises questions about authenticity and "real" nursing work.

In their work on nursing care, nursing scholars Sioban Nelson and Suzanne Gordon push back against connotations of "real nurses" and "emotional work" and the view that those nurses who work in administrative or highly technical roles are not considered authentic.[25] In the Soviet case the "authentic" nurse was often involved in doing emotion work, suggesting that "real" nurses did not spend most of their time doing administrative or technical work. Emotion-based narratives of care and compassion make it all too easy to overlook a nurse's hard-earned skills and knowledge.[26] Such associations belittle the nurse in a myriad ways, on both a professional and a personal level. Stereotyping nurses as kindly caregivers can marginalize them within the broader healthcare profession, affecting their self-esteem and sense of identity. The self, after all, does not exist in a vacuum but interacts with other individuals and communities who shape identity.[27] These are problems that confront nursing, past and present, but they often assumed different levels of intensity in the Soviet Union, usually according to a topical propaganda campaign. Ironically, the altruistic and philanthropic roots of Russian and international nursing were anathema to the young Soviet state, and yet it too ended up characterizing nurses in a similarly simplistic way.[28]

I argue that over the course of the 1930s–1950s nurses in the Soviet Union became increasingly professionalized, although there is a lack of consensus today about what "professionalization" constitutes. Sociologists and some healthcare experts have considered this term problematic and unhelpful.[29] Before the rise of sociological definitions of the professions from the mid-1950s to the 1980s, nursing was a legitimate form of profession or occupation.[30] One nursing textbook published in 2001 examines the following characteristics of the profession: "A body of Specialized Knowledge," "Use of the Scientific Method to Enlarge the Body of Knowledge," "Education Within institutes of Higher Education," "Control of Professional Policy and Professional Activity," "A Code of Ethics, "Nursing as a Lifetime Commitment," and "Service to the Public".[31]

The term "professionalism" can connote striving for "excellence in performance" and a "sense of ethics and responsibility in relationship to [nurses'] careers."[32] My use of terms such as "professional" and "professionalization" denote recognition and prestige afforded to nurses and nursing. This might entail higher levels of training and education, growing authority within a healthcare setting, or access to knowledge through conferences and publications. Professionalization terminology acts as a foil to simplistic portrayals of nurses as kind, caring workers, a reminder that nurses are also skilled workers engaged in complex tasks.[33] It helps move us away from the kind of "sentimentalized caring rhetoric" that we see today and that the Soviet state and nurses also deployed.[34]

Marginalization and Morality

In a 2001 US nursing textbook first published in 1980, students learn that their work is hard to define, straddling the borders of art and science, profession and occupation.[35] Prospective nurses are informed that their work is about caring for a person's health, whereas medicine is "concerned with the diagnosis and treatment (and cure) of disease."[36] The authors of a review of nurse theorists provide a "widely accepted definition" of nursing from Virginia Henderson for the International Council of Nurses (ICN) in 1958: "The unique function of the nurse is to assist the individual, sick or well, in the performance of those activities contributing to the health or its recovery (or to peaceful death) that he would perform unaided if he had the necessary strength, will or knowledge. And to do this in such a way as to help him gain independence as rapidly as possible."[37]

A definition from nurse theorist Martha E. Rogers in 1984 defines nursing as "an art and a science that is humanistic and humanitarian directed toward the unitary human, and concerned with the nature and direction of human development."[38] In addition to the many definitions of nursing from figures such as Florence Nightingale, Hildegard Peplau, and Myra Levine, US-based nurses could also look to the American Nurses Association and the National Council of State Boards of Nursing for further guidance on how to define and understand their role.[39] The limitless interpretations suggest that nursing escapes easy definition. This was similarly the case in the Soviet Union.

A 1979 Soviet textbook for junior nurses defined care work as "assisting in satisfying basic life functions: ingesting food, bowel and bladder emptying, personal hygiene, helping the nurse or doctor during manipulations with acute patients—vomiting, phlegmatic cough, incontinence [involuntary defecation, or *neproizvol'naia defekatsiia*], and also supporting the sanitary-hygiene conditions of a patient's bed, wards and departments, etc."[40] In a section on general patient care and the "moral character and norms of behavior for the junior nurse," students learn that they are the "first aide to the ward nurse and doctor" and that "in communist society the basic medical morality is humanism."[41] Although there was no specific equivalent to the code of ethics introduced in the United States in 1950, the ICN Code of Ethics of 1953, or even the Florence Nightingale Pledge of 1893, Soviet discussions about the "moral character" of the nurse infused Soviet nursing in the 1950s and 1960s. By the early 1980s Leonid Brezhnev had inspired concern about humanity, fueling discussion on deontology and ethics in nursing.[42] As the 1979 Soviet textbook indicates, an entanglement between love and duty prevailed. Junior nurses "[were to] have defined medical knowledge and professional skills to help the patient," while "successful treatment" often depended on her "skill, attention and love."[43] They were to be sensitive and disciplined workers who also had practical personal hygiene rules to follow, such as bathing once a week and showering after every shift.[44] A sense of humanity imbued nursing work in the Soviet Union, a fact that allowed nurses to be cast as clean heroes and moral leaders.

Paradoxically, nurses were also marginal figures or people marginalized by the Soviet project. To be sure, many engaged with processes of transformation and constructed identities that fit into a broader socialist story (Nechkina, Lenin's nurse, perhaps being one such example), but this book is more an examination of nursing work, that is to say, the public and professional face of Soviet care. How did nurses adapt to Bolshevik ideas about nursing and care? What did care mean under socialism—was it not a time of incessant repression and misery? The following case of a middle medical worker is illustrative of some of these issues.

Six years after the revolution a feldsheritsa wrote to *Medical Worker* (*Meditsinskii rabotnik*) about the May 1 holiday. Her family was excited about attending the festivities, but she was too physically exhausted to take her place among them.[45] This woman made known her support for the revolution and regime but did not conceal her dissatisfaction with her job. She worked a twenty-four-hour shift without a break and returned home at ten in the morning to find that her daughter had already left for the holiday celebrations. At work she had spent "every hour, every minute" caring for patients without time to eat or drink. When she finally returned home, she could not even summon the energy to prepare breakfast. Yet this tired feldsheritsa had to "find the strength to go back to the hospital the following day." She wrote about how she would meet people the next day and hear them say that everyone participated in the May 1 celebrations except "backward" medical workers. "Is this fair?" she asked and suggested that people help medical workers out of their awful predicament rather than "judge" them.[46] The revolution had done nothing for these workers, and the suspicious, critical attitude of others only made them feel more aggrieved. The lingering dissatisfaction medical workers felt was an ominous sign of things to come.

The sense of marginalization manifested in different forms over the entire Soviet period. To be sure, nursing was stripped of its religious associations, but care, ethics, and notions of the good nurse made their way into socialist discourse. We can understand that much of this had to do with a compulsion to "conceptualize nursing as a fundamentally moral act."[47] But morality in the Soviet context was not quite the same as the "moral agency" found in more modern conceptions of nursing—the "agency" part was problematic.[48] Soviet nurses were to be doctors' assistants, and their moral role was often more closely connected to being "good" communists.[49] In the Soviet Union morality was frequently politicized and relocated from the private to the public sphere: ideology consequently forms the "background picture" for the "moral and spiritual intuitions" of Soviet citizens.[50] Nurses and indeed other medical workers navigated ideological and professional codes or scripts that characterized their relations to the patient.

As the Bolsheviks attempted to move away from religion, they imparted a strict moral and ethical code on the behavior of nurses and other medical workers. Comprising a mix of revolutionary trained Sisters of Mercy and newly trained Soviet nurses, nursing inhabited a somewhat awkward position in the new worker-peasant state. The state elevated science and medicine as rational and objective pursuits during the entire Soviet period—they were ideologically sound fields of expertise to lead the revolution forward—but nursing lagged behind as a shadowy occupation that the new authorities at first seemed unable to fathom. The Bolshevik conception of nursing came to reflect ethical and moral ideas around "the good life" and the sense of "the importance of the everyday in human life" and "the importance of suffering."[51] While these ideas might seem to go against the grain of an authoritarian society such as the Soviet Union, nursing and, more broadly, healthcare became spheres defined by a dialogue about care of the person.

While it is clear that later narratives of kind and caring nurses produced predominantly in Soviet nursing literature reflected official ideological lines, especially after the 1961 Moral Code of the Builder of Communism, the work of contemporary authors on nursing care suggests that nurses can be complicit in the construction of such a narrative.[52] Some nurses describe their work as caregiving and humanistic rather than medical or technical—this is the role and function they see themselves inhabiting.[53] Soviet nurses saw themselves occupying a similar kind of caregiving space and conceived of their work as a type of moral duty to support the emotional and mental well-being of the patient. But that did not mean that they were not also hungry for knowledge and professional recognition. Attendance at advanced training courses required every three years offered them a chance to improve their skills and knowledge. As others working on nursing have argued, nurses themselves often foreground their role as caregivers: to use a modern expression, they see this as their "unique selling point."[54] The compulsion to constantly redefine their role suggests an ongoing sense of alienation and marginalization born of a lack of public and perhaps official understanding of what nursing work means and entails. This is something that affects nurses past and present, Soviet and non-Soviet.

Chapters

This book's nine chapters span the nineteenth and twentieth centuries. Our story starts with the origins of organized nursing care in Russia and goes full circle to the end of the Soviet Union. The Crimean War (1854–1856), perhaps best known in medical history for the work of Florence Nightingale, was also fundamental to the establishment of Russian nursing. After Crimea, Sisters of Mercy cared for wounded soldiers at times of war and during epidemics and continued their work during peacetime in hospitals and nursing communities across the empire. In chapter 1, I contend that Russian nursing developed along similar, though not identical, lines to European nursing. I show that the experience of the First World War changed Russian nursing when the old imperial system began to fragment under the pressure of increasing conflict and chaos. Nursing organizations felt this fragmentation. The establishment of professional nursing unions, the most prominent being the All-Russian Union of the Society of the Sisters of Mercy, established in August 1917, signified a drive for greater independence and professionalization within nursing. The impetus for change gained pace during the February and October Revolutions when Bolsheviks and leading Sisters of Mercy worked together to shape nursing care through the development of a new education and training program.

In chapter 2, I focus on the period of transition during the civil war years, 1918–1921, and the effort to establish a Soviet system of nursing in the early 1920s. Revolutionary tensions did not dissipate but continued to shape attitudes to nurses and nursing reform well into the 1920s and even the 1930s. While the Soviet public health authorities pushed for a new type of socialist nurse, divested of any former religious associations, many Sisters of Mercy remained working as before. In fact, despite resistance from "new" cadres, prerevolutionary nurses formed the backbone of the nursing service during the early Soviet period. The civil war years were also marked by battles between various Soviet authorities—inter alia, public health, the Red Army, and the medical union—all trying to seize and reclaim nursing infrastructure and assets from the Red Cross. The fraught transition process receives attention in this chapter, as do the complicated conditions on the ground. Lack of resources, personnel, medicines, and food affected the treatment and care of patients as well as working conditions for medical staff.

In chapter 3, I argue that many of the issues confronting the Soviet government with regard to nursing care and in particular nursing education were to an extent universal. I consider how nursing care and education, as envisioned by the Commissariat of Health, connected to broader international trends.

During and after the First World War large-scale medical relief work was undertaken in Europe. This formed part of the general humanitarian effort conducted by primarily US charitable organizations and philanthropies. The Soviet government, as this chapter shows, was open to negotiation during the course of the 1920s. Conversations and connections with those involved in foreign healthcare also helped shape Soviet ideas about nursing and public healthcare that might work in 1920s Soviet Russia. The growing attention paid to mother and infant care exemplifies this effort. In this regard, I examine Quaker attempts to establish a nurse training school in Russia, an effort that reveals much about both Western and Russian attitudes to public healthcare in the 1920s. The attempt to establish and operate the school illustrates the nature and extent of the Western "superiority" complex.

Chapter 4 places nurses in the broader medical worker experience and situates them within the context of the New Economic Policy (NEP) and the introduction of the Five-Year Plan. How did these policies affect public healthcare as well as the reality of daily life for middle medical workers in the Soviet Union? One of the main problems during the 1920s was unemployment, and I analyze this topic in relation to medical workers. Here a huge paradox existed—despite an urgent need for professionally trained medical workers, the unemployment rate for medical personnel was high. One of the primary reasons was their low pay, and the resulting flight from the profession led to fears over a loss of medical specialists. This raises the question: Who, exactly, was caring for Soviet citizens? Also assessed in this chapter are the associated problems of poor living and working conditions for medical workers, which sometimes created tensions in the workplace. Accusations of unprofessionalism and press scandals further served to frustrate and alienate medical workers. One of the other alarming features during the late 1920s was violence against medical workers, who often lived in fear of assaults by patients. Tensions increased between the state and medical workers as a result and continued to mount during the late 1920s and early 1930s.

Joseph Stalin's Constitution of 1936 prioritized the well-being of all citizens, but cases of violence and tensions in the workplace threatened to undermine this goal for patients and medical personnel. Chapter 5 considers how Soviet healthcare met the needs of patients. While workers called for improvements in their salaries and living conditions, major reforms were under way in nursing and medical education. Soviet commissariats underwent restructuring after 1936, and these changes took place in healthcare too. The Commissariat of Health set about revising nursing curricula and discussed the role of nurses in hospitals and clinics. These reforms coincided with a period of medical advancement that raised questions about the level of nurses' professional autonomy. Discussion about nurse qualifications, experience, and autonomy also connected to the government's ideological agenda. As state mechanisms of terror moved into action in the second half of the 1930s, nursing and healthcare narratives reassured citizens that the party-state cared about them.

Threat of war, looming large since the end of the 1920s, led to increased militarization of Soviet nurses by the 1930s. Training nurses to cope with battle wounds, blood transfusions, and chemical weapons attacks became a standard component of nurse training. Propaganda campaigns also attempted to overhaul the image of the nurse's role from passive and caring to active and paramilitary. Central to this training and increased militarization was the work of the SOKK and KP USSR in the 1930s, examined in chapter 6. Hundreds of thousands of medical workers trained through the Red Cross and Red Crescent in the 1930s and 1940s (and again after the Second World War). The beginning of the chapter focuses on the relationship of the Red Cross and Red Crescent with the Communist Youth League and efforts to promote the former. The initial goal was to shed its prerevolutionary image. Films and the press stressed the proletarian nature of SOKK and KP USSR. Patriotism played a significant role in mobilizing first communist youth and later the general public through state initiatives such as the Get Ready for Sanitation Defense (GSO) norm, introduced in 1934.

Soviet women's contribution to the war as medical workers was no less important than their role on the field of battle or on the home front. Soviet women medical workers suffered trauma, injury, and death when tending to wounded soldiers and shared the horrors and disillusionment of soldiers hospitalized behind the front lines. Chapter 7 highlights the important role of nurses during and after the Great Patriotic War, as the Second World War is called in Russia, and examines the narrative that developed around Soviet nurses. I also analyze the general preparedness of the Soviet Union's efforts to meet its healthcare needs. With the sheer scale of the war placing unprecedented pressure on the medical services, how did nurses and the healthcare system respond to the challenge? And what happened after the war? The war saw the loss of more than twenty-seven million Soviet citizens and widespread destruction. Consequently, in this chapter I am as interested in what happened in nursing and healthcare after the war as during it. Was there a direct continuity with prewar policies, or did the wartime experience and postwar challenges precipitate a change of direction?

In chapter 8, psychiatric care receives closer examination, and here I maintain a focus on assessing the late Stalinist years. A new emphasis on psychiatric nursing emerged on the eve of the war and continued and expanded in the 1940s and 1950s. I pay particular attention to psychiatric handbooks published for middle medical personnel and how forms of therapeutic care in the Soviet Union compared to broader international developments in psychiatry. How much autonomy did middle and junior medical workers wield in psychiatric institutions? What kind of training did they have? What were their working conditions like? This chapter also takes us through to the end of the Soviet period but with a specific focus on psychiatry and social rehabilitation in particular. In the late Soviet period a political and ideological turn toward "being human" was especially evident in nursing care for psychiatric patients (though this does not relate to political psychiatric institutions). Psychiatric nursing also affords us the opportunity to explore how changes in Soviet nursing paralleled international trends toward framing nursing as humanistic.

Chapter 9 brings us to the end of the Soviet period. Here I concentrate on questions of ethics, activism, and morality. Even though the experience of war elevated Soviet nurses into patriots and helped to raise their prestige in the public eye, life remained very difficult for nurses and other medical workers in the immediate postwar years. But this was also a period of increasing professionalization, a process hastened after Nikita Khrushchev's ascent to power in 1956. The ideological tenor of the 1960s, especially the 1961 Moral Code, had a crucial impact on nursing and medical ethics. Under Khrushchev an emphasis on social activism also made itself felt in nursing, with the SOKK and KP USSR once again involved in public campaigns to train nurses, except this time the focus was on taking care of the disabled, infirm, and older people. But how did nurses fare during the Brezhnev years? Brezhnev's government wanted to make communism human, and nurses were constantly reminded of their mission in this regard. This chapter assesses official pronouncements on morality and how these translated into nursing care in the 1970s and 1980s.

This book is a history of nursing in the Soviet Union. It principally considers urban nursing, and in particular the hospitals and clinics in Moscow and Leningrad. The focus is also largely on Russia, although nursing in other parts of the Soviet Union is also featured. While I discuss nurses in factories or in the various national republics in places, I devote more time to assessing psychiatric nursing, mother and child nursing, nursing in sanatoria, and other forms of nursing practice in the Soviet Union. My overall aim is to provide a representative picture of Soviet nursing.

The sources that I draw on are wide and disparate: they include a number of archives in Moscow, St. Petersburg, Sochi, and Tambov as well as sources in the United States, the United Kingdom, and Ukraine. I also use online archival repositories, such as the invaluable, but not unproblematic, Harvard Project on the Soviet Social System Online (HPSSS) and I Remember / Ia pomniu.[55] The Harvard project consists of interviews with refugee Soviet citizens arriving in the United States in the late 1940s and 1950s, and so the broader context of the interviewee's experience is important. The I Remember project deals largely with memories and testimonies gathered long after World War II. As we know with first-person testimony, political, social, and cultural factors can shape the experiences and understandings of events, often imbuing these narratives with layered or hidden meanings.[56] For these reasons I tend to combine such sources with a wide range of other published and unpublished material. Likewise, the Soviet press is an indispensable source but one that requires critical reading—periodicals and newspapers conveyed news and information, but the state organs published these as part of a broader ideological mission to educate readers.

Finally, nurses were part of the socialist project, but they also belong to the wider international history of nursing. Most chapters feature comparisons with other countries, primarily the United States and the United Kingdom. Chapter 3 does this most explicitly. Nursing was and is an international profession, and I wanted to capture this to showcase commonalities between countries as well as to highlight the idiosyncrasies of socialist nursing. Through their everyday work caring for socialist citizens, nurses changed people's lives. When the socialist state asked nurses to be moral ambassadors for socialism, many of them took on the ideological and professional role with enthusiasm. The story of Soviet nursing is a history of socialism through humanism.

CHAPTER 1

War and Revolution

War and revolution wreak havoc on society, and Russia saw its fair share of both in the nineteenth and twentieth centuries. With war came violence and a desperate need for personnel to care for the wounded. The development of Russia's nursing profession corresponded with the outbreak of war and calls for medical workers. Aristocratic and religious women became involved in establishing communities of nurses, or Sisters of Mercy, in the nineteenth century, building on a model of care and charity established a hundred years before.[1] The rise in radical and revolutionary politics in the nineteenth century together with increased urbanization and industrialization led to changes in how imperial Russian society viewed women; it was within this context that Sisters of Mercy communities expanded and developed.

This chapter introduces Russian nursing before the revolution and foregrounds the many challenges confronting nurses. During war and revolution nurses had to navigate gender boundaries, lack of professional regulation, and a changing society. The key figures responsible for shaping the nursing profession in Russia were Grand Duchess Elena Pavlovna (1807–1873), Ekaterina Mikhailovna Bakunina (1812–1894), Nikolai Ivanovich Pirogov (1810–1881), and, on a more symbolic level, Dasha Sevastopolskaia.[2] These protagonists arrived in Russian nursing at about the same time as the march of modernity and the demands of war.

Almost twenty years after the Crimean War, in 1876, the eminent surgeon and pioneer of Russian nursing Nikolai Pirogov wrote that nursing would be neither tethered to the conservative Russian Orthodox Church nor developed along Western lines.[3] Russian nurses would be women with a "practical mind," "good technical education," and a "sympathetic heart."[4] In placing professionalism above religion, Pirogov shared the view of other international pioneers of nursing such as Florence Nightingale.[5] But such a process was far from complete by the time the Bolsheviks came to power, and a hard-fought battle over the future of nursing took place in 1918 and into the bitter civil war years. This endeavor was long and arduous, highlighting the incredible difficulties that nurses faced as both professionals and women. The early history of Russian nursing also shows that war was a crucial factor in its development, by forcing nursing work to become more organized and vitally molding public and state perceptions of nurses. Above all, we see that women were active agents who identified problems and sought ways to address them, even if that brought them into direct conflict with authority figures.

The Saint Troitsky community (*obshchina*), established in 1844 by the Grand Duchesses Aleksandra Nikolaevna and Maria Nikolaevna and Princess Teresa Oldenburgkaia, was Russia's first Sisters of Mercy community. The English Quaker Sarah Biller (1794–1851) was at its helm, overseeing the community's Sisters of Mercy, probationers, a medical and educational department, and a women's school.[6] One historian of Russian nursing notes that it resembled convent life "in form and spirit."[7] The Saint Troitsky community's first charter in 1848 stipulated its goal to "care for the poor sick, comfort the grieving, direct fallen people along the right path, raise homeless children, and correct children with bad habits."[8] Pirogov, N. F. Arendt, E. P. Pavlov, B. E. Ekk, and the first female physician in Russia, N. P. Suslova, were some of the luminaries who taught and worked in the community. From its outset, nursing was infused with a spirit of compassion and humanity as a tight-knit group of devoted medical professionals and philanthropists steered its development.

The desire to care flourished in the late nineteenth century, a time when monasteries and the Red Cross established nursing courses and new Sisters of Mercy communities.[9] Two of the most well-known communities were Duchess Shakovskaia's Soothe My Sorrows community (Utoli moi pechali obshchina), founded in 1866, and the Order of the Exaltation of the Cross community (Krestovozdvizhenskaia obshchina), founded by the Grand Duchess Elena Pavlovna at the beginning of the Crimean War in 1854. The former, numbering 250 Sisters of Mercy by 1877, was the largest community.[10] Some attribute to the latter the first formation of female medical aid to the wounded during war; others argue that this accolade belongs to Nightingale.[11] Irrespective of who got there first, by the end of the nineteenth century, the groundwork for a philanthropic form of nursing, present in western Europe and the United States, was being laid in Russia. The work was not yet systematically coordinated or centralized but depended on communities and their patrons.

Despite the lack of centralization at this point, the number of Sisters of Mercy grew as the communities expanded across the Russian Empire. The women in the communities often represented a cross-section of society and had some level of "elementary education."[12] The beginning of nursing in late imperial Russia depended on the goodwill of a host of individuals: those who established and funded the communities, the physicians who taught there, and the women who joined them to help take care of those in need. But when the Crimean War broke out, a new context was given to nursing care.

War and Peace

When Elena Pavlovna established the Exaltation of the Cross community, the Grand Duchess "called on all Russian women to serve for one year as military hospital nurses" and to wear a brown habit and serve without pay to identify their work with religion.[13] Their reward would be the fulfillment of their patriotic duty through "self-sacrifice and spiritual devotion."[14] The language of both patriotism and religion no doubt caught the attention of those fearing the threat of war. Mother Superior Ekaterina Bakunina pressed for permanent deployment of Sisters of Mercy in military hospitals, and the Ministry of Defense passed a decree to this effect in 1863.[15] This decree also instituted a pension for Sisters of Mercy, and some scholars of Russian nursing history consider it to be *the birth of the professional nurse in Russia.*[16] While this claim depends on one's definition of professionalization, the move contributed to formalizing nursing.

The success of the Sisters of Mercy in Crimea was central to a growing recognition of nurses' important role during times of peace and war. Sisters of Mercy actions in Crimea brought the nursing communities to the attention of soldiers and the wider public. Terrible wartime conditions also tested the Sisters of Mercy. Although the over one hundred Sisters of Mercy serving in the Crimean War had won soldiers' respect, internal squabbling forced Bakunina to stop nurses "spreading rumors and malicious gossip."[17] The challenging experience of Crimea proved to be formative for the Sisters of Mercy. Increased organization, recognition, and development helped to professionalize Russian nursing.[18] Indeed, the outstanding work of Sisters of Mercy in

Crimea served to show that women could make important contributions to Russian society—an achievement that led to calls for nurses to have access to university education.[19] One need only look to Florence Nightingale to appreciate how the Crimean factor also played a role outside of the Russian Empire.

And it was not only the Crimean War that widened the sphere of Russian nursing activities. The Russo-Turkish War of 1877–1878 again exposed Sisters of Mercy to military nursing. This time, 1,288 Sisters of Mercy went to the front to nurse the sick and wounded.[20] By the outbreak of the Russo-Japanese War in 1904 about twenty-four Sisters of Mercy communities existed.[21] Indeed, as the twentieth century dawned in Russia, war became an important influence in shaping the Sisters of Mercy communities. It functioned as a rallying call, and volunteer numbers swelled as female interest in playing an active role in military conflict increased. Women's growing interest in serving at the front lines during war also endowed them with "new professional and social status."[22]

As the Russian Sisters of Mercy presence extended to the war between Serbia and Turkey in 1876, the role of women became a point of discussion. The Russian Society of the Red Cross (ROKK) forerunner, the Russian Society for the Care of Injured and Sick Troops during War, had organized medical help to the wounded in Serbia.[23] Although the society included a large number of women among its members, its governing synod only agreed to allow "women's committees" following public pressure. Noblewomen drove these committees that ensured the society's liquidity, curriculum development, and nurse training.[24] Their involvement was testament to the intense interest in women's medical education and wider discussion of women in Russian society post-Crimea.[25]

Women's position in Russian public healthcare distinguished both Russian and later Soviet medicine.[26] Russian women entered medical courses in universities in "unprecedented numbers," demonstrating a thirst for education and independence and a desire to help people that lasted long into the twentieth century. Changing political and social conditions as well as the desperate need for doctors, especially in rural areas, helped to convince people of the need for women physicians.[27] Women's involvement in Russian medicine was "unrivaled in any other country."[28]

Shortages of medical workers in general posed a problem. Care was frequently left in the hands of the *sidelki* and Sisters of Mercy because feldshers were "too preoccupied with statistics, prescriptions and other work not concerned with patient care."[29] This was also a criticism of women who "were illiterate and from different professions, temporarily staying in the hospital while searching for better work." The feldsher-midwife was often fused together, despite the fact that the *"poval'nye babki,"* or midwives, were generally "known to be illiterate and without qualifications, familiar only with a very limited knowledge of childbirth and care for newborns."[30] Concern about medical personnel and qualifications cast a shadow that followed public health leaders and educators deep into the twentieth century. But this was an issue already identified in the nineteenth century as nursing pioneers set their sights on improving standards of care and establishing nursing as a respectable profession.[31]

Just as Florence Nightingale organized a nurse training school at St. Thomas's Hospital on her return to London, Bakunina set about making Sisters of Mercy a more prevalent feature of Russian society during peacetime. After the Crimean War, Bakunina's Order of the Exaltation of the Cross community expanded its activities in healthcare and education, opening a women's hospital and a school in 1860.[32] As the Sisters of Mercy communities increased in the second half of the nineteenth century, so too did medical institutes for feldshers and midwives.[33] Those entering a school for women feldshers were to have a certificate of middle-level education, and competition for places was so fierce that "medalists often made up a large portion of the intake."[34] Efforts to develop medical education for nurses reflect broader developments in late imperial Russia, when women became a real force in Russian medicine.

The last decades of the nineteenth century saw a great deal of change in the structure and organization of the nursing communities. Much of this was owed to Pavlovna, Bakunina, and Pirogov, who made the Sisters of Mercy indispensable during times of war and peace. But with the imperial powers showing little interest or direction, the communities were not a unified or centralized force—until the formation of ROKK in 1867.

A New Era

Some historians herald the establishment of ROKK as "a new era in female care for the sick in Russia."[35] It oversaw the work of the communities, but a degree of independence continued as each community had its own goals and study programs.[36] Some 232 committees and sixty-two Sisters of Mercy communities and their hospitals came under the remit of ROKK.[37] Not only did the ROKK play a greater role in the Sisters of Mercy communities, but it was also involved in broader social endeavors that included first aid courses for the general population.[38]

At this point, it is important to note the role of the Brothers of Mercy. Officially established by ROKK in 1897, Brothers of Mercy played their part in the Russo-Japanese War in 1904–1905. They had the same two-year program of study as the Sisters of Mercy.[39] Brothers of Mercy, and indeed feldshers, did not leave a particularly good impression. Some nurses and physicians claimed that Brothers of Mercy were drunk much of the time, had little medical knowledge, and "discredited their title."[40] Relations between the Sisters of Mercy and both the Brothers of Mercy and feldshers (male and female) were often strained. Feldshers, for example, might respond "with indignation" (*negodovaniia*) to ROKK orders if nurses were not in a "subordinate position to them."[41] Class, education, and gender already played an important role in the medical world. Nurses—the main protagonists of this story—had to contend with colleagues' superiority complexes from the outset. There were occasions when men did not seem to take too kindly to women giving them orders.

By 1903 ROKK had drawn up a set of regulations (*ustavy*). The head doctor, priest, mother superior, treasurer, and representatives from ROKK formed the Council of Patrons.[42] This council and a committee were at the top of the new structure, ahead of the mother superior, senior nurse, and Sisters of Mercy. Under ROKK regulations, training and education included theory and practice and took place over a one-and-a-half- to two-year period.[43] A doctor or mother superior supervised students as they undertook practical work in a medical institution.[44] The new regulations imparted a greater structure and coherence on the nursing communities—another important move toward some form of professionalization. The increasing organization and the rise in demand for nurses and other medical workers were part of a more expansive shift in late nineteenth- and early twentieth-century Russia that saw the rise of workers and professionals to support the growth in Russian industry and government services.[45]

Writing in the *American Journal of Nursing* in 1946, US nurse Ellen Albin asserted that the ROKK schools "made a great step forward in developing nursing as a profession," were completely secular, and had a much more advanced curriculum that required passing an exam "before the title 'nurse' could be bestowed."[46] This move toward greater secularization, Albin claims, allowed women to become nurses rather than nuns.[47] While religion and priests were an important part of community life in the nineteenth century, the twentieth century saw the ROKK and the physician play more prominent roles.[48] The increased secularization of nursing became even more pronounced during the First World War. By the time of the October Revolution in 1917, Russian nursing's reach had spread beyond its religious influences.

Conditions for Change

The move toward increased secularization might also have resulted from the difficult life for women in a Sisters of Mercy community.[49] Those who entered had to conform to strict codes of behavior and assume a life of subservience.[50] Young Sisters of Mercy struggled the most with the harsh conditions and feared for their future; some women "ran from the communities."[51] Growing problems in the communities and generally awful living conditions meant that the beginning of the twentieth century was a trying time for Russian nursing. Sisters of Mercy were often women with limited options and little or no education.[52] Only war seemed to rejuvenate the profession by drawing women volunteers.

Although the Russo-Japanese War was another example of mobilization, the women who served in it endured terrible conditions. As one Sister of Mercy from the St. George community (Georgievskii obshchina), O. A. Baumgarten, wrote in her published diary, *In Besieged Port Arthur*: "With the help of God, nobody will ever see or live through what we have seen and lived through. It was so awful that at times it seemed the world was coming to an end."[53] Such conditions seemed either distant or unknown to women interested in training as Sisters of Mercy and joining the war effort. A doctor working in the military hospital noted that many of the women drawn to nursing in the Russo-Japanese War were "young, educated women who wanted to experience the world, widows who wanted to escape the boredom of life, married women who were unhappy, officers' wives who wanted to be near their spouse, and aristocratic ladies who often did not have much interest in nursing work per se."[54] And they continued to come from an array of social and educational backgrounds.[55] The reputation of volunteer nurses as "little sisters," wearing silk skirts and perfume, and fraternizing with the opposite sex began to emerge in 1905 and was not all that dissimilar to the First World War narrative of Russian nursing.[56] One volunteer nurse recalled her shock at the wedding of a nurse and a military officer in the hospital.[57] War reshaped the contours of Russian nursing in different ways.

Notwithstanding the increasing diversification of nursing personnel, the Sisters of Mercy experience of war in the nineteenth and early twentieth centuries was traumatic; the exposure to the dangers of war, disease, and generally dreadful living, working, and travel conditions not only helped to shape these women into nurses but also meant that they had a shared experience of the horrors of war, theretofore an exclusively male domain. Given the demands and strain of the Russo-Japanese War, those involved in the upper echelons of the ROKK and Sisters of Mercy communities realized that Sisters of Mercy and volunteers needed additional medical training to prepare for what awaited them near the front lines.

The Red Cross thus continued to train limited numbers of reserve nurses between 1905 and 1912.[58] Similar peacetime moves for war service were undertaken in the United States at around the same time; indeed, a meeting about ROKK work discussed this very issue in April 1909.[59] Nurses around the world mobilized. Delegates at the International Council of Nurses (ICN) congress in France in 1907 and Cologne in 1912 discussed state registration and nurse involvement in social work, although only a handful of Russian nurses, from Madame Mannerheim's organization in Helsingfors, were present.[60] Still, lack of presence did not signal stagnation.

By 1913 ROKK had an impressive 109 communities with 2,438 Sisters of Mercy, 1,004 probationers, and 750 reserve nurses.[61] This compared to 27 feldsher schools in the Russian Empire in 1911, 12 of which were for men only, 8 for women only, and 7 mixed sex. The figure had risen to 80 feldsher and feldsher-midwifery schools in 1915, with some 9,500 students enrolled.[62] The prospect of war and ROKK coordination boosted the number of Sisters of Mercy communities to 150 and 10,000 trained nurses in 1914.[63] This growth in the number of communities led to increasing demands for organization and pushed nurses closer to professionalization.

As Russia endured rebellions, riots, revolution, and war in the first decade of the twentieth century, modernization and challenges to the political status quo rocked the empire and its tsar, Nicholas II. Russian nursing was changing too, although the communities generally remained conservative.[64] The greater liberalization in relations between men and women went against the strict moral standards of community life. The Red Cross influence saw priests, and ipso facto religion, play a less important role in the life of the communities; instead, medical doctors assumed more influence and authority as nursing professionalized.[65] Developments in the seeming binary of science and religion had led to changing dynamics in medicine and nursing in Russia and abroad.[66]

Whether the revolutionary foment in Russian society radicalized Sisters of Mercy is not clear. Examples of female physicians who were also revolutionaries are well known, but the matter is harder to assess in relation to nurses at the beginning of the twentieth century. While many of these women—who straddled the border of professional and worker—might not have had the time for revolutionary activity, they might have engaged in low-level revolutionary activity in the hospital or community.[67]

By the early twentieth century, people in the Russian Empire had begun to see themselves as independent from monarchy and church.[68] Nurses and other medical workers, especially those who had been through a wartime experience, developed new worldviews that were not exclusively defined by religion and the sphere of the Sisters of Mercy community. War, professional independence, and the rise of revolutionary sentiment—exemplified by the formation of medical unions—now competed with religion as a way of life within the community. Sisters of Mercy were not cut off from society; they trained, treated patients, and worked alongside doctors. They saw the changes that marked Russian politics, society, and culture.

The First World War

When World War I broke out, Sisters of Mercy and thousands of volunteers demonstrated a great urge to help the wounded. These "white angels"—inspired by the example of Empress Aleksandra Feodorovna, her two eldest daughters, and the tsar's sister, Olga Aleksandrovna—became popular in the media. At the war's outset the severe shortage of nurses led to the introduction of short-term Red Cross courses for nurse volunteers, as was the case in other European countries that also called on women to fulfill their "patriotic duty."[69] In 1916 17,436 nurses went to the front, with "2,000 of these serving in field hospitals and at the rear."[70] Red Cross volunteer nurses continued to represent a cross-section of society, from well-to-do ladies swayed by press appeals to volunteers, ordinary working women, and young girls seeking adventure. The sight of these volunteer nurses created different impressions on those whom they encountered.

Nurse memoirs of the First World War illuminate how women perceived themselves as nurses and how others perceived them. Although ego documents are largely romantic and heroic in style, they nevertheless provide a window into the nursing war experience and the nature of Russian nursing. While nursing work is often depicted as the "romantic ideal," some accounts portray a more variegated perspective of nursing at the Russian front that suggests underlying tensions and divisions.[71] One drawback of nursing memoirs is that they can be "unconvincing either as literature or as historical records," with few of them resolving the "tension between the rhetoric of noble suffering and heroic sacrifice and the reality of dirt, pain, fear, and fatigue."[72] Many memoirs of Russian nursing also evince signs of this problem, with the rhetoric of noble suffering and heroic sacrifice usually dominating the narratives. Nonetheless, the accounts of nursing offered in these memoirs provide important insights into the nursing war experience in Russia.[73]

Among the most informative accounts of the Russian nursing experience of the First World War are those of two British nurses (Florence Farmborough and Violetta Thurston), two Anglo-Russian nurses (Mary Britnieva and Sophie Botcharsky), and three Russian nurses (Lidiia Zakharova, Tatiana Alexinsky, and Tatiana Varnek). Of these women, three received medical training prior to the outbreak of war: Thurston; Alexinsky, a trained physician; and Varnek, who trained in the Kaufmanskaia Sisters of Mercy community for a few weeks in 1912 and then continued her training in a short course after the war broke out. Alexinsky's, Zakharova's, and Thurston's accounts were published in 1915 and 1916; Botcharsky's and Britnieva's in the 1930s; and Farmborough's in 1974. Varnek's account was published in 2001 as part of Aleksandr Solzhenitsyn's All-Russian Memoir Library series.[74]

The diaries and memoirs of the volunteer nurses in Russia are very much expressive of the sheer enthusiasm and willingness to help in the war effort. What the women might have lacked in medical knowledge, they compensated for in compassion and self-sacrifice. Initial doubts and fears appear to have been overcome on encountering their first wounded soldiers. Sophie Botcharsky recalled terrifying initial encounters with surgery—one friend exclaimed in the operating room: "But we haven't ever seen operations, nothing, just little ones!" To that the doctor replied: "Ah, you just came to wear the pretty caps. Eh? Six weeks training in Petrograd, I suppose, and before that, High School? Well, you must have some sense!"[75] The frightened recruits were then made to pass instruments, administer anesthetic, and hold ligaments.[76]

For those volunteer nurses who had never worked in a hospital or medical environment, their first encounter with surgery was often frightening, sometimes involving extreme cases such as amputation. They had to learn on the job and overcome their fears. Not only does the above recollection show the nervous state of the new recruits, who in this instance did not even attempt to disguise their anxiety, but it is also suggestive of the skeptical and sometimes misogynistic attitude of male doctors toward volunteer nurses. Would the doctor have remarked on the pretty caps and taken the new workers more seriously had they been men? The dynamics of the relationship established between the medical personnel was important. Nurses discussing the surgeons and physicians with whom they worked valued their professional competence over their personalities. They saw this as crucial in establishing a trusting working relationship. For those with considerable medical experience who disagreed with or challenged physicians, the relationships were not so harmonious. When physician Tatiana Alexinsky questioned the decision to keep two critically ill patients on a train instead of leaving them at a station for transfer to a nearby hospital, the male doctor told her, "I know better than you."[77] Gender and power dynamics shaped the relationship between male and female doctors as well as between doctors and nurses.

The Good Nurse

The qualities of a "good" nurse were often ambiguous and enmeshed in ideas of "feminine care" and "kindness." Some patients showed pride in the fact that the nurses in their unit were good-looking as opposed to skilled medical workers. A patient showed his gratitude to Botcharsky by saying: "Our sisters are beautiful. Look how tall they are, some units have short sisters."[78] The dual narrative of femininity and competence seemed characteristic of European nursing discourse of this period. In some of the military hospitals in France doctors demanded "thoroughly professional staffs" but also accepted that "a nurse's womanly qualities were as important as her technical training," with "women's voices, their way of moving, bending over, or sitting at the bedside" a comfort to patients.[79] In the harshness of war, some men seemed to value the physical characteristics of women over their professional competence.

The nurse narratives usually do not elaborate on the vision of what a nurse should be or touch on feminist or emancipationist issues—the memoirist's main concern was with her personal journeys or caring for the patient. There were some exceptions. Alexinsky, as a socialist and feminist, referred to her transport train as a "feminist train" because the majority of medical personnel on board were women.[80] Botcharsky portrays herself as a fast learner who adapted well to the conditions of war and medicine. She endeared herself to patients, including German patients whom she could comfort in their own language.[81] Likewise, Florence Farmborough focused on her personal development, which she tied very closely to her ability to adapt to nursing in Russia. In their outlook many of the nurses show that war acted as a leveling device for those at the front.

Nonetheless, class and status mattered. Sanitary personnel such as orderlies were delineated from other medical personnel. The Red Cross identified these women workers by their uniforms, a plain gray cotton dress with a white apron and headscarf, and a bandage with a cross that they wore on their left arm while on duty.[82] The uniform made it clear that they were not Sisters of Mercy. Divisions were especially evident in the writings of nurses whose memoirs were not in the romantic mold. Trained Russian medical workers, such as socialist Tatiana Alexinsky, who was about thirty years old in 1916, did not take to some of the volunteer nurses. On seeing the "society benefactresses," she admitted: "I don't know why, but I felt a certain feeling of irritation against these ladies and all their kind."[83] Swedish Red Cross nurse Elsa Brandstrom expressed similar sentiments based on her experience in Petrograd. She wrote that little-trained "society women" were "often a parody on the sister of mercy."[84] This attitude is somewhat reminiscent of the class antagonisms that arose among British nurses who reported tension between the privileged but relatively untrained Voluntary Aid Detachments and the professional nurses who worked for a living.[85] Brandstrom wrote that the primary duty of the "society women" was "to shake pillows, dry the foreheads and comb the hair of the wounded," but "when the novelty wore off they fled back to their dinners, bridge-parties, and dances." After they left, only the genuine nurses—"simple, kindly women"—remained.[86]

This description draws into sharp relief the existence of two types of nurses, as called in the French context, the "true" nurse and the "false" nurse.[87] True nurses, as depicted in the French press and volunteer nurse memoirs, were maternal, feminine, and professional, whereas false nurses, if referred to in memoirs, were socially ambitious, self-interested, and lacking in true devotion.[88] This delineation is not so straightforward or clear-cut in the case of the image or perception of Russian nursing, but such differences existed. It is also clear that this was not limited to nursing in the First World War. In her memoir written in 1909, Sister of Mercy M. I. Deviz recalled the negative impressions left by society women volunteering in hospitals after the Russo-Japanese War. Soldiers had informed her that these society ladies sat and talked with the healthy officers, leaving the sick and wounded soldiers alone.[89] Like the British nurses who "resented any kind of 'playing at nurses' by amateurs" during times of war, the Russian nurses similarly resented some of the volunteers who entered their field.[90] The anger elicited by the volunteer nurses indicates that Sisters of Mercy were demarcating their professional territory.

The diaries and memoirs of trained Russian nurses show levels of resentment that seem largely absent in the narratives of the volunteer nurses. Perhaps this is because they did not encounter such "society ladies." But the distinctions between Sisters of Mercy, wartime-trained reserve Sisters of Mercy, and volunteers were not clear, especially as the last two categories assumed more responsibilities over the course of the First World War. As a result, they came to perceive themselves differently and as no less qualified. In an interview conducted by the Imperial War Museum years after the war and the publication of her memoir, wartime nurse Florence Farmborough, when asked, "Were you treated as though you were a qualified sister with several years of training?," replied, "We were qualified." The interviewer pressed further, "But some sisters [had] a few years rather than a few months," to which Farmborough replied: "That [was] in England. But in Russia if we passed our exams and had six months of training with the wounded and dying soldiers—not with the ordinary sick people—we were qualified. I was made a Town Sister once— *Goradskaya sestra*. And that was a great compliment and that meant that I could be really at the head of the profession in the town and go to any of the hospitals as a Town Sister."[91] Farmborough considered herself a trained nurse, in spite of having had no formal nursing education or training aside from the six months' prewar training course she attended. But she was not alone in holding this view, and after the war there were wartime nurses who considered themselves fully qualified. Many of them went on to work in the Soviet health-care system.

By 1917 an effort was made to closely monitor volunteer nurses—those with no training as opposed to wartime-trained nurses. Sisters of Mercy communities would provide only a "moral" recommendation to voluntary nurses that allowed them to work at the front or in military hospitals.[92] Nurses completing short-term nurse training courses were assigned a Sisters of Mercy community, and representatives from that community (or ROKK) were to be present at exams.[93] Those nurses who had completed a three-month course but had not received a recommendation from the community were now threatened with expulsion from the rural and urban unions.[94] These changing perceptions of the nurse were perhaps informed by mixed appraisals of nurses earlier in the war.

Volunteer nurses were criticized as early as 1915, when contrasts drawn between Sisters of Mercy and volunteer nurses highlighted the perceived ignorance and carelessness of the latter. Readers of *Ladies World* (*Damskii mir*) were left in no doubt about the superiority of the "genuine" community-trained Sister of Mercy after the publication of an article describing nurse uniforms and conduct. Readers learned that Sisters of Mercy wore only linen or cotton dresses, which collected less dirt than woolen or silk dresses, and that they wore headscarves and aprons for hygienic purposes.[95] Experienced nurses kept their uniforms clean by leaving them in the hospital, but volunteer nurses "flaunted" their new uniforms on the street, where they became covered with dirt.[96] On streetcars volunteer nurses were in close quarters with people whose clothes had not been washed since the "day they were made," and so the volunteers walked among patients wearing uniforms "covered in microbes."[97] Such horror captured a mood that was current in some circles at the time. But it also showed that there was no singular nursing experience. Nurses could elicit any number of emotions from others as they went about their work.

To be sure, the diaries and memoirs are not wholly representative of the wartime experience, and they do not explain the full history of Russian wartime nursing, but they do shed light on many aspects of nursing. For one, they insert the Russian nursing experience into the wider European experience, showing that Russian wartime nurses shared many commonalities with their nursing counterparts in Britain and France. They also show the different self-perceptions among the nurses and how these varied according to training and class. Finally, they confirm the importance of the female contribution to the war and the immense sacrifice of women in war, as well as point to the significance attached to more traditional notions of "womanhood" as perceived by men at war. Positive press reports of women at the front galvanized the image of nurses as patriotic and hardworking. In 1915, for example, an article titled "Women and War," published in *Women's Herald* (*Zhenskii vestnik*), celebrated women awarded medals for their work and acknowledged those who had died in the line of duty.[98] Positive accounts featured in *Women's Affairs* (*Zhenskoe delo*) that same year, highlighting the sacrifices and efforts of women at the front.[99] But press recognition of their sacrifice did not seem to lead to improvements in their professional status. At one nurse congress organized at the Minsk front, as reported in a 1955 publication about ROKK, Sisters of Mercy proclaimed: "Many speak lately of freedom; for some this is already happening, but not for us Sisters of Mercy."[100] Not for the first or last time, nurses found themselves on the margins and in need of greater material support and recognition.

Even though the image of the Sister of Mercy became modish, some historians argue that the widespread dissemination of the fashionable nurse also served to partly diminish the traditional sense of respect and moral authority associated with Sisters of Mercy.[101] This seemed to be the case with nurses or nurse volunteers irrespective of political affiliation. The moral standing and reputation of nurses was in an apparent state of decline. Such perceptions remained long after World War I ended. In her book on Soviet healthcare published in 1928, the American Quaker Anna Haines noted that the "general attitude toward nursing . . . was not such that would induce women to undertake the work unless under some religious motivation."[102] She added that "nurses who did not wear the uniform of some order were not apt to receive very courteous treatment from the hospital staff or the public at large, and it is true that they were often not the type of women to command much respect."[103] This ambiguity created different images of the Russian nurse during the First World War—the religious nurse, maternal nurse, prostitute nurse, and patriotic nurse.[104] Wartime experiences transformed the demands on nurses as well as the public perception of the nurse, and women, whether for good or bad.[105]

Nursing Revolution: The All-Russian Union of the Society of the Sisters of Mercy

The First World War accelerated much of the change that had been under way in the first part of the twentieth century. During the chaos of war, and particularly after the abdication of Tsar Nicholas II in March 1917, a host of professional organizations and unions sprang up across the former Russian Empire. Nursing was no exception, and unions of nurses formed in Russian towns and cities.[106] In the uncertain political times, nurses—like those in other countries during and after the war—were keen to assert their professional rights and defend their interests. While Sisters of Mercy and wartime nurses took care of the injured near the front and across the country, in Petrograd moves were being made toward professionalization. In August 1917 the All-Russian Society of the Union of Sisters of Mercy (Vserossiiskii soiuz obshchestva sester miloserdiia), or for brevity, the Union of Sisters of Mercy, emerged from the First All-Russian Congress of Sisters of Mercy.[107] Nurses thus joined a host of other recently formed local medical unions—a sign of the times.[108] According to the onetime head of the Soviet medical union, A. Aluf, the over one hundred delegates were predominantly wartime nurses, but there were also many representatives from the Sisters of Mercy communities.[109] The journal publication following the congress, as well as archival transcripts of union discussions, shows that the Sisters of Mercy communities, not the military nurses, dominated proceedings and later the organization of the union.

Nurses at the congress remained politically neutral but agreed to work with the Provisional Government.[110] The Petrograd-based communities had two overarching aims: first, to organize nursing along professional and secular lines and, second, to help improve conditions for nurses.[111] In these uncertain times the nursing communities were in such a precarious financial position that they recruited no new students.[112] Nursing and medicine reflected the chaos of war and revolution.

Some of the nurses in the Union of Sisters of Mercy claimed the communities did not want to join their union because its members included wartime nurses, whom they apparently did not consider to be bona fide community nurses.[113] In January 1918, in discussions about the role of the union and the reorganization of the Red Cross, one union nurse underlined the importance of finding a "common language" that included the different interests of full-time (staff / community) and temporary (wartime) nurses.[114] Other nurses agreed with this position.[115] One of them was Sister Bazilevskaia, who argued against such a divide between "genuine and not genuine sisters." In her words,

"All worked well and the same." She wanted nurses to show a united front so that "midwives and orderlies would not replace them in hospitals."[116] But six months after these discussions, in July 1918, those in the Union of Sisters were unsure about who would be in control of the nursing schools.

In spite of their efforts to organize nursing, the union nurses seemed to be fighting a losing battle against the rising tide of Bolshevism.[117] Sister Arkhipova-Khilkova, the chief editor of *Pervyi vestnik sestry miloserdiia*, complained: "We do not have in our hands a decree from the Bolsheviks that outlines a program for the reorganization of the Main Administration [of the Red Cross]; they have said nothing about the Sisters of Mercy."[118] The Sisters of Mercy felt an acute awareness of their responsibility to their members, having "a whole army of sisters who without them would go hungry and cold."[119] But at the same time, they felt their control lessen and feared losing their links to the Red Cross since its reorganization by the Bolsheviks in August 1918.[120] Although rights and freedoms were terms often used in Russia during war and revolution, attaining these seemed to constantly elude nurses. The Sisters of Mercy communities had made great advancements in delivering a nursing service since the middle of the nineteenth century, but now a core group of nurses was leading their fight for survival.

The Bolshevik Way

The establishment of the Commissariat of Health (Narodnyi komissariat zdravookhraneniia) in July 1918 signaled Bolshevik intent to push ahead with plans for a socialist form of public health.[121] Meanwhile, the Union of Sisters was faltering. Diminishing influence in light of the commissariat's increasing grip over public health combined with continued internal divisions threatened the union's existence. Despite its initial hopes, the Union of Sisters never managed to attract all the community nurses; as a result, there was an uneasy relationship between the Union of Sisters (claiming to represent all nurses) and the communities (which were still also under ROKK).[122] The situation was not helped by the Union of Sisters' stipulation that the communities join wholesale, as opposed to nurses joining on an individual basis.[123]

In October 1918 the Union of Sisters, the Commissariat of Health, and the Committee for the Reorganization of the Red Cross approved the nursing schools. All three authorities agreed that the goal of nursing schools was to "train experienced cadres of nurses to care for the sick" and help junior personnel whenever possible.[124] Training nurses was a "state concern" and based on the principle of a "free school system with one common lecture program ratified by the Commissariat of Health."[125] ROKK reorganization required the Union of Sisters to furnish information about the possibility of reorganizing the communities as schools.[126] At this point, it seemed as though the nurses and the Bolsheviks might find some common ground—perhaps the Sisters of Mercy could develop a program that would be acceptable to all parties. But that was not the case. The Bolshevik health authority was happy to have the nurses develop a program, but not happy for this relationship to be publicly acknowledged. Needless to say, the nurses, having fought so hard to be in this position, did not want to be sidelined.

But sidelined they were. The Commissariat of Health and the Red Cross committee deleted the phrase "and the regulations on schools, accepted by the Union of Sisters" in the proposal for schools, and this amendment irked the nurses, who feared that it might lead to future "misunderstanding."[127] The Union of Sisters of Mercy considered the schools "one of the most important questions for the existence of the entire nursing organization" and thus took immense interest in their future development.[128] For now, the nurses were able to maintain a presence, but their future still seemed uncertain.

Further disappointment prevailed on the Union of Sisters in November 1918 when their position again became unclear after the conference of medical workers convened to discuss the merger of all medical unions.[129] The Sisters of Mercy seemed to be dependent on the decisions of other groups, with little say in determining the fate of their own organization and profession (in spite of their best efforts). With the Commissariat of Health taking control and with the Union of Sisters divided, the demise of the All-Russian Union of the Society of Sisters of Mercy appeared imminent. By March 1919 the nurses joined the newly formed union for middle medical personnel (All-Russian Medical Sanitary Work [Vsemedikosantrud], organized in March 1919; renamed Medical Sanitary Work [Medsantrud], in 1924), based on the understanding that there would be nurse representation.[130] That was not to be—the Bolsheviks disbanded the union and nurses lost leadership autonomy.

The committee for the reorganization of the ROKK and the Commissariat of Health held discussions about the reorganization of the Sisters of Mercy communities. A small group of Sisters of Mercy joined Y. M. Sverdlov, Z. P. Soloviev, and Nikolai Semashko in attempts to work out a system of nursing.[131] Semashko wanted graduates of the new nursing schools to be "qualified workers." He also wanted to reconsider the plan to merge the hospital and the school for practical classes and argued that it would be "no harm for students to gain practical experience in a range of medical institutions, because remaining in one institution could not guarantee enough practical experience." Soloviev considered a three-year course to be sufficient to produce nurses who would specialize in "the nature of care" in special medical institutes, not "confining the school to the community."[132] The nurses also supported the three-year course but favored specialization in the third year.[133] Ultimately, the commissariat established a commission that included Popov, Soloviev, representatives of the Sisters of Mercy, and representatives of the Military-Sanitary Administration to work out a detailed project for the schools.[134] I examine these Bolshevik approaches to nursing education and organization in chapter 2.

Despite having established a seemingly good working relationship with the new health authority and continuing to contribute to the development of nursing in Russia, the tumultuous nature of power and politics in postrevolutionary Russia provided no guarantees of safety. Nurses who had worked in tsarist institutions occupied a precarious position, and in 1921 the new government incarcerated the Commissariat of Health–employed nurses.[135] Sisters of Mercy struggled to gain a foothold in the corridors of power after this brief period in the immediate postrevolutionary years. Still, their medical training and strong work ethic made Sisters of Mercy ideal candidates to help with the public healthcare crisis unfolding in Russia.

Many women continued their nursing work after the war and revolution. The patriotic and humanist calling that had drawn women and men to work in public healthcare remained in spite of who was in power. Motivations were also largely secular, and irrespective of their religious title—Sisters of Mercy—Russian nurses had already started down the road of secularization many years before the Bolshevik revolution. Russian society nonetheless associated them with the "old way of life." The battle between the old and the new continued long after the revolution. War and revolution did not end in 1918. Nurses and medical workers continued to fight for their rights and lives during the terrible years of civil war. At the same time, the new Bolshevik government busied itself with consolidating power and setting up a socialist state.

CHAPTER 2

Creating Order out of Chaos

The brutal and violent three years of civil war that started toward the summer of 1918 saw a reshaping of Russian nursing and public healthcare as part of the broader effort to establish a Marxist-Leninist state. To nationalize industry, ban private trade, and forcefully requisition grain, the Bolsheviks introduced the controversial economic policy of war communism. The policy was "an attempt to leap into socialism."[1] Institutional changes took place amid chaos, violence, and famine. Medical workers, especially nurses, were desperately needed as the country was ravaged by a conflict that saw seven million people perish.[2] A key objective of the Bolsheviks right after the revolution was the creation of a healthy society, free from disease. To help achieve this aim and deal with the desperate public healthcare situation unfolding across Russia, the new government immediately started to train medical workers.

The public health front was crucial strategically in creating economic and political stability but also ideologically as part of "a quest to protect the health and welfare of all citizens."[3] In circumstances of civil war this endeavor was particularly fraught. In this chapter I track Bolshevik efforts to establish a revised system of education and training during the years of the civil war, highlighting the disjuncture between center and periphery in conditions where authority and control were lacking. The challenges of reorganizing nursing serve as a useful reminder of the extreme difficulties presented by state and institution building in the midst of national/international conflict.[4] While trying to establish a system of care that would provide proletarian nurses for the worker state, administrators in the newly formed Commissariat of Health were also struggling to meet the urgent healthcare needs of the time.

The efforts to forge a new, socialist nursing profession during this turbulent period of Russian history illustrate how various stakeholders—the state and its institutions, the healthcare administration, medical workers, and patients—came to understand the revolution. They had different expectations of what the revolution meant, what form it should take in practice, and what rights and responsibilities it would bring. But there were no clear guidelines to explain how socialist nursing should work—this would be figured out along the way.

The new leaders struggled to deal with the challenges that followed the revolution.[5] While those charged with working out a new system of nursing for the first socialist state seemed to have a tabula rasa on which to map their vision of socialist nursing, that was not the case. The new public healthcare authorities overseeing nurse training and education during the period 1918–1922 had to work with what they had inherited—a damaged infrastructure, a decimated workforce, and a divided profession. Nursing in Russia was also subject to a range of internal and external forces interested in shaping the direction and form it should take. As the country descended into a bloody civil war and general disorder, the battle for communist care began in earnest.

Chapter 1 showed how difficult it was to construct a system of nursing before the revolution. When the chaos of war and revolution turned to civil war, the situation became even more complex. Once the Union of Sisters of Mercy joined the medical union, nurses more or less lost control of their professional representation. Gone were their hopes of building a strong professional cohort of Russian nurses with rights and professional development. Their interests were instead left in the hands of the Commissariats of Health and Education (1922–1930). And while eager to improve medical standards and nurse training, these agencies were often pulled in different directions; one could hardly describe them as patrons.[6] Nurses, without leadership or patronage, were in a vulnerable position and hopelessly susceptible to the political vagaries of the emerging Soviet state. This context defined nurses and nursing: as civil war raged across the former Russian Empire, nursing confronted questions of education, duty, care, and professional values.

Medical Education and Mobilization

At the end of October 1917, the Bolshevik government established the Medical-Sanitation Department in Petrograd with the aim of organizing medical help for workers and soldiers.[7] The department would then tackle the reconstruction of medical and sanitation institutions across the country. In July 1918 the Russian Red Cross, under V. M. Sverdlov and, starting in July 1919, Z. P. Soloviev, organized short-term courses for red nurses and orderlies. Courses usually ran for two weeks for the former and three days for the latter, although some of these were extended to five months in 1919.[8] The Commissariat of Health still planned to run short, two-month courses to train nurses and "red assistants" in Moscow, Petrograd, and regional towns in 1919.[9] Red nurses learned about the theory and history of the class struggle, the Red Army, and Soviet power.[10] Their task was not only to care for Red Army soldiers but also to provide political enlightenment.[11] While hardly useful for nursing, political instruction was integral to Soviet education and customary for Soviet citizens. It also became a keystone of nursing education during the Soviet period.

Away from the new offices of government, nurses continued to suffer on the front lines of civil war. Many of the red nurses, along with orderlies, could face torture or death if captured by White Army forces at the front.[12] Aleksandra Stepanovna Bystrova worked in a military infirmary in Tomsk after completing a short-term nursing course in 1920. Bystrova felt she was a true comrade and soldier only when at the front. She recalled—albeit in a 1960s Ministry of Defense publication—that many people attended meetings in the hospital square, where they would hear about the Red Army and medical personnel shortages. At these meetings a girl would be "plucked from the crowd and, to cries of approval, would affirm her desire to go to the front." In this way, Bystrova claimed, many medical workers decided to become involved in the civil war.[13] The daughter of another nurse who volunteered for the White Army during the civil war wrote that her mother was "deeply worried about human suffering and wanted to help."[14] During the civil war Sisters of Mercy were the "only exceptions" to the rule to keep women away from the battlefield.[15] Whether voluntary or coerced, many medical workers were on the civil war fronts, Red and White; the historian A. G. Katsnel'bogen puts the number of red Sisters of Mercy at six thousand and the number of orderlies at fifty thousand.[16] The state awarded the Red Cross medal to nineteen Sisters of Mercy and orderlies.[17]

The civil war and epidemics dictated emergency medical measures, and short-term training programs continued apace. A demographic catastrophe had already occurred after the loss of 2 million people from tuberculosis during World War I, more than the number of soldiers who died from wounds or disease (1.7 million).[18] Internationally, 40 million people died of Spanish flu in 1918. The English Quaker Muriel Payne wrote that illness or semi-starvation killed or invalided some 50 percent of the Russian medical staff in 1921.[19] Rampant disease as well as awful conditions in clinics and hospitals endangered the lives of many public healthcare workers. Nurse Zinaida Mokievskaia-Zubok, who had short-term training, recalled seeing the injured in corridors because of medical personnel shortages and the lack of wards.[20] She also noted that orderlies and *sidelki* were "good assistants" to the nurses.[21] In Voronezh, reports from the field in 1919 indicated that all medical workers in the area shared a 60 percent mortality rate.[22] But middle and junior medical workers seemed to suffer the most. The mortality rate for doctors infected with typhus was 60 percent in parts of Tambov; the rate for Sisters and Brothers of Mercy was 100 percent.[23] In other Russian towns hunger, cold, and lack of adequate healthcare led to high mortality rates and the spread of disease in 1918 and 1919.[24] The epidemics that spread during the civil war years spared neither medical workers nor their patients.

Given the attrition rate, the state called on anyone with medical experience to help fight against epidemics and work in medical institutions. One of the main authorities responsible for recruiting medical workers was the medical union. But the union experienced immense difficulties and struggled to mobilize Sisters of Mercy, a major problem given the "catastrophic situation" of the sick and injured in infirmaries and the absence of middle medical personnel.[25] Mobilization proved so difficult that in May 1919 the Main Military-Sanitation Administration called on the All-Russian Extraordinary Commission for Combating Counterrevolution and Sabotage (Cheka) to apply "a range of repressive measures to medical workers (especially Sisters of Mercy) who concealed their professional titles."[26] The nature of these repressive measures or their implementation is not clear. Nor is it clear whether they were effective. The Bolshevik approach to care, although aggressive, was characteristic of the time. Care would be ruthlessly enforced. A June 1921 Commissariat of Labor and Defense decree made it "obligatory for all medical workers, irrespective of age, to work in their profession."[27] This order was to take effect in September 1921.[28] The excessive discipline that came to characterize the Soviet home front during the Second World War was already evident during the civil war years. But the measures had some effect: by the end of the civil war sixty-six thousand women were serving in the Red Army, and almost 40 percent of them were medical workers.[29]

Nursing Schools

While the medical union was busy trying to send medical workers into the field, the Commissariat of Health turned to setting up nursing schools.[30] Beginning in August 1919, the Commissariat of Health's Department for Medical Schools and Personnel, led by L. Raukhvarger, would be the main authority charged with overseeing middle and junior medical education.[31] One of the department's first tasks was to determine how many nursing schools were actually open and functioning.[32] It was also supposed to establish "a relationship" between the schools and medical institutions as well as between medical and educational staff.[33] That was not all. The commissariat also charged this department with assuming the responsibilities of the Red Cross section for medical education and overseeing the establishment of new, socialist nursing schools. None of these were easy tasks. Taken together, the department had a substantial workload. The schools for which it was responsible were initially opened in medical departments of the Russian Red Cross (since transferred to the commissariat), and the first one opened in Moscow in 1920.[34] In 1922 the Main Committee for Professional-Technical Education (Glavprofobr), which was under the Commissariat of Education, took over middle medical education from the Red Cross (the Commissariat of Health took over middle medical education in 1930).[35]

The Commissariat of Health faced a formidable task. Its leaders, keen to get started, worked quickly with the Red Cross medical section to compile and issue the first socialist nursing textbook in February 1919. With a preface on the "basic rules of the organization of training in Sisters of Mercy schools," by V. M. Mikhailov, head of the Training Section of the Medical Council of the Central Board of the Russian Society of the Red Cross, the textbook set out the study plans and function of the nursing schools. The schools would "educate caring personnel for the patient's bedside" who were "able" and "conscientious." In the hospital the nurses would be the "closest person[s] to the patient, whose health was their primary interest." As those "at the beds of patients," nurses were to be "clever" and "honest," with a "correct understanding of relations toward the sick and their role in the life of the medical institution," and had to "execute all duties exactly as instructed by the attending doctor." Nurses were not to consider any kind of work beneath them, and "shirkers had no place in the hospital."[36] As the civil war continued, the new authorities began putting plans in place for the development of socialist nursing and what a socialist Sister of Mercy, or nurse, might look like.

Given the circumstances of civil war, the new healthcare authority managed to devote considerable attention to reshaping the nursing system. In

May 1920 a Commissariat of Health decree stipulated a complete takeover of the Sisters of Mercy schools by the new health authority; they were to have no religious connections, and political literacy was to be part of the study program.[37] No longer Sisters of Mercy, they were simply sisters.[38] By 1922 the Soviet Union had thirty-one reorganized nursing schools. Instruction in the schools placed an emphasis on practical hospital training.[39] The curriculum included "the new subjects of psychiatric illness, infectious diseases, factory medicine, and the basics of hospital management."[40] According to N. I. Propper, a key contemporaneous commentator on middle medical education, the new study program of 1922/1923 was not all that different from the Red Cross community program.[41] The Commissariat of Health's initial interest turned out to be more focused on changing the structure and organization of Sisters of Mercy schools. When it came to the content of nurses' education and training, healthcare officials seemed willing to leave well enough alone, at least for the time being.

The literature that new nursing students were to read, perhaps unsurprisingly at this stage, consisted of prerevolutionary texts. The majority of the over eighty or so recommended books were Russian medical textbooks, but some (about ten) were German translations. Only five textbooks were specifically for "sisters" and one was for "women"; most were medical textbooks for doctors, medical assistants, and feldshers.[42] Nurses, it seemed, did not merit their own literature. The course program made clear the importance placed on care and practical training. Theoretical training did not "illuminate any changes in the condition of the patient" and made nurses perform their duties in a "mechanical" fashion.[43] To avoid such an outcome, practical training would ensure that nurses emerged from the schools not as "third-rate doctors" but rather as "first-rate caregivers."[44] This stance was almost identical to that taken during the interwar years in Britain, where nursing establishments "feared that an emphasis on theory over practice would result in nurses becoming second-rate doctors and losing touch with the essential qualities of nursing."[45] As nursing schools were set up, ambiguity remained around the role of the Russian nurse. While nurses navigated the new terrain, the hospitals and institutions in which they worked were subject to change and restructuring.

Transition, Takeover, Reconstruction

Organizational challenges were a key feature of these years. The "countervailing pulls" of central and local actors identified in other professions, such as the printing industry, also applied to public healthcare.[46] Reorganizing the

Sisters of Mercy communities sometimes showed that the Commissariat of Health and local actors did not always have the same aims. Years of war had destroyed many hospitals and medical facilities, but not all, and local authorities valued those that remained in good condition.[47] By the end of 1919 the Bolsheviks, believing the civil war won, shifted their focus to "rebuilding and strengthening the Soviet state."[48] Such reconstruction efforts took place in nursing. But rebuilding infrastructure and institutions was not an easily surmountable task.

As the Commissariat of Health was setting out its agenda for the future of socialist healthcare, the situation on the ground was less orderly. The Red Cross Sisters of Mercy communities and their hospitals did not always experience a smooth transfer of power to the new Bolshevik authorities. Sometimes it was not even clear which authority would be taking over a given community, training school, or hospital. Although the process of transferring monies from the former Red Cross communities to the Commissariat of Health was relatively clear-cut because it involved only these two bodies, that was not the case with property. Any organization could use for military or medical purposes the buildings and premises belonging to the communities.[49] These organizations were ultimately answerable to the Commissariat of Health, as were all medical personnel.

This rather loose arrangement led to a struggle for control in some places. In Astrakhan, for example, the Red Cross infirmary was the victim of several attempted takeovers. The Union for Invalided Soldiers, the Provincial Commission for Health, and the Red Army all attempted to use the hospital for their own purposes. The Red Army tried to take charge, despite having an "excellent and well-equipped" 250-bed infirmary of its own.[50] This was of concern to the local Red Cross. It wanted to preserve the infirmary to serve the needs of the local population (all the more so because the infirmary had a department for women and midwifery).[51] The Red Cross authorities hoped to emerge victorious in this power struggle for the infirmary, claiming that the Sisters of Mercy community and the infirmary would be "destroyed" if taken over by the Red Army or the Union for Invalided Soldiers.[52] The struggle underscored the importance of property, with local authorities vying for control of buildings and equipment and sometimes using the interests of the local population as a form of collateral. This picture was broadly illustrative of the administrative situation affecting various organizations and professional groups across Russia, with "all sorts" of personnel mobilizing to protect their status and interests.[53]

Similar transfers took place in Yaroslavl', where the regional (okrug) Red Cross administration attempted to return the community hospital to the Russian

Red Cross but was unsuccessful, and indeed the Commissariat of Health wanted the hospital to be at the disposal of the health insurance fund.[54] While the administration of the hospital was under discussion, it still had to function as a teaching hospital, and its Sisters of Mercy worked in provincial and district medical facilities.[55] Sowing the seeds of a new state was deeply complex and dependent on social dynamics and societal relationships.[56] And as these power struggles and takeovers played out, medical workers had to continue to deliver care.

Sometimes the transfer of Red Cross nursing community property to the new Bolshevik authority (usually the health insurance fund) did not seem successful initially. The prolonged sense of confusion and impermanence among those involved in nurse training continued well into the 1920s. In discussions about the transfers, one Red Cross committee representative worried about the uncertainty of using buildings restored by the Russian Red Cross. The scenario "posed a serious threat to the successful development of local Red Cross activities," "harmed work," and "created unnecessary complications in the localities."[57] To eliminate the confusion, the new, Soviet Red Cross petitioned the Council of People's Commissars (Sovnarkom) for complete control over Russian Red Cross property and facilities, which were in any case "practically under its control."[58]

The transition from the tsarist-era Sisters of Mercy community schools to the new Soviet schools was a slow process that often encountered obstacles and required a good deal of negotiation between the relevant authorities. The ease of the transfer also depended on the size and location of the school. Discussions about transferring the large Aleksandrovskaia community to the Red Cross were quite complex.[59] A wealthy community, it possessed a 120-bed hospital (operating at a 100-bed capacity at that time) and a Sisters of Mercy training school for 120 students (82 at that time).[60] The authorities did not want to separate the Aleksandrovskaia community's hospital and school.[61] Moscow's Iverskaia community and its school also remained open (its hospital had 120 beds and its school had 36 students).[62] Sorting out the financial particulars and how the new schools should operate independently of the former communities was a major concern. The archive files suggest that transitions were also largely managed on a case-by-case basis.

That some of the Sisters of Mercy communities continued to function as such until the 1920s is testament to the difficulties of transfers and the protracted nature of discussions between the various parties involved. Also taken into account was the impact a transfer might have on nurse training. The head of the Medical Department, A. S. Puchkov, considered training experienced cadres of nurses to be one of the primary objectives of the Society of the Red

Cross.[63] It was important that the Aleksandrovskaia community did "not interrupt work in producing such nurses during the revolution" (in May 1922
the number of nurses would be nineteen and was set to increase to thirty in
1923).[64] Puchkov wanted the school and hospital handed over to the Red Cross
so that they could become a model institution.[65] The welfare of Sisters of
Mercy in the communities seemed to be of secondary interest to the process of transferring property and limiting disruption to producing nursing
graduates.

Once the new authorities took control of hospitals and schools, the issue
of maintenance became a problem for the cash-strapped Bolsheviks. Students,
staff, and patients needed food, bed linen, medication, and other essentials.
The Aleksandrovskaia community's school, which organized a two-year nursing course for seventy students in 1922, was to provide accommodation, food
rations, and administrative support for these students.[66] Glavprofobr and the
Moscow Health Department had to pick up the tab. The new proletarian
nurses were not in a position to pay for their studies or live under the "protection" of the community and thus became another expense for the public health
authorities.[67]

Such was the case in the handover of some of Moscow's hospitals. The Red
Cross was to have control over these so that it could have well-trained nurses
for its expanding activities. These hospital nurses could also work in military
hospitals, and, in this case, the Military Department "might subsidize the con-
tents of the school and hospital."[68] In the case of the Aleksandrovskaia community (and community hospitals and schools more generally), the Red Cross
could "break even" (bezubytochno) through the transfer and appropriation of
the former hospital.[69] Financial and economic considerations were foremost
in the minds of those overseeing medical education and organization thanks
to the exigencies of war communism.[70] Building the new socialist state was
expensive. It came as a serious shock for rural healthcare when the Soviet government issued a decree to transfer the funding of public health to local bud-
gets on May 1, 1922, thereby forcing the reintroduction of fees and the layoff
of medical personnel in some places—measures that put medical workers in
a precarious position (see chapter 3).[71]

A brief study of nursing schools in the Don Territory, back under Red Army
control since early 1921, exemplifies the problematic nature of the transfer of
power from one authority to another. Seven years of war, revolution, and civil
war left 5 percent of the population dead and 2.5 percent invalided.[72] When
the Red Army moved into Rostov in 1920, the nursing communities in the area
were reportedly closed and converted to schools for red Sisters of Mercy or
red nurses.[73] The new school for red nurses, with its thirty students, opened

under the Don Health Department (Donzdravotdel) in 1920, but the Don Department of Professional Education (Donprofobr) was due to take it over at
the end of 1921.[74] The transfer was "dependent" on the school merger with
the midwife-feldsher school, and "the two coexisted for a year." But unprepared
students left when they could not get to grips with the nursing program.[75]

Many of those entering the school were apparently only interested in a
"temporary place to stay" before "moving on once they had found somewhere
better," perhaps not an unreasonable attitude under the circumstances.[76] Those
who remained were "insignificant" in number and had nowhere to go.[77] Students showed a "complete indifference to study"—hardly surprising in the context of emerging famine after disastrous Bolshevik policies wreaked havoc on
the countryside.[78] Although the midwife-feldsher school had 160 applicants by
the end of the summer, the school for nurses received no applications.[79] Despite the dire need for nurses in Rostov-on-Don, few found a career in nursing
attractive.

The authorities in the Don Province reported that the nursing courses were
"undesirable" because of limited demand for medical personnel other than orderlies and *sidelki* to care for the sick and wounded. They closed the courses.[80]
These authorities also confirmed that the Donprofobr struggled to financially
support the school for red nurses under its authority since November 1921.[81]
In fact, it "proved difficult to force the remaining students to attend lectures
and undertake practical work," and they only did so under constant threat of
losing their "miserable ration" and "the right to live in dormitories" and even
expulsion." "Only in this way" did the school manage to produce nurses.[82] Survival and desperation motivated participation in the construction of the new
Soviet society. The period of transition and takeover saw individuals and institutions scramble to gain a foothold in the new society that was being created around them.

Defining the Soviet Nurse

While nursing schools were being set up, short-term courses to train "nurse
assistants" continued to address the shortage of medical workers. As matters
stood, untrained, "overwhelmingly illiterate" personnel cared for the sick.[83]
Junior medical personnel with little or no training cared for patients.[84] With
medical personnel falling ill, sometimes no personnel were available for shift
changes.[85] Raukhvarger argued for the short-term courses in 1920, saying that
it was better to have someone "partly trained" than "completely untrained."[86]
Short-term courses would continue in tandem with the two-and-a-half-year

courses. The latter would lay a "solid foundation on which to train cadres of genuine workers to care for the sick."[87] Until these schools started to produce nurses, the sick would have to make do with little-trained medical personnel. From the government's perspective, poorly trained nurses were better than none at all.

The medical union supported this short-term training arrangement as well as the commissariat's efforts to restructure education more generally.[88] The union kept busy: it organized new schools, and its central committee liaised with regional and provincial union branches when opening medical institutes, including nursing schools. It also oversaw both nursing schools and short-term courses for nursing assistants. The union and the Commissariat of Health agreed on the subject of education. As one union doctor noted, personnel to care for the sick were needed and short-term, six-month courses were the first step; thereafter, students could complete a two-year or two-and-a-half-year course in a nursing school.[89] The arrangement, supposedly temporary, appeared to meet with broad support. Power was not yet consolidated, and civil war conditions necessitated immediate and short-term measures.

Grander visions and practical realities coexisted and collided. Dreams of a socialist future but, more importantly, also planning for present needs characterized discussions about nursing and medical education. The indefatigable Raukhvarger envisaged the new school system as training medical students who were above all practically equipped to work in medical institutions. The school courses would familiarize young nurses, orderlies, and nannies with hospital life in ways that remained "unknown" to doctors and administrators.[90] Already possessing a good general educational background, they would learn about the biological sciences, caring for the sick, and hospital economics in the junior courses to help them be less "awkward around patients." The program covered a range of subjects such as social diseases, social hygiene, and epidemiology, as well as pharmacy and pharmacognosy—two "morphological subjects" that were included in the course in botany and pharmacology to avoid overloading students.[91] Presumably these downgraded subjects were to be restored to their longer formats once circumstances permitted. For now, the Commissariat of Health engaged in fire-fighting measures rather than strategic planning.

Raukhvarger and his colleagues in the Commissariat of Health had lots of ideas on how best to organize a Soviet healthcare system, but in conditions of civil war and famine, how could they expect to attract students to the nursing profession? Anna Haines, the American Quaker with a keen interest in Soviet nursing, claimed that the nursing profession was so unattractive to young women that "all ambitious and intelligent girls" instead opted for a career as feldsheritsas or midwives. As a result, Haines surmised that "hospital patients suffered from the lack of good nursing care, but usually neither they nor the doctors treating them had ever known what this might mean."[92] Nursing was an unknown entity to large swathes of the Soviet population and an occupation many associated with the aristocracy. The World War I portrayal of the tsarina and her daughters as kindhearted, gentle, and devoted was most likely an image that the Bolsheviks were not willing to be identified with, particularly as narratives of femininity were becoming displaced by the rhetoric of militancy and masculinity during the civil war years.[93]

Moreover, the role and status of the nurse was difficult to define. Midwives had a historical role in Russia and functioned on a semiprofessional basis. But the nurse was relatively new to Russia, at least in the trained, professional sense. The Sisters of Mercy had training that, according to Haines, was "more social than scientific."[94] The Commissariat of Health leaders were not discouraged by the somewhat ambiguous figure of the nurse. In fact, they seemed confident in their approach to creating the ideal Soviet nurse. Haines wrote that, having more or less all traveled abroad, they had ideas about how to introduce modern nursing to Russia.[95] Or, rather, they were eager to introduce what they understood to be modern nursing to Russia. As a result, Haines described how "enthusiastic medical men" across the country attempted to start training courses for nurses, though these were often disorganized. The majority were "miniature medical courses with most of the art of nursing omitted."[96]

Haines was not too far off in claiming that nursing was an unattractive profession for young Russian women. The new nursing schools sometimes struggled to draw and keep students. In Yaroslavl', for instance, the school for nurses had twenty-six students in 1920, but nine dropped out, partly for personal reasons and partly because of general economic conditions.[97] Two others were expelled for "indecent behavior" and violating dormitory rules. That left fifteen nursing students; after exams, thirteen remained. The following year, only five enrolled, with four turning up. This low figure was put down to "public ignorance" about the new program and the purpose of nursing schools.[98] Feldsher-midwife schools were more attractive options—as Haines had observed—and were "less demanding" with regard to general education qualifications.[99] Feldsher-midwife schools were already familiar to many Russians, who considered these professions to be more grounded in medical training. In Ufa many young people preferred the three-year feldsher-midwife courses to the nursing courses.[100] The health authorities validated this common perception, with Propper claiming in 1927 that midwives did not belong to the category of middle medical workers—their greater general medical knowledge base elevated their status.[101]

Another obstacle for schools was the lack of teaching staff. Doctors were already busy teaching courses for medical students, feldshers, and midwives. Even during school holidays, they taught short-term courses for disinfectant workers and orderlies.[102] They did not have the time to teach student nurses. There were some incentives. One doctor in Novgorod volunteered to become head of a nursing school to avoid active military service. He requested a transfer from his position in water transport, hoping that by heading a nursing school he would be ineligible for service.[103] It was probably not the kind of motivation the Commissariat of Health anticipated.

Some problems not only were practical in nature but also struck at the heart of who Soviet medical workers should be and how they could contribute to Soviet society. In its plans to dispense with the old system, the Commissariat of Health was keen to eliminate feldshers (field feldshers in particular), largely because of their generally bad reputation.[104] This plan caused considerable confusion in practice, not just for feldshers but also for local health boards, medical schools, and employers.[105] In Yaroslavl' the health authorities wanted to liquidate the feldsher school and reclassify it as a nursing school in the medical college (*tekhnikum*).[106] The reclassified nursing school would include an intake of men. This raised some eyebrows. Some commission members (a female doctor, three male doctors, and a female union representative) worried about Brothers of Mercy graduating from these nursing schools. They feared the schools would be "a poor surrogate, destroying feldshers and moving from caregiving staff to attending staff" (*perekhodia iz ukhazhivaiushchego personala v personal lechashchii*), where they would serve a "rural, uncultured population."[107] The urgent need for medical personnel and the drive for institute takeovers precipitated cursory discussions and hasty, ad hoc decisions about men and women as caregivers. Amid the practical and organizational changes taking place, those involved in medical matters used a language that differentiated between "care" and "medicine." Much of the debate about nursing over the next seventy years would be an attempt to reconcile the two.

After a rather terse discussion, the befuddled commission members charged with overseeing the enrollment of students at middle-level medical institutes in Yaroslavl' decided not to admit men to the nursing schools. These were a replacement for the feldsher schools, producing nurses instead of feldshers.[108] In the Smolensk health department (*guzdravotdel*) officials discussed whether field feldshers should attend lectures in the nursing schools but worried that they would gain an "incorrect interpretation" of their role because the schools aimed to train "caring personnel-nurses" to assist doctors, a role that would not overlap with that of the field feldshers.[109] As local officials adjusted to the new socialist reality, the center seemed to provide little in the way of clear instruction.

The gender lines dividing caregiving and the transfer of power between nursing and feldsher schools revealed confusion and discomfort among members of organizing committees, some of whom did not see men in a nursing (read caregiving) role. And still, as far as I have found, no discussion of Brothers of Mercy and their role as caregivers took place among Soviet healthcare planners. Nurses were women, even though small numbers of men qualified as nurses (Brothers of Mercy and then medical brothers) during the Soviet period. Men seemed more drawn toward becoming schooled feldshers while these courses still existed, and as the medical profession became feminized, men assumed the most senior positions in the medical profession. One advocate of women's rights writing shortly after the revolution noted that the few men working in medical institutions occupied a privileged position but "did not like difficult work," leaving that to their female colleagues.[110] As nursing schools and titles were being established in the 1920s, those administering care would be women.

Nurses Speak Out

Women encountered immense difficulties in their work as nurses in Russia, a situation exacerbated by the horrors of civil war. Violence became a modus operandi for tackling political and social problems after Lenin called for mass terror in June 1918.[111] Some Sisters of Mercy fled this terror. French-born Sister of Mercy Natal'ia Annikoff had trained for two years in St. Petersburg's Kaufmanskaia community, graduating in 1914. She spent the First World War working in a military hospital in St. Petersburg. Between 1918 and 1920 she worked in hospitals in Kiev, Sevastopol, and Novorossiysk, as well as at the front and on a Red Cross train. But in March 1918 she "escaped" Russia via Turkey and France and in 1923 settled in the United States, where she worked as a nurse.[112] Some were not so lucky: the Red Cross nurse Andrea-Aleksandra Stegman (born Baroness von Foelkersam) served time in the Lubianka prison in Moscow, an experience she later wrote about in her memoirs.[113] Other Sisters of Mercy fleeing Bolshevik terror during the civil war went eastward into China, as well as west to Yugoslavia.[114] Zinaida Mokievskaia-Zubok also emigrated in 1923, moved through Russia and into Ukraine and finally to Gallipoli, leaving behind the "horrible days of the Russian civil war."[115]

But a great many Sisters of Mercy remained in the former Russian Empire in spite of the civil war violence and political uncertainty. In October 1918 the speed of revolutionary change and the language of violence in Petrograd led to confusion. Ideas of revolution had taken root in medical institutions. Medical workers challenged authority figures.[116] In the Holy Trinity community head nurses accused probationary nurses of making false allegations about "repressions," including threats to deprive them of their food and wages, and claimed they committed infringements against community rules and regulations.[117] Depending on the severity of their offenses, some nurses remained in the community, but others faced expulsion owing to their "harmful attitude [*nastroenie*]."[118] The probationary nurses in this instance did not have protection within the community or outside of it, and so speaking out did not help their cause.

A general picture of disarray emerged during the years 1918–1919. The transition from one power authority to another in conjunction with demobilization, civil war, violence, epidemics, and famine created a mobile and disorderly society. The authorities sent nurses to different hospitals, towns, and provinces, often just temporarily. Why this was necessary was not always clear. Red Cross officials in the Petrograd region seemed to have their hands full after demobilization and orders to close the Sisters of Mercy communities. Their reports to the demobilization authority noted that the "majority of nurses in the northern front did not want to obey the order to leave their homes and communities."[119] Elsewhere, one bewildered Red Cross official requested that all orders for holidays and "needless" work trips (*komandirovki*) of nurses "stop immediately."[120] The treatment of medical personnel seemed to be a problem too. A feldsher and two nurses wrote to the medical union's conflict commission requesting an investigation into the "unjustified" removal of medical workers in Kursk.[121] Changes in administrative personnel precipitated dismissals. The medical union dealt with these various complaints, although whether it ever managed to resolve them is not clear.

Certain disputes were quite serious and, it would seem, demanded urgent attention. One such case was a complaint brought to the medical union's attention at its members' meeting in Mogilev in November 1919. The 150 present heard various complaints, including how workers in the Second Soviet hospital were "terrorized" in the wake of a restructured and "ineffectual" administration.[122] Employees appealed to the union, believing that the matter would be addressed. By taking this action, nurses and medical workers understood that the revolution offered them rights and responsibilities. Many of them acted when they believed the new rules of equality granted by the socialist revolution were being transgressed. A similar kind of agency has been ascribed to factory workers in Petrograd, where in 1917 their struggle to survive elicited a growth in "revolutionary feeling."[123] Appealing to the union thus gave workers a say in running the Mogilev hospital.

Nurses and medical workers also appealed to various forms of authority for clemency and support. One Sister of Mercy with two young children wrote to the Borisoglebskii medical-sanitation branch in Tambov, stating that she did not want to do anti-epidemic work.[124] A "responsible and useful" worker in the Commissariat of Enlightenment (the Ministry of Education), she received a favorable outcome, as the commissariat was keen for her to continue her work there.[125] Medical workers able to show their commitment to building the revolution had some leverage. That the nurse had two young children was of less importance than her work in the Commissariat of Enlightenment.

Ample evidence shows that nurses wanted to have their say. In Moscow a group of nurses from the Aleksandrovskaia community, having already formed a council of nurses in the hospital where they worked, voiced their displeasure after a new head doctor was appointed in a closed competition and the council of nurses had not been informed of the vacancy. The nurses wanted the hospital to open a new competition.[126] Such instances of nurses acting in an independent manner were a relatively new occurrence. Before the revolution the appointment of a new head doctor, even if unpopular, would not have met with such challenges.

Nurses in Tambov also spoke out against perceived injustices. Problems with the Tambov nursing community came to the attention of the Union of Sisters of Mercy after four unemployed nurses, identified as working in a community, "refused" to go to the Volga District to treat epidemic victims.[127] Meanwhile, another group of nurses, identified as "wartime nurses" working in the community's infirmary, "categorically refused" to vacate their dormitory places for medical staff.[128] The medical and nursing authorities had their hands full dealing with personnel, training schools, and general reorganization. Civil war and epidemic conditions made their work much harder.

The difficult circumstances no doubt contributed to the frequent reports of problems in infirmaries and field hospitals. A military commission found that patients were rude to service personnel and suggested warning unruly patients that if they complained but subsequently made a full recovery, they would face "disciplinary punishment." The commission added that altercations with patients and obvious negligence would in the future count as "noncompliance" of their contract (*kak nesootvetstvie svoemu sluzhebnomu naznacheniiu*).[129] Sometimes nurses had to take matters into their own hands. At the behest of her nurses, the head nurse in the St. George community wrote to the head doctor of the Semenovskii-Aleksandrovskii infirmary to complain about the dirty conditions of the infectious disease department. She also told colleagues that her nurses did the work of orderlies and students (besides their own duties).[130] These nurses, as the head nurse claimed, tolerated the awful conditions out of feelings of "pity for the patients." When the nurses requested a transfer, the head nurse petitioned the head doctor, requesting an improvement in their working conditions; if this was not done, she threatened to "withdraw the nurses as soon as possible."[131] The head doctor replied, acknowledging the invaluable work of the nurses, and promised to improve their working conditions and ease their workload.[132] In the above examples, nurses identified as a group and took collective action to make their case to higher authorities. Their local, collective action formed part of the revolutionary zeal that characterized the times.[133]

Patients Speak Out

The terrible conditions for medical workers and patients were particularly apparent to outside observers. Friend Muriel Payne noticed that patients often slept "two in a bed and even on the floors," while in the provinces it was "common to find dead children among the living."[134] In a pamphlet on a proposed American hospital for Moscow, Quaker Jessica Smith wrote that wages were so low that some doctors and nurses served in two or three different hospitals (a situation that remained unchanged after the civil war).[135] Corpses lay in some hospital yards for two months due to the absence of coffins and transport.[136] Nikolai Semashko, as Commissar of Health, reportedly implored the American Friends Service Committee (AFSC) to "send ambulances, sterilizing outfits, instruments, and drugs sufficient to equip a large hospital in Moscow, where epidemics were taking a terrible toll."[137] The Bolsheviks opted to fund industry rather than public healthcare, thus gambling with people's lives. Even military hospitals and infirmaries in Leningrad lacked dishes, spoons, and plates for patients.[138] The Central Military Control Commission reported that medical workers also had no gowns, nor was there was soap for washing bed linen (and sometimes bed linen was not even available).[139] In some of the military hospitals, lice were "literally eating the patients."[140] By 1921 the Bolsheviks represented "a socialism of scarcity," where the needs of the individual were subordinate to economic development.[141]

That patients complained should come as no surprise given these conditions. Doctors meeting in Tambov's provincial hospital discussed "sabotage," while patients accused middle medical personnel of providing "insufficient care."[142] Nurses and feldshers were often absent from wards and left patients to their own devices.[143] Thus began a recurring pattern: blaming medical workers instead of abstract and often misunderstood forces such as the revolution or the government. By not prioritizing healthcare funding during the civil war and well beyond, the Soviet state turned its back not only on medical workers—who became easy targets of criticism—but also on the very citizens whose lives it sought to improve.

Some patients who were unhappy with the care they received wrote letters of complaint to the relevant authorities. Several patients, former soldiers, wrote to the Red Cross about their great need to receive care. They were in a Red Cross infirmary, where they claimed that nannies, orderlies, and nurses did not treat the sick and injured, told them they were all "crazy," and said that "if they complained, nobody would pay any attention." The group of former soldiers wrote that patients suffered and died. Those who could afford to paid nannies to clean and provide them with extra food portions. In this Red Cross infirmary, the patients lamented, only the bugs enjoyed freedom, and there was more freedom "in prison or under the old regime." These conditions were particularly hard for the mentally ill patients, who understood that they were being "laughed at and forced to be silent [*prinuzhden molchat'*]." The former soldiers saw patients' anxiety and agitation increase whenever a sidelka—a nanny who sat with and looked after patients—swore or laughed at them. They wanted the authorities to know what was going on and to improve the situation.[144]

To a degree, the provincial health department (*gubzdravotdel*) addressed the problem in February 1921 when it set about organizing three-month nursing courses for the care of the mentally ill.[145] This move was likely a response to problems in the area. A Comrade Lamberg, for instance, had noted a decline in labor discipline among junior personnel and wanted to raise their qualifications, especially with regard to psychiatric care, where caring for mentally ill patients required "more conscientious and intelligent workers" who could "calm patients and not disturb them."[146] While not particularly medical or scientific, this approach to the care of the mentally ill nonetheless recognized that psychiatric patients needed help. The proposed three-month courses would "focus on psychiatric institutions," and nurses who completed the study program would be able to provide better care.[147] This arrangement to introduce yet more short-term courses unfortunately only led to future problems in the quality of care, problems that would be felt some ten years later. But the move at least acknowledged the still grave problems confronting the Commissariat of Health, not to mention the appalling suffering of patients.

Challenges to Order: The Case of Lesnikov and the Soup

In 1918 a case from the Fourth Red Cross Infirmary for Red Army Soldiers, located in Vologda, in northwest Russia, demonstrates the difficulties patients and nurses experienced. The case involved the patient Lesnikov and the nurse Aleksandra Prokof'eva, but other patients and staff in the hospital became embroiled as the investigation ran its course. Problems in the hospital first came to the attention of the senior doctor when the head of housekeeping, Valentina Ivanovna Lipinskaia, complained that patients received food they did not want and therefore had to "starve."[148] At the center of the consternation was the twenty-two-year-old patient Lesnikov, accused of being rude and complaining about the coffee and food, especially the soup.[149] The practicalities of making socialism work in hospitals and clinics come to the fore in this case. That the Bolsheviks did not plan a clear strategy for workers' self-management or provide guidance becomes evident when examining medical institutions, where confusion indicated a battle for power and control on every level, as the following incident shows.[150]

Housekeeping had its hands full with young Lesnikov, who became unruly and smashed dishes when he was unhappy with the food or the service.[151] Rowdy patients would not listen to staff appeals for calm, responding only with "obscene swearing and insults." Lipinskaia stopped going to the ward and implored the head doctor to take measures to prevent such "undeserved abuse" and to inform superiors about the patients' behavior.[152] Another patient, thirty-three-year-old Alekseev, claimed that the nursing staff gave them oatmeal porridge instead of semolina, thereby more or less confirming Lesnikov's unhappy mealtime experiences. When the nurse denied this accusation, the patients smashed the plates. If fed in this way, and if this was "patient care," then there would be more "excesses," they claimed.[153] Alekseev added that when he inquired whether Sister Prokof'eva, who had come to dress him, had washed her hands, she retorted that "the nurse herself knows how to do a dressing."[154]

Another patient called on to testify in the case was the soldier Shakkel', who corroborated the other patients' testimonies but added that there were "among the caring personnel many good and attentive workers, although there were negative types, not suitable for their positions, such as Sister Prokof'eva." He claimed that Prokof'eva put diluted hydrochloric acid drops in his eyes on purpose to "make them [his eyes] ugly."[155] When he complained about the pain and requested boric acid to rinse his eyes, he was subjected to "gross abuse." Another patient made similar complaints about food and patient care. He also claimed that Prokof'eva spent all her time caring for another patient in the ward and never washed her hands after dealing with him (the patient had gonorrhea).[156]

When questioned, Prokof'eva claimed to know nothing about the Lesnikov matter, but she did defend herself against Shakkel''s accusations about the eyedrops. She said she made a mistake but claimed Shakkel' verbally abused her when she tried to remedy the situation.[157] She accepted that she was rude to patients but blamed the Red Army and Red Guard soldiers for bringing disorder to the hospital.[158] The investigation found that Lesnikov's behavior was due to his dissatisfaction with the soup, but more so to the food he received being contrary to doctor's instructions. Most important, the investigation commission concluded that the entire incident was but a "partial manifestation of the permanent misunderstandings between patients and caregivers more or less plaguing all medical institutions recently."[159] This damning indictment was a sorry reflection of patient care in the fledgling Soviet state.

The commission further concluded that the food in the hospital was "good and tasty." It blamed the "spirit of the times" for disagreements between patients and medical personnel, as well as between the middle and junior medical personnel. The patients were too demanding, considering it their right to meddle in the internal running of the medical institution; meanwhile, the caregiving staff was not always attentive to the sick.[160] The commission noted that even in the presence of the investigative officers, Lesnikov received a meat dish (likely also against the doctor's orders) and the service personnel abused him. To resolve the issue, the Red Army and Red Guard soldiers would move to the First Red Army Infirmary. The commission would deal with the Prokof'eva and Shakkel' incident separately. It had the unenviable task of deciding who to believe—the patient or the nurse.

Irrespective of this particular case, the commission found the overriding issue to be that almost all patients filed "allegations of negligence, mistreatment, and curtness" against Prokof'eva.[161] Consequently, the commission recommended that the local Red Cross administration dispense with the services of Prokof'eva. But Sister A. Krasnitskaia, a commission member and colleague of Prokof'eva (identified as a wartime nurse), stated that Prokof'eva "always met the medical requirements."[162] Krasnitskaia acknowledged the complaints against Prokof'eva but favored her transfer to another hospital and discharge from the Red Cross only if there were further incidents.[163] The final decision to dismiss Prokof'eva was unanimous. Her actions did not befit the "high title of nurse" and the "moral duty" of nurses "to serve their patients with love"

and to fulfill doctors' orders.[164] But because of her young age and long service, as well as words of support from Krasnitskaia and other colleagues, she
was not to be dismissed from the Red Cross unless found guilty of further
misdemeanors.[165]

Above all, the case indicated the poisonous atmosphere that could develop
as a result of poor relations between staff and patients. After the revolution,
both patients and medical workers believed they had the right to demand better conditions. But as the Lesnikov case highlighted, expectations were sometimes too high. The lofty ideals of the revolution led many to feel entitled to
a better life under socialism. When these ideals and expectations were not met,
as in Lesnikov's case, they became disillusioned and occasionally aggressive.
Those in administrative positions had identified a gulf between revolutionary
rhetoric and reality, but it had yet to become evident to some of the patients.
Also lacking was a clear moral or ethical code. Ethics was a considerable gray
area, and Lenin had been dismissive of morality's usefulness to the proletar-
iat.[166] The lack of clarity was not particularly helpful for medical workers navi-
gating the choppy waters of revolution.

In spite of problems and complaints, patient care seemed to be a priority
in most medical institutions, at least in principle. The references to "moral
duty" and "love" suggest a nascent ethical code. Senior personnel were willing to take action against complaints, and hospitals usually took measures to
improve the situation for patients and staff. Evidence shows that state actors
saw the revolutionary project as "humane and emancipatory" as well as "rational and modern."[167] Even in spite of the desperate need for medical workers, an attempt was made to maintain standards, with nurses such as Prokof'eva
called to account for their negligence. Patient care came first.[168]

Elsewhere, a Commissariat of Health inspection team conducted an investigation at the Zakharino hospital-sanatorium to hear patient complaints. The
initial plan was to interview certain patients to ascertain whether they had any
grievances, but in the end the inspectors walked around all the wards interviewing patients.[169] Complaints were generally about food, delays in changing bed linen, lack of shoes, and other problems. Investigators suspended a
nanny seen eating meat destined for a patient's soup as she walked from the
kitchen to the main building (there was no escaping the hunger of the times—
in her defense the nanny pleaded "starvation").[170] Patients and medical workers felt free to exercise their rights before the Commissariat of Health and the
medical union, believing that they deserved better. To their credit, the authorities made a genuine effort to sift through and respond to these issues. And
while they often did their best to improve conditions, sometimes they were

fighting a losing battle. Once again, the ideals of the revolution outpaced the realities of the present. The mismatch created conflict and tension for nurses and patients.

The attempt to establish a socialist healthcare system that prioritized the patient experience overlooked the habitat of medical workers, particularly newly trained nurses. The nurses called for by the state allegedly lacked the level of culture necessary to deliver the standard of care expected by the public health authorities. The civil war years and the possible "brutalization" of social life that accompanied them were more conducive to a "roughening" of behavior than to delivering a high level of care.[171] This applies to both medical workers and patients. And yet, especially from 1923 on, workers familiar with cultural revolution and the Bolshevik party's drive to promote manners and good habits came to expect better treatment at the hands of medical workers. This idealistic view of the revolution was evident even in 1918, as the case of Lesnikov shows.

To be sure, Semashko and the health authorities had good intentions for creating a socialist nurse and an effective public healthcare system. But in the early 1920s there was no real effort to popularize nursing and present it as an attractive and worthy profession. The restructuring that took place during the transition period created a great deal of chaos. Power vacuums and power struggles led to immense tensions in hospitals and other medical institutions as management changes and reorganization often had negative consequences for medical workers and patients.

What did care in an aspiring communist society actually mean? What was the moral duty of the nurse? These were questions healthcare workers asked after the revolution. While medical workers and patients wondered about the moral economy of the new socialist state and how this translated to patient care, the Commissariat of Health and its departments were busy overseeing institutional transitions and course programs. Although the Soviet state would later come to care a great deal about the morality of its people, upstanding behavior was not exactly a state concern during the civil war years. Local actors parsed the directives and worked things out for themselves. The ideological mission was on ice. Pressing political and economic circumstances meant that there was no definitive ethical guidance for medical workers. As Russian and, later, Soviet citizens died from starvation, disease, and conflict, major questions about nursing, and public healthcare more generally, went unanswered.

CHAPTER 3

Black Star, Red Star

Finding the Soviet Way

In 1921 the New Economic Policy (NEP) replaced war communism and its associated policies of state nationalization of industry and grain appropriation. Marked by a return to private trade and cultural experimentation, the more liberal NEP years were not roundly welcomed. NEP society was not popular among those who fought for the revolution and viewed the policy as a betrayal. Even though Lenin and the Bolsheviks envisaged the NEP as a temporary measure, for committed Marxists it seemed an ideological departure. It also led to the creation of a contradictory and pluralist society. While some, the so-called NEPmen and NEPwomen, profited during the years 1921–1927, others continued to endure hardship. Still, this period offered an element of relief from the horrors of war.[1] For medical workers, the NEP years also offered some respite, but life was still very difficult.

Training nurses and medical workers remained a key healthcare goal. But it became apparent that the Soviet authorities needed international help. Aware that vast swathes of the population were not enamored with the NEP or still suffering from the effects of years of famine and fighting, they had to tread carefully in accepting support from foreign entities. This chapter examines that delicate balance between providing care amid an overwhelming lack of resources and obtaining medical supplies and expertise without ideological and political compromise. Soviet interest in foreign healthcare was a step on the path to shaping a socialist system of care best suited to the needs of Soviet citizens and the state.[2] In some ways, working with foreigners helped senior Soviet healthcare figures build a clearer picture of socialist nursing.

Debates about the future of Soviet nursing were symptomatic of larger political discussions about the nature of socialism under the Bolsheviks and how Soviet leaders sought to position the state internationally. In spite of the political tensions present after the Bolshevik revolution, international groups discussed and coordinated medical relief and assistance. The chaos and horrors of world war, revolution, and famine met with a massive humanitarian response. Connections with foreign contacts continued, albeit on a lesser scale, during the 1920s, when the Soviet government was open to negotiation and the presence of foreign organizations operating within its borders.[3] But Soviet health leaders were also intent on pursuing their own agenda for public healthcare. In the 1920s this agenda principally focused on social hygiene, an area of public health that promoted well-being in the belief that disease was a problem of social as well as biological conditions.[4]

The foreign organizations' attempts to establish a nurse training school in Russia reveals much about both Western and Russian attitudes to public healthcare. Examining medical assistance and negotiations shows that "outsiders" dealing with Russia often found it more challenging to overcome social and cultural differences than the political or the ideological.[5] The attempt to establish and operate a school illustrates how Western agents assumed that their system of medical practice was better than the Russian. Such issues and attitudes were at the heart of establishing and running a Western-style training school. While dealing with foreign efforts to establish a nursing school, the Soviet government was also confronted with the mammoth tasks of improving the public health system and quelling economic crises and a host of other pressing issues. This chapter tells us much about how the Russians envisaged nursing taking shape in the first decade of Bolshevik power.

Foreign Influence and Exchange

The early 1920s saw the health authorities struggle to define and organize nursing education. The fledgling socialist state, while politically cast away from the wider international community, found itself drawn toward Britain and the United States when it came to matters of public health and nursing. These countries, standard-bearers for nursing education, were also grappling with nurse training. Good quality care depended on the training and education of medical workers. Those authorities responsible for medical education were still trying to figure out a system that would work. While the Soviet Union deliberated on nursing education in the early 1920s, other countries also were asking questions about the training nurses should undergo. In Europe and the United States, "one of the greatest impediments to reforming nursing education," notes historian Anne Marie Rafferty, "was the lack of agreement among nurse leaders as to what constituted a proper training."[6] In the United States the Goldmark Report (1922–1925) and its questions over the training of public health nurses and hospital nurses was evidence of this debate.[7]

The Soviets might have argued that a new type of communist approach was necessary to address particular local conditions, but, at the same time, there was no concealing the interest of the Soviet health authorities in British and US nurse training or the fact that Soviet debates fit into wider international debates during the interwar period.[8] But nursing occupied a liminal space on the edges of science and medicine; as a profession it was still reasonably young by international standards. Nursing thus represented a venture into the unknown for the new Soviet healthcare officials.

Diminishing the role of the Sisters of Mercy and advancing the cause of ordinary women to train as nurses should have complemented the Bolshevik campaign for female emancipation and helped meet the urgent need for medical workers. It would in principle have opened up a new field whereby women could prove themselves and become socially active, a central tenet of party policy and political rhetoric. Moreover, women had shown that they were capable of performing nursing duties during the First World War and civil war.

But the Bolsheviks were slow to arrive at this idea. After war and revolution, middle medical workers were not promoted but "inhabited an ill-defined and expansive territory."[9] Early Soviet policy regarding medical workers and gender was, if anything, conservative. Nurses, as women, were "natural caregivers," and men did not seem to have a place in this feminine world. In the context of the NEP, nurses might easily have struggled to identify as proletarian workers.[10] Indeed, in addition to the great need for physicians in rural areas, another reason for the ultimate retention of the feldsher might have been to provide men with a place in middle medical work apart from supposedly female nursing. Nursing in Russia followed the northern European and US trend whereby women dominated the profession. But care and compassion are not unique to women, and as Christie Watson, a former nurse in Britain's National Health Service, writes, "Nursing is seen as one of the most lowly (female) professions . . . and rather than integrating it along non-gender lines, the act of caring is not considered valuable."[11] The Soviet healthcare authorities did place value on care: the difficulty lay in transposing ideas around caregiving to the clinical setting.

Exchanging medical literature between the Soviet Union and the United States, Germany, and England was part of the process of learning about public healthcare, nursing, and caregiving.[12] The New York Medical Academy sent copies of *American Nursing*, the *Journal of Social Hygiene*, and the *American Journal of Public Health* to Russia between 1920 and 1923.[13] Representatives from the medical union wrote to communists working in medicine in North America and Great Britain, looking to establish contact. They also wrote to the British Bureau of the Red International of Labor Unions, or Profintern, and sent materials for publication in the organization's literature.[14] There were similar exchanges with the International Council of Nurses (ICN) in London and the Medical Association of Canada.[15] Medical workers elsewhere in Europe were of interest too; medical union correspondence with the Union of Catalonian Physicians in Barcelona inquired about medical workers in Catalonia and Spain. The union was also eager to disseminate its work abroad through the journal *Medical Worker* (*Meditsinskii rabotnik*). Other countries corresponding with the medical union included the United States, Belgium, France, the Netherlands, Japan, and Bulgaria.[16]

Commissariat of Health correspondence from the period 1923–1926 indicates a clear Soviet interest in British attitudes to healthcare, especially childcare.[17] Indeed, in July 1925 the Commissariat of Health correspondent in London sent a letter to Moscow suggesting that League of the Society of the Red Cross and London University's Bedford College–run courses to train nurses for administrative and teaching positions might be of interest to the commissariat.[18] The international courses, with the aim of training nurses to work in the fields of "visiting nursing, child welfare, school and TB nursing, prenatal and maternity nursing," addressed areas of public health in which the Soviet Union had a strong interest.[19] The emphasis on hygiene in the home, school, and factory would also have appealed to the Soviet proclivity toward prophylaxis, with lectures on hygiene and sanitation already featured in the Soviet nursing curricula from 1922.[20] In education, the Soviet government also concentrated its efforts on basic hygiene and cleanliness to help reduce infant deaths and disease.[21] Yet no Soviet nurse ever attended the courses.

The Soviet health authorities were keen to observe rather than necessarily adopt Western models of nursing education. There was still a lack of international clarity about nurse training, with considerable conflict between the British and US approaches to nursing.[22] Many European countries had only begun to establish their national nursing professions during these initial decades of the twentieth century, when nurses had started to seek greater professional rights and recognition. Predominantly male physicians looked down on the overwhelming majority of female nurses, with institutional and political policy reinforcing this gendered and hierarchical imbalance in the medical world. In an attempt to deal with such perceptions, the ICN characterized nursing as a "particularly female profession": nurses were reformers who "built upon a sense of nursing autonomy in which they claimed that nursing was not a medical profession and thus presented no threat to the authority of doctors, but that therefore neither [was] nursing [to] be controlled by doctors."[23] Parallel debates did not happen in the Soviet Union because nurses did not have their own association or leaders.

The "Art of Nursing"

When foreigners came into direct contact with Russian nursing, other issues overshadowed these broader debates about the profession. Western nursing was largely presented as well developed and generally more advanced than Russian nursing. Indeed, negative accounts of Russian nursing standards abound in First World War memoir and diary literature. The trained British nurse Violetta Thurston, for instance, who worked for the Russian Society of the Red Cross (ROKK) in a Russian hospital in Warsaw, observed: "The art of nursing as practiced in England does not exist in Russia."[24] The effort to "reform" nursing after the war began when US philanthropies such as the Rockefeller Foundation funded medical training schemes across eastern Europe. It established and funded nursing schools in Poland, Czechoslovakia, and other countries and set up training exchange programs in the 1920s.[25] Russia was also of interest to the foundation.[26]

In 1922 the English Quaker Muriel Payne and Lady Muriel Paget of the Save the Children Fund proposed setting up a training school for nurses in Russia to address the lack of knowledge about motherhood and infant mortality.[27] While the Russian health authorities signed an agreement for an English medical unit to train Russian nurses, sufficient international funding was not secured.[28] Payne, a registered nurse, considered nurse training and care in Russia lacking and claimed that "40% of the deaths among the children in the Emergency Children's Homes and Hospitals, were not directly due to Famine, but could have been prevented if the nurses in charge, had had some knowledge of Medical and Nursing care."[29] Paget shared Payne's concerns and blamed much of the infant mortality in Russia on its poorly trained personnel.[30] Payne and Paget had a point, but they overlooked problems with food supply and distribution.

The high rate of infant mortality also troubled the Soviet government, and the Commissariats of Health and Enlightenment both supported the idea of a nursing school.[31] The scheme was also proposed at a time of immense suffering. There are many examples of the horrors endured by families afflicted by famine and disease, with mothers abandoning or murdering their children to avoid witnessing their suffering from starvation.[32] The discussions between the Russians and relief organizations thus took place against a backdrop of extreme hardship for those in the famine-stricken parts of Soviet Russia.

It was hardly a surprise, then, that the Russians seemed to welcome the proposal for the training school and the presence of foreign nurses. The chief doctor in the Commissariat of Enlightenment hoped the British would hold a series of lectures on nursing in medical institutions.[33] While Paget believed that the commissariat wanted to improve child welfare, she considered it "handicapped by total lack of executive female personnel through whom to carry out a constructive health program."[34] In her plan to combat child mortality in Russia, Paget recommended establishing a hospital for mothers and children, organizing a child welfare center, and establishing a training school for Russian nurses, as well as eventually establishing nursing schools in different parts of Russia.[35] This plan spilled over into the remit of the physician Vera Lebedeva's Department for the Protection of Mothers and Infants (*Otdel Okhrany Materinstva i Mladenchestva* or OMM), established in 1918. Lebedeva (a strong candidate for "executive female") was already involved in recruiting young women interested in attending the OMM's ten-month courses on childcare.[36]

For its part, the Russian Commissariat of Enlightenment agreed to recognize the Russian nurses who would receive this training as a "special part of the Russian nursing profession" and continue their caregiving work after the British unit left Russia.[37] Payne devised a detailed syllabus for the training school, but she made it clear that English nurses would be in charge of the wards and would supervise training.[38] Such an arrangement left little doubt about which country had the "superior" nursing system, but the Russians nonetheless supported the scheme. The Soviet health authorities engaged in information gathering as part of their effort to acquire greater knowledge about nursing practice and how it might work in the context of socialist public healthcare.[39]

Foreign Flirtations and Soviet Exhibitions

A large part of the information gathering centered on the health of the mother and child. Maternal and infant care were considered a woman's domain and were associated with the *babka*, or midwife.[40] As much as the Soviet government might have disliked midwives, it could not afford to dispense with their services.[41] But perhaps the prospect of trained public health nurses and a move away from the image of traditional midwives, and connotations with the pre-revolutionary past, also attracted official support for the nursing scheme. Even so, the Soviet health authorities seemed content to observe the nursing scheme's developments from the margins while continuing to deal with public healthcare issues such as mother and child health. They also continued to develop new roles for the nurse: one early initiative was the creation of the Tuberculosis Section of the Moscow Department of Public Health and the Model Dispensary, which employed nurses to visit patients.[42]

As the Soviet state tackled various problems, US parties continued to express interest in helping it deal with maternity and infant care and the public health crisis more generally. Two US physicians, Elsie Graff, of the American Medical Women's Association, and Esther Lovejoy, arrived in Moscow to provide support in the areas of motherhood, infancy, and childcare, as well as tuberculosis and venereal disease.[43] Payne, in the meantime, continued with her plans for the nurse training school.[44]

The Russian government, the Commissariat of Health, and the ROKK continued to support Payne's efforts.[45] They also remained interested in US and British approaches to childcare and maternity.[46] The plan for the international school of nursing, which was to be under the purview of the Commissariat of Health, was essentially the same as that proposed in 1922 and entailed sending about eight fully qualified English nurses to Russia to train Russians in the care of mothers and infants and the sick and in disease prevention.[47] It would have a training center with a hospital for children "suffering from dietetic diseases" along with "an Infant Welfare Clinic, Milk Dispensary, and ward for mothers." Such a scheme would have been significant for mother and child health in Russia. Vera Lebedeva no doubt welcomed the foreign support, all the more so since the OMM had to close a third of its facilities and accept budgetary cutbacks in 1922.[48] Unfortunately for Payne, in early 1923 she admitted with "great sorrow" that the international school had not succeeded in obtaining the necessary funds.[49] But once again, others stepped into the fold.

At around that time, Lillian Wald—a major figure in US nursing and human rights—took an interest in Russian nursing.[50] The interest was mutual. In February 1924 public health officials invited Wald to Russia to inspect activities in public health and nursing.[51] For the new Soviet state, the trip in late spring of 1924 held considerable potential. The Commissariat of Health noted that Wald and the other delegates had "immense experience in the area of public health" and could "demonstrate for the Soviet audience how public health in America was conducted." Health officials invited her to do just that at a touring exhibition; it would feature material on nursing and public health in the United States, including "two posters, six copies of 'The Public Health Nurse,' miscellaneous pamphlets," and other material on social hygiene.[52] (Wald had also sent ahead several thousand dollars' worth of films, charts, books, and other materials, funded by Mrs. John D. Rockefeller and US nurses, but the Russians mislaid these items.)[53]

Wald's trip to the Soviet Union was also designed to familiarize Americans with Soviet public health and childcare.[54] The Russians did not show Wald a Potemkin village: from 1924, part of the Soviet strategy when receiving foreign guests was to demonstrate socialist achievements and tailor their visits accordingly.[55] Wald saw the best and the worst that Soviet public healthcare had to offer. She was generally unimpressed by the lack of organization and the Soviet inability to put theories of child welfare into practice. Nonetheless, the efforts of Lebedeva and her department heartened Wald, even if they seemed unable to "initiate intelligent interesting nursing" and send trained nurses to the countryside.[56] For his part, the Americans' host, Nikolai Semashko, seemed to take great pleasure in informing his guests that socialism had given proletarian women the opportunity to become nurses, which "never would have happened under the old regime." Wald saw similar challenges confronting Soviet and US public healthcare, and her most pertinent concern was the lack of medical workers drawn to work outside of the major cities. To remedy this problem she suggested establishing a school of nursing in the Samara region.[57]

Wald's trip took her to Soviet hospitals, clinics, factories, and other institutions. A highlight was a factory preventorium—in Wald's opinion, one of "the best establishments of its kind for tuberculosis . . . seen in any country."[58] In her reflections on Russia, recounted in her book *Windows on Henry Street*, Wald did not always see Soviet socialist medical practice as different to that before the revolution or in the West. Having already visited Russia in 1910 and armed with a deep knowledge of social and public health work in the United States and abroad, Wald was often hesitant to view changes in organizations and structures as "Soviet initiatives" or innovations. Yet, Wald's interest in Russia and the Soviet approach to public healthcare would soon be cemented by her role as one of the vice presidents of the American Russian Society for Cultural Relations with Russia, established in 1926.[59] More importantly for nursing in Russia, Wald's trip drew attention to nursing and the importance of establishing training schools to provide modern standards of care to Soviet citizens.

New Soviet Nurses

Vera Lebedeva was working toward the same goal. Her motherhood and infancy clinic hosted Anna Haines when she returned to Russia as a qualified nurse in the summer of 1925. Between 1918 and 1927, the OMM had three divisions: women's outpatient clinics (*zhenskie konsul'tatsii*), Soviet women's homes (*patronazh*), and homes for mother and child (*doma materi i rebenka*).[60] Although it sought to improve mother and child health, the department also wanted to change peasant perceptions of the world and took a pronatalist position.[61] Through their interest in training and education, Haines and the American Friends Service Committee (AFSC) made a valuable contribution to Lebedeva's department. They helped to fund the training of several nurses, some of whom came from Samara and Mongolia.[62] Lebedeva's clinic itself had a school for three hundred student nurses training in infant welfare.[63] Once they graduated, the nurses, largely from rural areas, would return to work in the countryside. This kind of arrangement would fit with state propaganda campaigns to educate and inform village mothers about infant care, acculturating and enlightening the masses.[64] It also indicated that some of Wald's ideas about rural nursing might have had some influence.

The Commissariat of Health engaged in an ongoing process, begun back in 1918, to determine the best way to organize and administer care. By 1924 the Russian Soviet Federated Socialist Republic (RSFSR) had 35 midwifery colleges, 28 feldsher-midwife schools—although some of these were subject to closure—and 24 nursing schools, from which 587 students had graduated, including a further 120 schools in maternity and infant care.[65] Two evening schools with three-year courses for training nurses opened in Moscow in 1925.[66] Two middle medical workers' conferences, the first held in 1922 and the second in 1926, played an important role in determining the shape of middle medical education and specialization.[67] New roles for an educational nurse for maternal and child care (*sestra vospitatel'nitsa*) and nurses for patient care and midwifery were also created—by the mid-1920s a multitude of very specific nurse titles and roles existed.[68] In an article about middle medical education, N. I. Propper questioned how the medical college would cater to these specific types of nurses and middle medical workers. This was logistically challenging but also, as Propper deduced, expensive and likely limited to specialist centers in major cities. In the end, Propper concluded that four types of middle medical workers were necessary: midwives, nurses, motherhood and infancy nurses, and nurses for social assistance.[69]

Discussions about middle medical education presaged further restructuring in 1926–1928, when the authorities overhauled the system of middle medical education to create departments to train three basic types of workers in the medical college: midwives, nurses for the protection of motherhood and infancy, and general nurses.[70] Social assistance nurses were not trained in the new program.[71] Medical education was general in the first year, and by the final year training was quite specialized. Certain medical colleges in Moscow and Leningrad had already started to train nurses in psychiatry, pediatrics, surgery, gynecology, and other subjects, as well as introduce new nurse specialists in x-ray, dentistry, midwifery, pharmacy, and other areas.[72]

The state instigated further changes to the role of personnel and medical education to meet the needs of industrialization and collectivization (see chapter 4). The structural reorganization, according to the Soviet medical education writer, A. P. Zhuk, was to significantly raise the quality of middle medical training and bring the middle medical college closer to the Institute of Higher Education (Vysshee uchebnoe zavedenie).[73] The move was also supposed to raise the nurse above the feldsher.[74] It was clear that the Commissariat of Health was still trying to figure out the best way of organizing medical and nursing education as well as structuring the public healthcare system. As Soviet society moved from civil war to the period of NEP, the demands of Soviet citizens and their healthcare needs also changed. To this end, the commissariat revisited nursing and the kind of nurse required for present conditions in the Soviet Union (the tuberculosis nurse being one example).

Through the structural changes in training and education, the healthcare authorities aligned nursing more closely with science, perhaps hoping to elevate it somewhat in the eyes of Soviet citizens.[75] Still, gendered roles within healthcare tended to associate men with science. Although female physicians were on the rise in Russia (by late 1926, 39 percent of registered physicians were females), the tendency to associate women, especially nurses, with gender stereotypes of feminine kindness and gentility (as was the experience of the First World War) often remained.[76] Women medical workers also performed some of the most physically exhausting and menial jobs.[77]

Nurses played an increasingly prominent role in people's lives, and demand for them grew. In 1925 the Commissariat of Health called for courses for public health nurses (aged eighteen to twenty-five), accepting candidates with some prior knowledge of sanitation and administration and a familiarity with economics and sociology.[78] Public health nurses had several functions: to care for preschool-age children living in rural districts; attend the child and mother consultation centers to "advise mothers on a range of issues related to the care and upbringing of their children"; provide medical care in schools under the supervision of a doctor; and visit tuberculosis patients.[79] A memorandum on nursing courses sent to Semashko emphasized that the public health nurse should be "trustworthy" and have "common sense," as well as "sufficiently educated to deal with potential problems."[80] Additionally, the "memorandum underlined the importance of practical hospital experience, knowledge of midwifery, as well as a good understanding of the public sphere in which she would work."[81]

Reflecting on the 1920s, Anna Haines wrote that midwifery courses improved significantly during the NEP period. Well-trained midwives sent to the provinces helped stem the high infant mortality rates.[82] The OMM-run midwifery institute in Moscow was to serve as a model for all other institutes and schools throughout the country. In many ways the midwife replaced the need for having a physician or nurse deliver normal births, "giving a service" that was "efficient and economical."[83] The authorities created the role of patronage nurse (*patronazhnaia sestra*) for this reason. She visited single mothers in their homes, investigated their living conditions, and offered them instruction and assistance. Creating new roles and reimagining old ones became an integral part of the commissariat's efforts to make healthcare "Soviet."[84] Such visits also functioned as important spaces for acculturation and instilling Soviet values.[85] Home visits, including issuing dispensary orders, were another form of domestic control.[86]

Lebedeva's clinic offered Haines the chance to teach Russian student nurses. Despite enjoying the experience, Haines felt a palpable sense of frustration—she found the narrow focus on infant nursing too restrictive but could not convince those in charge to provide students with a more basic medical training to equip them to care for adults rather than infants.[87] Yet Haines was not completely despondent and praised Lebedeva's clinic. She considered the standards of care in Lebedeva's clinic to be high.[88] Still, this was a model institution, with standards lower elsewhere. In the 1920s, the Bolsheviks invested in prestigious scientific institutes that received much public attention and endorsement. Lebedeva's clinic was one of these.

Given the high levels of infant mortality in Russia, the new Soviet government placed much emphasis on instructing new mothers in how to care for their newborns. But Haines, coming from a different social and cultural background, favored taking a more traditional Western approach to medical training that bypassed the "rudimentary" elements provided by Lebedeva's clinic. Haines envisioned introducing a Westernized system of nurse training to Russia, whereas the Soviet government favored training that it saw fit for addressing current needs as well as its political and ideological plans for molding Soviet society. Medical workers, as valuable state intermediaries caring for Soviet patients, had to comply with Soviet rather than Western plans for nursing.

Haines realized that nursing improvements would not happen "without the equipment and desire on the part of the officials in charge."[89] She later recognized that the Commissariat of Health was "not convinced as yet that American methods of nursing" were "the best methods."[90] In her approach to Soviet nursing, she perhaps overlooked the ideological and political factors at play. For example, nurse consultations with mothers, especially those that took place in the home, presented officials with an opportunity to inspect households.[91] Training nurses to visit homes and meet with new mothers thus allowed the state to shape people's habits and practices, helping them conform to new Soviet standards of health and hygiene.

The Quakers read the situation from an outsider perspective. Soviet nurses did not hold a high position within the medical hierarchy: they did not have a national nursing association, nor were they members of an international nursing organization. The nurse may have occupied a position of power and authority during home visits, but in the wider healthcare sphere the nurse was inferior to the doctor.[92] Similarly in France "the modern nurse was to use her innately feminine skills to balance the emotional, spiritual, and physical needs of the patient with the professional and scientific interests of the doctor."[93] While nurses in the Soviet Union lacked equipment, politics and ideology as much as nursing technique would inform their training. They were also expected to balance the maternal and the scientific facets of their professional role.

Despite differences in attitudes to nursing, Soviet healthcare officials continued to benefit from their relationship with the Quakers. When Lebedeva needed linoleum for the clinic, she turned to Haines for help to procure it in England.[94] In Samara, the head of the Buzuluk District health authority approached the AFSC for help in purchasing an x-ray machine from Berlin.[95] Through their presence in hospitals and clinics, Quakers made valuable contributions to Russian healthcare and became important intermediaries between Russia and the West at a particularly difficult time. This achievement was notable given the strained international relations and changing domestic climate in Russia after Lenin's death in January 1924. Both the Quakers and the Russians wanted to improve Soviet public healthcare, but they had differing visions of how to tackle it.

West Is Best

To the AFSC, "one of the greatest needs of the peasants and the workers in Russia [was] for a type of health service represented by the Public Health

Nurses in America and England."[96] It did not consider why the Western system was better than any Russia could offer. Instead, its plans for a training school in Moscow would be modeled on "the most modern foreign schools." Although Anna Haines made no reference to Muriel Payne's scheme, there were similarities in the proposals for a nursing school, most probably a reflection of their Western experiences of nursing in Russia. The school would have a total of sixty students enrolled across three years. Russian doctors would oversee theoretical classes, while English and US nurses would be in charge of practical nursing and general administration. In the final months of the course, students would receive training in midwifery so that as nurses they "could command more respect."[97]

The school was set to open in 1928, allowing the AFSC enough time to raise funds.[98] The Commissariat of Health approved the nurse training school. Although the Russians endorsed the scheme, they were not convinced that US methods of nursing were any better than Russian methods.[99] Nonetheless, in the mid-1920s the Soviet health authorities maintained a general interest in mother and child healthcare abroad, collecting information on children in Britain suffering from rheumatism and disease (with notes about the high price of quinine).[100] They were also interested in Glaxo, a dry milk produced in New Zealand with a "very good reputation in Britain."[101] The Commissariat of Health, with Lebedeva as its representative, welcomed the nurse training school as an "experiment," but the Soviets only considered it as such because they were not "sold" on the idea that this type of system was of value to them.[102] Indeed, the precise function of the public health nurse was still debated in the United States, considered by some to be an instructor "bringing the message of prevention and hygiene to the masses" and by others a practitioner "providing direct patient care."[103]

In any case, and as the Wald visit had demonstrated, the Soviets wanted to learn more about the US experience of public health nursing. This was an area of great expansion in the United States during the interwar years, increasing from three thousand public health nurses in 1912 to almost twenty thousand by 1938.[104] Still committed to the foreign scheme, the Russians agreed to provide a building (albeit one in an extreme state of disrepair), with the AFSC shouldering all other costs.[105]

While the nurse training school scheme was to serve philanthropic and humanitarian purposes, there was no doubt of a disconnect between Russian and Western intentions. Both wanted to improve medical conditions in Russia, but their means to this end differed. Haines and her colleagues wanted to establish a nursing school along Western lines, whereas the Russian approach did not regard Western standards as either better or appropriate. It was clear that those in Soviet healthcare such as Lebedeva and Semashko did not consider that the United States or the West knew the only route to modernizing nursing. From their perspective, US and British nursing did not necessarily represent modern or correct methods of care. Ideas of modernity are, after all, not exclusively Western.[106] When it came to modernizing healthcare, the Soviets were above all pragmatic. If funding and support were forthcoming, Russian authorities were hardly in a position to refuse. They would take what they considered to be both intellectually and practically useful to meet their needs.

Perhaps the Soviet healthcare authorities were also skeptical about securing a firm foreign commitment to running a nurse training school. The Quakers were still pursuing their nursing school project in 1927, this time undertaking a massive fundraising campaign in the United States after the Rockefeller Foundation rejected the nursing school scheme in February of that year.[107] Haines, undaunted, claimed that "wrong ways of educating nurses" were under way in Russia.[108] Quaker Alice Davis, at that time training in the Commissariat of Health's school for nurses in Moscow, felt that a lack of teachers and the political education hindered nurse training.[109] Davis claimed the political and social education led to "constant interruptions," even though an understanding of the Marxist-Leninist system was a baseline of Soviet education.[110] In spite of the setbacks, Haines continued her efforts to obtain the remaining funds in the United States, deciding not to return to Russia.[111] For the Russians, setbacks were not unusual. The delays and problems involved in setting up a school may have frustrated Haines, but Soviet healthcare officials often had to wait several months for accommodation and funding to come through for various schemes.[112] Even if the scheme had received funding, it might have come too late.

The End of an Era

By the late 1920s, Joseph Stalin's emergence as leader of the Soviet Union resolved the power struggle that followed Lenin's death. The political landscape of the Soviet Union was changing rapidly. At about the same time that the First Five-Year Plan came into effect in 1928, Quakers turned their attention to developing a hospital to train nurses in Yasnaya Polyana, the former estate of the writer Lev Tolstoy. It would be a joint effort by the English and American Friends, with Alice Davis at its helm to retrain Russian nurses in Western methods for the hospital.[113] The scheme had received permission to go ahead from the Tolstoy Committee (of which Semashko was a member), and Semashko had written a letter of support to the British Foreign Office for the visit of an English nurse.[114]

It was then a "bombshell" when Semashko told Quakers that this was the first he had heard of an English nurse going to Yasnaya Polyana, that Yasnaya Polyana was not a suitable location for a nurse training school, and that Russians had "their own system of nursing and so did not require a foreign nurse there."[115] Quaker headquarters recognized that there had been no written acceptance of the scheme.[116] The political situation in Russia at this time, and the end of the NEP, no doubt had immense bearing on how events transpired. In 1928 Stalin's Russia was a very different country from the one Western visitors encountered in the early 1920s. Massive campaigns of industrialization and collectivization were under way or in the works, and the political climate within Russia was perceptibly changing. The 1927 war scare no doubt increased tensions further.[117] Semashko was likely already under pressure to strictly regulate the movements of foreign agents, and his commissariat was also dealing with budgetary restrictions.[118]

Irrespective of financial and political circumstances, the AFSC still believed in a hospital scheme and remained on friendly terms with the Commissariat of Health.[119] While disappointed, the AFSC understood the rejection to be "natural," since "no hospital in America would accept a foreign nurse as a matron in a hospital that was to be run on nationalistic lines."[120] It had a valid point, and one that reinforces the extent to which the Soviet government had generally been willing to stretch to accommodate foreign medical help on Russian soil.

As one door closed, another opened. In 1928 the professor A. Speransky, who replaced Lebedeva as director of the OMM's research institute and who was also president of the Scientific Council in Moscow, sent a proposal for a clinic to the AFSC. The clinic would study the prevention and treatment of mother and infant diseases.[121] Because it would be part of Speransky's institute, the scheme would be Russian- and not Western-led. Semashko and his commissariat signed off on the agreement on July 12, 1929. The Commissariat for Health required two foreign nurses to work as assistants to the matron, and they were to be responsible to Speransky.[122] Before this they were to have spent some three months in the physiology department and in children's consultation to learn about "the Russian methods of care of healthy children."[123] They were also to have some knowledge of the Russian language to help train local nurses.[124] Foreign nurses would not be imposing their own style of nursing and would adapt to the Russian medical setting. By July 1929 Russian health authorities were "most anxious" to have the foreign nurses begin work at the clinic.[125] In September the AFSC approved the scheme.[126]

As the Quaker Dorice White explained, placing two foreign nurses in the hospital was not to be part of any "scheme of nursing" but simply the "expression of friendship through service and the value of personal international contacts."[127] Nurses would be working together. Speransky's clinic, as White understood it, was never to be a stepping-stone to establishing a nursing school. The Russian health authorities impressed the Quakers—as White acknowledged, "No English or American medical Institution would be willing to take two unknown foreign nurses on such favorable terms." Speransky's clinic represented a final chance for foreigners to shape Soviet nursing and maintain international connections. But at the end of August 1931, Haines had not received her visa and the AFSC closed its center in Moscow after failing to have its lease renewed.[128] Political changes in Russia led to conditions wherein the AFSC presence was no longer acceptable. Both Semashko and Speransky lost their positions. A new era was dawning and Soviet nursing would have to make its own way forward.

The Russians never admitted that standards of nursing care were inadequate or that the training system was inferior to that in the West; they were happy to test out Quaker ideas as an experiment. They never considered Western methods of nursing to be better than Russian, but they were glad, no doubt, to accept the help, expertise, and personnel that Quakers brought with them. Negotiation about the nursing school proved to be significant in illuminating Russian and Western perceptions of "right" and "wrong" forms of care and their connection to social and cultural conditions. Had Payne or Haines managed to win enough financial support or had the Rockefeller Foundation become involved in Russian nursing in the early 1920s, one wonders what impact a nursing school might have made. In such a huge country undergoing vast political, social, cultural, and economic changes, the influence of a model training school for nurses would likely have been short-lived or limited.

Soviet conditions were simply not conducive to the kind of systematic nurse training envisaged by Payne and Haines. Although the long-term importance of establishing a nursing school and setting high standards of care were clear to the Quakers, and indeed appreciated by some of the health officials in Russia, the "long-term" benefits of such an endeavor weighed less on the minds of those struggling to deal with a population ravaged by war, disease, and famine. The AFSC was primarily engaged in medical relief and reconstruction work in Samara and Moscow, but for the Russian government, developing an internationally endorsed system of nurse training was far from a priority. The significance of these foreign encounters did not, in the end, translate into a systemic change in approach to Soviet nursing policy. But the encounters showed that "public health was one of the few channels of communication left open between Russia and the West for a decade."[129]

The sweeping political changes at the end of the 1920s, touched on in this chapter, were of great professional import to medical workers. While the Commissariat of Health engaged with foreign medical workers during the NEP years, it was dealing with a whole host of other issues at the same time. In the context of the massive crises confronting healthcare, it is surprising that Semashko and his colleagues in the commissariat devoted such attention to the Quakers and their ideas for a nursing school. The serious challenges that confronted Soviet nursing after the civil war were not addressed during the NEP period, when propaganda was often used as a substitute for rather than a supplement to health and hygiene campaigns. Soviet nurses and middle medical workers remained in a very uncertain position during the NEP years, unsure of their exact role and still lacking a sense of professional identity after the revolution.

CHAPTER 4

Proletarian Paradise
Medical Workers Rise Up

The Soviet project had unintended consequences for medical workers, who struggled to define their professional identity after the revolution. Were they scientific workers or caregivers? Were these categories mutually exclusive? The medical authority Vasili Mikhailovich Banshchikov's claim that the "revolutionary process" had still not finished creating a new type of middle medical worker by 1928 was on the mark.[1] The revolution had up-ended but not resolved nurses' and feldshers' understandings of their role, rights, and responsibilities. As the First Five-Year Plan and collectivization began to take hold of Soviet society, middle medical workers still seemed to be in professional limbo. The revolutionary process was so incomplete that middle medical workers were not even sure of their proper job title. Were they doctors' assistants or technical workers?

The ambiguity also spoke to the amorphous role of the nurse. This chapter is about medical workers, and the sources it draws on feature doctors and feldshers as much as nurses. This is because nurses and nursing were very much in the shadow of doctors and medicine during the 1920s. Nurses, feldshers, and doctors worked together, and their roles often overlapped. Sources frequently discuss "medical workers" as opposed to nurses. The chapter therefore views the nursing experience through the eyes of a spectrum of medical workers.

In the new Soviet world, medical workers required new roles and job titles reflective of science and medicine rather than care and mercy.[2] But deciding on a title for Soviet middle medical workers proved challenging. "Doctor's assistant," "medical technician," "medical sister" or "social assistance nurse" were not popular among medical workers and students.[3] Medical workers were seemingly at a less advanced stage than others in their revolutionary process of transformation. Consequently, the Cultural Revolution and the Great Turn that occurred in the late 1920s and early 1930s under Stalin would—in the eyes of the state—be crucial to reshaping the medical profession and bringing medical workers into line with broader industrialization trends.

Indecision about job titles hardly helped the already battered morale of medical workers. Nor did such debates help to elucidate the core function of middle and junior medical workers. If the early Soviet state was committed to improving care for patients, then it needed to focus more attention on clarifying the role of medical workers and raising their standard of living. In their current situation, some medical workers lived in awful living conditions, and their working conditions were not much better. Although the state continued to advocate for better standards of care for patients, medical workers became increasingly disillusioned with their lot. In a growing divide, medical workers and the state collided in three key areas during the period 1928–1932: (1) employment, where medical workers always felt they were treated unfairly; (2) concerns about medical negligence and state accusations of unprofessionalism, or, in Soviet parlance, a lack of labor discipline; and (3) the spate of violent attacks that placed medical workers' lives in danger.

Two different narratives were running in opposition: one told of a state that cared for its people and tasked medical workers—especially nurses—with providing a cultured medical experience. The other vilified medical workers and blamed the problems in the healthcare system on their callous, insensitive behavior. Although the state espoused cultured relations between medical workers and patients in an effort to provide the high standards of care befitting the first socialist state, the overwhelming majority of medical workers were from the working class and the peasantry. In this respect they were similar to working-class printers, for whom "rudeness was a way of life."[4] In trying to make medical workers adopt a more sensitive and caring demeanor at work, the state was essentially asking them to overhaul their proletarian and peasant identities.

Working and Living Conditions in the 1920s and 1930s

A huge population increase in urban centers, but particularly in Moscow, led to a severe shortage of housing during the 1920s and 1930s. In 1926 the party described the situation as catastrophic.[5] Such was the shortage of apartments and decent housing that many workers ended up living in overcrowded barracks or dormitories, a feature of proletarian life before the revolution. A 1924 article in the fortnightly journal *Medical Worker* provided insights into everyday life for medical workers in the Botkin and Sokol'nicheskaia hospitals. The Botkin hospital, formerly the Soldatenkovskaia, was one of Moscow's largest, with a staff of 500, including 32 doctors, 15 feldshers, 16 pharmacists, 97 nurses, and 110 *sidelki*. The remaining 230 personnel were orderlies and other manual labor workers.[6] Party members—mostly unqualified workers—numbered about 40.[7] The Sokol'nicheskaia hospital's 150 middle-level and some 300 junior medical personnel, about half of them women, experienced a similarly bleak housing situation.[8] Union membership reflects the gender breakdown, with female membership consistently rising, from 56.9 percent in 1921 to 64.1 percent in 1927.[9]

Medical workers' complaints about housing were particularly pronounced in the early 1920s but continued over the course of the NEP.[10] In general terms the amount of living space per person in Moscow declined in the 1920s.[11] And outside of major cities, medical workers often had to endure awful conditions. In a report that made it to Sovnarkom, one correspondent from the Chuvash Republic wrote that orderlies slept alongside patients in wards because they had "nowhere else to go."[12] In the Cheboksarskaia hospital fifteen orderlies lived in the wards, although not in the infectious and venereal diseases wards (there were limits to medical workers' desperation).[13] Some made direct connections between low salaries, living and working conditions, and the high death rate among medical workers.[14] Compared to statistics for those working in crime or security or in correctional facilities, death rates among medical workers were higher, especially among feldshers.[15] Unsurprisingly, conditions led medical workers to perceive of themselves as set apart from other groups of workers.

Tight living arrangements in dormitory accommodation revealed stark contrasts between past and present, or between the "old" way of life and the new. The state attack on religion and tradition led to tensions among workers and peasants living in shared accommodation.[16] In a Poltava hospital, *sidelki* decorated their dormitory accommodation to reflect the new way of life (lots of red, five-pointed stars, and portraits of party leaders) and regularly attended party talks at the club for medical workers. The union secretary removed icons from nurses' dormitories (identified as Sisters of Mercy). The author, P. I. Nemkovskaia, described the nurses as much more "passive" in their social lives, as well as "old," "quiet," and used to the "better times" of the past.[17] In the new world of the Bolsheviks, religion was losing ground to science and medicine.[18]

But some nurses seemed unperturbed: as one Sister of Mercy said of political literacy, "I, as an older person, don't understand any of this," while she was "reading an essay from Boccaccio's *Decameron* with pleasure."[19] Hospital accommodation revealed how ideological and physical boundaries could be constructed between class and generations, or pre- and postrevolutionary worlds (figure 1).

Indeed, the health authorities worried about the social and class background of the approximately ninety thousand middle medical workers, who were men and women of all ages and from various class, ethnic, and national backgrounds.[20] The majority of nurses working in 1926 had less than two years' training, having only attended short-term courses during the years 1916–1923,

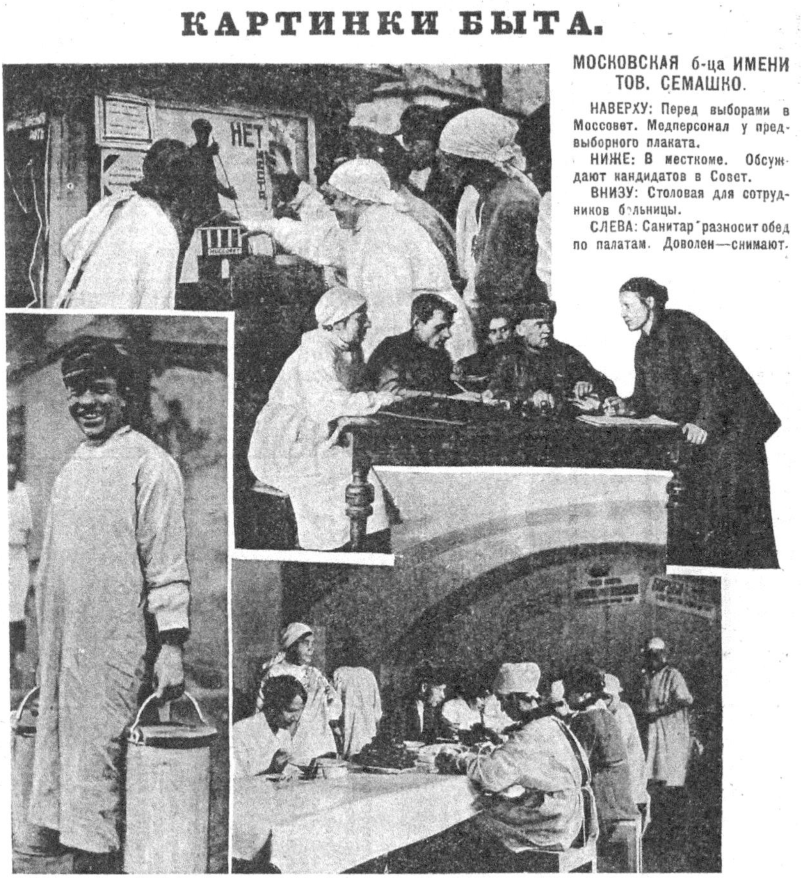

КАРТИНКИ БЫТА.

МОСКОВСКАЯ 6-ца ИМЕНИ ТОВ. СЕМАШКО.

НАВЕРХУ: Перед выборами в Моссовет. Медперсонал у предвыборного плаката.
НИЖЕ: В месткоме. Обсуждают кандидатов в Совет.
ВНИЗУ: Столовая для сотрудников больницы.
СЛЕВА: Санитар разносит обед по палатам. Доволен—снимают.

FIGURE 1. "Pictures of Everyday Life." From Moscow's Semashko hospital. Source: P. I. Nemkovskaia, "Kartinki byta," *Meditsinskii rabotnik*, no. 15 (1925): 10. Russian State Library.

and the largest contingent of middle-level medical workers (24.5%) were those who had trained between the years 1916 and 1920.[21] While some claimed that prerevolutionary Sisters of Mercy working in medical institutions were few in number, others feared that those trained before the revolution undermined efforts to create a new Soviet system of nursing.[22] Those writing on the subject worried that Soviet medical workers graduating from the technical colleges were more likely to assimilate with, rather than actively fight against, "class enemies."[23] But the statistics were moving in the right direction for the authorities, and the percentage of workers and their children entering the medical colleges in the RSFSR increased in the later 1920s (29.8% in 1927, 49.1% in 1928, and 53.9% in 1929).[24]

Class tensions affected relations between medical workers. Even though Leningrad doctors were "sovietized" in 1926, middle and junior workers in the party and on local committees did not trust them.[25] There were also tensions between hospital managers, party members, and nonparty members.[26] This process was a clear reversal of what was supposed to happen. Medical workers were divided within, a mixture of Soviet and non-Soviet citizens—in the ideological sense—who struggled to gain a foothold in the new Soviet system. Such fears chimed with more general calls for greater vigilance against "class aliens" supposedly infiltrating factories to agitate against Soviet power at the end of the 1920s.[27] Class tensions and the terrible living conditions could hardly have engendered fealty to the new regime or the medical profession.

The poor living conditions also led to huge worker turnover. One medical union worker conveyed to Sovnarkom head Vyacheslav Molotov in 1932 that lack of access to decent food and accommodation often resulted in an exodus of medical workers from the industrial centers where they were sent to work ("*razverstka*").[28] Disgruntled medical workers left their profession because they felt treated unfairly—why choose to live and work in these conditions if better pay and housing could be found elsewhere? Having qualified and found employment, the hardship of everyday life might have understandably proved too much for healthcare workers. Similar to other professionals such as teachers, medical workers often resorted to finding more comfortable or profitable employment and so moved to industry.[29]

Unemployment and the Final Throes of the NEP

But such options were not available to all medical workers. During the 1920s many medical workers were without work. The scale of unemployment almost precipitated a panic, though one not unique to the medical profession.[30]

Unemployment was rife in the 1920s, and in Moscow the number of unemployed exceeded 200,000, or 20 percent, by 1929.[31] In the printing industry workers' unemployment levels increased in the period 1921–1924, and between late 1925 and the start of 1927 unemployment stood at 18 percent of union members.[32] Statistics for November 1, 1923, showed that the highest unemployment numbers for medical workers were 3,044 Sisters of Mercy, followed by 4,435 orderlies and nannies. These figures were increasing; one month later they showed 3,296 unemployed Sisters of Mercy and 4,860 unemployed nannies and orderlies.[33] Unfortunately, the picture is incomplete owing to a lack of statistics on the total number of nurses, nannies, and orderlies working in these provinces.[34] But figures for 1924 confirm the trend: there were 4,000 unemployed nurses (out of 10,000) and 2,500 unemployed feldshers of 15,500 in the RSFSR.[35] Unemployment and labor shortages were characteristic of the NEP and "reflected both the influx of an unskilled urban and rural population into the labor market and the shortages of skilled labor."[36] No doubt these factors also had a bearing on the medical workplace.

The growing unemployment rate among medical personnel did not tally with the shortage of medical workers. The problem was that the unemployment figures represented a disproportionate number of wartime nurses and field feldshers, who worked in rural healthcare centers.[37] In the mid-1920s there was demand for middle medical workers with a different set of skills, for example, pharmaceutical or surgical training, and therefore these wartime nurses and field feldshers were no longer needed.[38] The following case highlighted in a *Medical Worker* article illustrates the problem. In 1927 the 150-bed Narimanovskaia hospital in the town of Gyandzha, Azerbaijan, did not have enough qualified middle medical workers with surgical training. The situation was so bad that a sign on the door of the operating room read: "Due to the absence of trained surgical nurses the department is temporarily closed." The administration turned to nurses in another town, but nobody had come by the time the *Medical Worker* article had gone to press.[39] This example also illustrates the perennial problem of attracting educated doctors and nurses to rural locations. A higher education resolution of June 23, 1936, sought to resolve this problem by stationing fresh graduates in rural areas for three to five years, as a kind of service or repayment to the state.[40]

It was clear that the medical institutes were not yet producing a sufficient number of graduates with a high level of specialist training, such as surgery, as in the Gyandzha case. And yet the lack of medical-sanitary institutes created high unemployment rates, a pattern also discernable in the printing industry in Moscow, where training was scaled down to a single school.[41] It was a vicious circle—medical workers without work experience were not hired, but they had no possibility to gain this experience.[42] This was part of a wider NEP trend. A rationalization campaign that began in 1924 aimed to reduce production costs, and this included reducing any unnecessary workers.[43] Yet the biggest employment challenge for workers was their lack of skills and work experience.[44] Medical workers, especially field feldshers and wartime nurses, who found that their particular set of skills or qualifications were not needed in the 1920s, would have to either leave their profession to find other work or try to find a way to complete their education. The latter was the harder option, for financial and family reasons.[45] By now medical workers were probably conditioned to their ongoing struggle to survive. But unemployment and uncertainty about the future undoubtedly dented their morale, dealing a severe blow to their identity as workers and professionals.

An attendant problem was the low pay, a clear contributory factor to the poor working and living conditions.[46] Medical workers' wages were behind prewar levels and were "lower than the average wage of industrial workers." The union claimed the low pay was not a fair reflection of medical workers' contribution to the healthcare service.[47] Of course, the problem here, too, was that medical workers, especially nurses, were by and large women, who typically earned less than their male counterparts and suffered the most from unemployment.[48]

Once again the tension between the state's desire to modernize public healthcare and its lack of commitment to improving conditions for medical workers came into play. A July 1926 plenum of the All-Union Central Council of Trade Unions (VTsSPS), heard discussion about the public healthcare services and the position of medical workers. Those present emphasized the need to raise wages for healthcare workers.[49] The Commissariat of Labor received reports about the flight of medical staff earning particularly low wages; doctors often left their jobs to move to better-paying work.[50] The Commissariat of Labor realized the potential loss of a large number of specialists. Even before the Shakhty Trial of 1928 led to a decline in the status of technical specialists across the Soviet Union, medical workers, but especially physicians, were leaving their profession.[51]

The position of doctors was still precarious in 1920s Soviet Russia, and mixed attitudes toward them led the state to depend on feldshers.[52] Although the Commissariat of Health held a poor view of feldshers, continuing its campaign against "feldsherism" throughout the 1920s, it realized that demands for medical workers warranted the use of schooled feldshers in most localities.[53] Feldshers, despite being in official disfavor, remained crucial figures on the rural healthcare scene. As one former refugee doctor said of feldshers, they were so close to the peasantry that doctors tried to get along with them, but in some cases the feldsher could "incite the population against the doctor since the majority of the population trusted him more than the physician."[54] Under such circumstances, who could blame doctors for trying to conceal their status?

Surely aware of this situation, the Soviet healthcare authorities wanted schooled feldshers and nurses to replace all field feldshers working in health-care facilities. These plans were part of a broader effort to retrain unemployed field feldshers, turning them into more qualified feldshers to serve in rural areas.[55] A special school with three-year courses facilitated field feldshers requalifying as schooled feldshers. Schools and medical colleges with two-year courses of study facilitated the requalification of wartime nurses. The medical union encouraged unemployed medical workers to enter medical colleges because they had medical experience often gained in the civil war, that is, during the "most difficult medical conditions," when there was a need for "skill, composure, and other qualities."[56] But unemployed feldshers and nurses who wanted to attend the courses had no financial support apart from unemployment benefits.[57] Feldshers taking a three-year feldsher course in the medical college did not receive a full stipend, and Medsantrud worried that lack of funding did not allow these feldshers to finish the courses.[58] The union therefore asked the Commissariat of Labor to provide a stipend for the final nine months of the course, allowing field feldshers to work and study.[59]

Similarly, wartime nurses were also supposed to retrain by taking a six-month course, where they would receive a stipend or unemployment benefit of 15 rubles a month, not enough to survive at a time when the average industrial monthly wage was 91 rubles.[60] The Commissariat of Labor provided a budget of 50,000 rubles for the RSFSR for the fiscal year 1926/1927 with the purpose of retraining unemployed field feldshers as schooled feldshers and raising the qualification of wartime nurses.[61] But the low stipend was hardly an incentive for medical workers to attend these courses, particularly if they had dependents.[62]

Indeed, the number of unemployed feldshers and nurses lacking the required qualifications, "rendering them useless to the public health organs," caused some concern for the Medsantrud Central Committee.[63] On October 20, 1927 the Medsantrud secretary, A. Aluf, appealed to the Commissariat of Labor to release funding for workers in need of further training in 1927–1928.[64] The Commissariat of Labor realized the benefits of retraining unemployed middle medical workers and wanted to grant this funding, but it was contingent on reports detailing how money was spent.[65] There were at least three state agencies now involved in trying to improve medical workers' employment opportunities and living conditions. Some of those writing on medical education supported these efforts and acknowledged that neither the health authorities nor the labor exchange could employ workers with no proof of complete medical education.[66] New initiatives would support those nurses and other medical workers who were unemployed and becoming less employable the longer they remained out of work.

Financial limitations remained a point of contention between state bodies. One disgruntled commentator criticized the Commissariat of Health for its lack of interest in retraining junior and middle medical workers and its unwillingness to ask the government for money.[67] Even the general public noticed problems in the sector. The editorial offices of *Medical Worker* received a letter titled "Ne uluchshenie, a ukhudshenie" (Not improving, but worsening), which underlined Soviet citizens' lack of confidence in the training and professional qualifications of medical personnel. Signed "Gor'kii—not Maksim," an embittered I. M. Zhukovitskii, who worked at a railway hospital in Ekaterinoslav, wrote that the medical service was deteriorating in spite of recent attempts to raise the qualifications of medical workers.[68] Another letter criticized the chronic shortage of medical workers, especially the lack of specialists in the countryside.[69] Striking the right balance between education, training, and pay was a major challenge and a constant source of disquiet among medical workers, the authorities, and concerned citizens.

Given these circumstances it would seem unlikely that the problems in public healthcare went unnoticed by the party-state leadership. But these high unemployment figures and the efforts to retrain personnel came at a time when Stalin tightened his grip on power and the NEP was wound down. The political climate was such that the commissar of health, Nikolai Semashko, was not in a sufficiently strong position to wield effective control over public health. The Commissariat of Health was now a much-changed body after the late 1920s shakedown in the wake of Stalin's success in the leadership struggle.[70] In 1930 Mikhail Vladimirskii replaced Semashko as commissar of health. The State Planning Commission (Gosplan) and Sovnarkom were critical and demanded "radical" changes to healthcare planning—indeed, the "stage was set for institutional conflict."[71] In August 1930 A. S. Tsikhon replaced N. A. Uglanov as commissar of labor. A month later the Commissariat of Labor, under Uglanov, was accused of "having squandered tens of millions of rubles on unemployment benefits."[72] A commissariat announcement in October stated that benefits were terminated because there was no unemployment—yet three hundred thousand workers were on the unemployment register.[73]

Violence against Medical Workers and Transition to the First Five-Year Plan

Perceived inequities and poor living conditions created a sense of growing disillusionment among medical workers. Additionally, the growing demands placed on medical workers and medical institutions in the 1920s led to deteriorating relations between medical workers and patients. The situation came to a head in 1927 when A. Aluf published an article about the increased number of "abnormalities."[74] Some of the abnormalities included people "insulting, assaulting, and even murdering medical workers"; "cantankerous, unjust relations" at an organizational level; and "false accusations in the press" that fostered mistrust. Hospitals seemed to be generally chaotic spaces. In a typical workday, orderlies going about their duties endlessly moving trolleys and patients between wards and buildings would encounter scenes of convulsing epileptic patients in corridors or nervous patients "shaking like leaves" in wards.[75] But that was just everyday disorder. Medical workers were also likely to encounter serious violence and assault.

It was a rather grim picture for medical workers. In addition to low wages and awful living conditions, medical workers also feared assault. Violence against doctors occurred in the nineteenth century and had not abated in the early Soviet period.[76] While the main reason for violence prior to the revolution had been fear, attacks against workers in the 1920s and 1930s mostly came down to a lack of trust. Medical workers had the support of the authorities, who considered the physical and verbal threats against them to be serious offenses. Aluf reassured medical workers that the "organs of the state stood behind them" and that no crime would go unpunished. [77] Still, the threat of violence in the workplace made the already difficult circumstances for medical workers much worse and added another layer of stress to their working lives.[78]

The Commissariat of Justice considered insults committed against medical personnel trying to fulfill their work obligations a serious attack on authority. It recommended a period of incarceration of "no less than six months" for this crime.[79] Nonetheless, accounts of trouble in various provincial hospitals continued to make their way to the Medsantrud Central Committee.[80] Patients in clinics and hospitals beat and tried to kill medical workers.[81] The press reported on the seemingly high incidences of violence against medical workers, especially doctors.[82] Apart from calling for reinforcing discipline in medical institutions and warning publications to get their facts straight before publishing any revelations about medical workers, Aluf suggested that medical workers become more "active" in the community to improve relations with the local population. This, he surmised, would help increase their authority and establish trust.[83]

Yet trust was continually undermined. The historian Samuel C. Ramer asserts that the murders of medical personnel were unrelated to the specialist baiting of the late 1920s that culminated in the Shakhty Trial, and I tend to agree.[84] But in some medical contexts the trial was a possible basis for patient mistrust. Patients in a Communist Red Army military hospital in Moscow were apparently "disturbed" by the miners' trial in Shakhty, a town in the Ukrainian SSR, and it "created a wave of distrust against specialists."[85] While the party activists in the hospital pledged to improve political and ideological work among "old doctors," they were at the same time keen to avoid any "unnecessary bullying." But others in the Red Army dismissed the Shakhty Trial factor and considered that it had "almost absolutely no impact on hospital specialists" and that there was no "Shakhty counterrevolution" in the hospital.[86] Party activists in this particular Red Army hospital wanted to mobilize a group of specialists to improve work in the hospital, but they wanted "conscience rather than fear" to be the basis for their motivation.[87] At the time there was evidently some debate and discussion about medical workers, especially doctors as specialists, and how to handle perceived problems arising from their status as specialists. And because this was a military hospital, Red Army soldiers might have been more attuned or sensitive to political currents than patients elsewhere.

The Bolsheviks had gone to great lengths to convince large swathes of the population to seek medical assistance from trained medical workers rather than approach traditional folk healers (*znakhari*). To an extent, the propaganda campaigns promoting the benefits of embracing modern science and medicine worked, because people evidently went to the hospital or clinic. The problem was that, once there, they reacted in ways that showed they still did not fully trust medical workers. Violent attacks were also occurring at a time when the Soviet press "was engaged in its own full-blown hooligan panic, which dovetailed nicely with other crime scares . . . [and] merged with the move toward, and the rhetoric of, the First Five-Year Plan.[88]" In this light, the crime scare among medical workers fits into the broader political context of the late 1920s transition period.

Yet violence against medical workers seemed to be more endemic. The psychiatric hospital, for example, was a frequent scene of violence against medical workers. Staff working in a regional hospital in Irkutsk were constantly at risk. Data from a table on occupational hazards show that between October 1926 and April 1928 patients punched 31 ward attendants, 18 nurses, 11 *sidelki*, and 3 doctors in the arm, leg, chest, or back. Spitting in the face was another common occurrence, with 10 nurses, 9 ward attendants, 3 doctors, and 2 *sidelki* targeted. Other, less frequent, incidents saw mentally ill patients pour soup and tea on workers, smear feces on them, bite them, and pull their hair. Most at risk were ward attendants, with 63 attacks against them. Next were nurses at 36, followed by *sidelki* at 15, and, finally, doctors at 9. These statistics, the head doctor noted, accounted for only the worst cases of violence.[89] Presumably lesser offenses occurred on a regular basis. In Leningrad, psychiatric hospitals registered mentally ill patients committing over 4,500 attacks against doctors, sanitary workers, and *sidelki* in 1929. Overcrowding and staff shortages were the main reasons given for the attacks.[90] Medical workers needed to be more vigilant and better equipped to cope with a range of situations in psychiatric institutions. Patients, meanwhile, needed better conditions and higher standards of care.

The medical union was, unsurprisingly, concerned about the attacks on medical personnel. At the Medsantrud Central Committee second plenum on October 22–26, 1928, secretary of the medical union's central committee, F. M. Seniushkin, stated that the medical system had many "weaknesses" and patients experienced "rudeness," "inattention," and a "formal" attitude at the hands of medical workers.[91] Seniushkin called for "public control," that is, generating public empathy by telling people about the awful conditions medical workers endured. He hoped it might also lead people to trust the doctor, protect medical workers, and improve standards of care.[92]

At the same meeting, a worker from Kostroma noted that patient complaints were often the result of a "lack of culture." The worker wanted to run an "explanatory campaign" to inform workers how to behave in a medical institution.[93] Medical officials and authorities spoke about the violence in a way that played on the rhetoric of uncultured, backward workers who did not understand the basic etiquette of the modern hospital. In some ways, this was unusual because workers were to have a degree of proletarian consciousness. But officials had lower expectations of peasants, traditionally viewed as "backward," and there were many workers of peasant origins in Soviet cities and towns.[94] Despite living in a worker and peasant state, Soviet officialdom often regarded peasants as culturally inferior.[95] Relations between medical workers and patients were still "unsatisfactory" by 1931, irrespective of the committee's suggestions.[96]

Trust and expectations are crucial to the image of public healthcare. Experts acknowledge that, although definitions of trust vary, "all embody the notion of expectations: expectations by the public that healthcare providers will demonstrate knowledge, skill, and competence; further expectations too that they will behave as true agents (that is, in the patient's best interest) and with beneficence, fairness and integrity."[97] In light of scandals and media scrutiny in the United Kingdom in the 1990s and 2010s, the issue of trust remains critical to how people perceive healthcare systems and medical workers. Trust can play out in two ways: confidence in the medical worker and confidence in the system. In the Soviet case the problem, at least publicly, seemed to lie in the former. Negative media attention exacerbated the breakdown of trust. But the bureaucratic healthcare system was also a problem that undermined public trust.

Tales of Compassion, Tales of Suffering

The press and some in the upper echelons of the Soviet government noted the poor healthcare service and lapses in care. Sensational articles about medical workers fit into the broader moral panic about NEP society. Care, love, and humanity were under attack in the NEP period, and the medical profession became a metaphor underlining the crisis of morality at the time. The revolution itself was on trial as the NEP came undone.[98]

At the Fifth All-Union Congress of Trade Unions in June 1924, head of the Soviet state, Mikhail Kalinin, reflected on his experiences of medical care.[99] He claimed that, when working-class people, or the *narod*, were admitted to a hospital in the 1920s they did not receive a warm welcome and therefore developed a "hostile relationship" with medical personnel. Kalinin believed medical ethics in the Soviet Union was underdeveloped and placed the onus on the medical trade union to help "develop a feeling of humanity." Medical workers were to have a "maternal" and "human" instinct to win the trust of their patients.[100] Senior figures in the Soviet state not only wanted trained personnel to provide citizens with good quality healthcare, but they also wanted people to feel that medical workers cared about them.

Kalinin's comments came at a time of debates on ethics in the Soviet Union; Emel'an Iaroslavsky, Nadezhda Krupskaya, and others also weighed in on party discussions about ethics and morality.[101] Pronouncements on the topic were vague, touching on behavior rather than providing a strict code for healthcare workers.[102] Nurses and medical workers had no definitive party line even though they had to care for Soviet citizens and contribute to building a new socialist society through their daily work and interaction with patients.

Medical workers who failed in their duty to provide care were shamed in the "court and life" (*sud i byt*) section of the medical and popular press. Medical workers from the First Moscow Maternity Hospital had their mug shots splashed across the pages of the "court and life" section of *Medical Worker* in

1926. Their crime was the death of the child Lidia Golovacheva on the night of August 16–17.[103] No details of the gruesome death were spared. The report informed readers about how rats attacked the child, printing in boldface type that they "scratched the skin of the entire face and chin" and removed "the upper lip, nose and right eye to the base of the eye socket, with further injury to the skin of the forehead, right cheek and right temporal parietal region."[104] The cause of death was asphyxiation: Golovacheva had "choked on her own blood." The author portrayed the doctor, Baron, as busy and callous. After the nurse called her, Baron "briefly examined the child" and then left, in spite of the child's shocking condition. The doctor claimed that she was already dealing with a difficult case and could do nothing to save the "dying child."[105] The suffering of the child clearly invoked shock, horror, and compassion among readers.[106] Medical workers reading the article would understand that the state would not tolerate neglect and mistakes.

Four years after Kalinin's call for greater humanity in the medical profession, negative portrayals of medical workers and the terrible suffering of patients continued. In 1928 women workers read about the problem through a case in the "court and life" section of the journal *Working Woman (Rabotnitsa)*.[107] Readers learned that a heavily pregnant Borisova went to a maternity hospital, where the doctor, Katz, was on sick leave. The midwife, Skliarskaia, told Borisova that she was not close to giving birth and asked her husband to take his wife away. The husband, a worker, protested, but to no avail; Borisova suffered a stillbirth on the street and died in the hospital later that night.[108]

The investigation that followed found the midwife and the absent doctor guilty.[109] The article showed readers, regular workers like Borisova, that their lives could be in danger owing to the callous nature of medical workers. Readers were also to be reassured that the state took any kind of medical negligence and lack of care very seriously. Medical workers who failed to deliver appropriate care would face consequences. While the gross misconduct of the guilty was rightly condemned, the moral of the story was skewed against medical workers. Their plight—working long shifts without sufficient relief or assistance—was not subject to discussion.

If the judgment of responsibility is usually shaped by laws and institutions, in the Soviet case medical workers were blamed.[110] The state was not publicly called on to address the serious problems afflicting the healthcare system and medical workers. The mixed portrayal of medical workers in the press did not help to improve their public image. Cases such as Borisova's represented a reversal of the ethics of care. Women medical workers, meanwhile, were clearly depicted as uncaring, even toward helpless babies and pregnant mothers—an apparent undoing of the natural order.[111]

There was no denying that some medical workers were rude and uncaring. But when called to account for their behavior, medical workers advanced a number of reasons for their misdemeanors. Sometimes it was inexperience, other times it was lack of culture. Workers explained that sometimes it also boiled down to circumstances within the hospital or clinic. Gritsuk, a *sidelka* working in a Moscow hospital, was accused of having a "rude and insensitive" attitude to patients. The hospital administration wanted Gritsuk dismissed, but the workers wanted Gritsuk to remain. The latter believed there to be extenuating circumstances, including the "absence of internal rules, the absence of any kind of instruction or guidance in the work of nannies, the low literacy and generally low cultural level of Gritsuk, and also the lack of patient discipline in the venereal department." In the end, the district health department (*uzdravotdel*) had to deal with the stalemate.[112]

Medical scandals also pointed to problems within the system itself. The publicized fatality scandals of 1926 and the Commissariat of Health's "excessively 'bureaucratic' control system," with its health branches that limited the authority of hospital administrators, led the medical union's central committee to pass "a series of resolutions" allowing for more local autonomy.[113] Although this move showed that the authorities were responding to the problems plaguing healthcare, it was not necessarily clear how exactly an increase in local autonomy would resolve problems with resources and training. If anything, it cynically removed responsibility from the Commissariat of Health.

Taking a Stand

Economic centralization and the state focus on forced industrialization for the development of defense and heavy industry led to the end of the NEP and limited private trade at the end of the 1920s. The First Five-Year Plan, launched in 1928, was in full swing by the early 1930s. Collectivization, introduced in late 1929 to forcefully gain a hold of grain supply, was similarly in full force by 1931, the year that workers in sixteen major medical institutions threatened a walkout if they did not receive a wage increase.[114] Medical workers were as outraged as industrial workers at rising grain prices and falling wages. All workers had felt the pinch of the grain crisis that led to food rationing in major cities and a decrease in workers' real wages in late 1927, with rationing in Moscow further extended in 1929.[115] Rising bread prices led to a threat of strikes in some factories. Soon rumors about war, famine, and even a coup began to spread among workers, who also believed Russia sold its grain reserves to foreign countries.[116]

By the summer of 1930, food shortages affected all workers, but closed shops were set up for industrial workers.[117] Workers privately expressed their anger about price rises and food shortages.[118] Access to closed stores with lower-priced goods was largely off-limits to lowly medical workers, who also felt the effects of rising prices for basic foodstuffs. Workers discussing the price rise in the Babukhina hospital commented, "Abroad goods are sold for a pittance, [so] it is necessary to make up for losses" and added that the local committee was inactive.[119] The local committee members in Moscow's Kashchenko and Semashko hospitals redirected workers elsewhere for support, advising them to "go to Narkomzdrav."[120] Dissatisfied medical workers connected the price rises to their low salaries, which were not increasing at a commensurate level with other professions.

In private conversations medical workers were heard saying they would "soon starve" and that they were "still confused, because they themselves [did] not know their situation." How long before frustrated medical workers would strike? Disaffected workers faced with starvation could be quite willing to air their grievances in public.[121] The disparities in the healthcare sector drew the attention of the press, including the major national newspapers *News* (*Izvestiia*) and *Red Banner* (*Krasnaia znamia*). The latter commented on the extreme inequity in rates of pay, where newly qualified doctors or nurses might receive the same pay as a colleague with greater skills and experience.[122] Growing unease and dissatisfaction among medical workers was evidently a talking point for those outside the public healthcare sphere. Medical workers were attuned to wider economic issues affecting Soviet society. Similar to other social groups, they found different ways and means of expressing their frustration with perceived injustices. This was part of the political culture created in revolutionary Russia, and the practice continued into the early Soviet period.[123] Consequently, the socioeconomic predicament of medical workers, rather than political consciousness per se, shaped the social identity of medical workers.

Workers in the large Botkin hospital complained about their "pauper's existence." Some actually invited dismissal from their jobs because they could not survive on 85 rubles a month (at the beginning of 1930 the average worker's monthly wage was 60–90 rubles).[124] Other workers threatened to leave.[125] Anger spread among medical workers of all rank. In the VTsSPS ambulatory doctors grumbled about their low wages, bemoaning that they studied for the same amount of time as engineers and worked similar hours but earned 100–200 rubles less a month. This forced them to "engage in private practice" (*nevol'no zaimesh'sia chastnoi praktiki*).[126] Junior personnel in the Medsantrud hospital, "knowing they could be dismissed for breaches of labor discipline, intentionally violated the rules in the hope that they might get a different, higher paying job."[127] Medical workers pursued collective and individual methods of resistance such as absenteeism and dismissal.[128] Indeed, forty junior medical personnel from Medsantrud demanded payroll cards of the first category instead of the second; they threatened to quit if their demands were not met.[129] The instigators were "old workers" in the hospital, some for "30–35 years."[130] Historians have written about the tensions between old and new workers at the end of the 1920s.[131] In the case of medical workers, the story is more complicated owing to the different professional and social histories of nurses, physicians, feldshers, orderlies, and nannies. Medical workers also possessed a mixed skill set and were of proletarian, bourgeois, and peasant origins. Such a divided group did not pose the same kind of threat as older industrial workers, who had a greater sense of class solidarity.

A similar story of discontent unfolded in the Ostroumova hospital, where middle and junior medical personnel demanded a pay increase. These workers "had a tendency to leave their jobs" (*imeiutsia tendentsii k ukhodu s raboty*), and "many negative conversations" were heard in the hospital, leading to the collapse of negotiations about wage increases.[132] The "unhealthy mood" of medical workers was increasing because of their low wages, the insecurity of food supply through closed canteen and distribution systems, and the incorrect allocation of their category of "payroll cards" (*zaraboti kartochki* [*sic*]).[133] The head of the Marynskaia hospital, A. Lotz, reported a lack of discipline among the medical personnel, who greeted each new instruction with "deafness" followed by "open opposition" (*nedovol'stvo*).[134] In the end, workers did not walk out, even when prices in Moscow rose. Instead of protesting, workers wanted an explanation so they could understand the reasons for the price increases. These hospital workers engaged in a form of activism known as "workerism"—petitioning trade union leaders to address their material needs.[135] Even after the desperate hardship of the civil war years and the disillusionment of the NEP period, medical workers' living and working conditions were unacceptable to them and did not equate with their understanding of how socialism should work. Their plight also spoke to broader trends in industry in 1929–1930, when there were calls for egalitarianism (*uravnilovka*) and a leveling of workers' wages.

Some medical workers turned to private practice, bribes, and tips to supplement their income. A nanny in the Sklifassovskaia hospital threatened the father of one patient; if he did not pay her 100 rubles, it "would be reflected in the care his sick son received."[136] In the same hospital junior medical workers, when not on shift, provided extra care to patients to supplement their income. Some doctors argued that it was "against the principles of Soviet medicine" and worried that the practice would interrupt regular hospital work, especially when medical workers were already so overworked. The head doctors from several major Moscow hospitals (including the Ostroumova, Babukhina, and Semashko) confirmed that they did not tolerate this practice in their hospitals.[137]

The head doctor of the Semashko hospital, G. M. Gershtein, stated that there was an increasing demand for special paid care. He added that it was unreasonable for patients to expect this given that medical workers already were *"extremely busy"* and in light of "the *shortage* of medical help" and "patient dissatisfaction with the quality of care" (emphasis in original).[138] There were similar problems with so-called tips (*chaevye*). Although illegal, tipping medical personnel frequently occurred. When leaving the maternity hospital after her most recent birth, one hospital administrator's wife gave a ruble to about ten to fifteen of the junior medical workers.[139] In the Ostroumova maternity hospital new mothers wanted to give money "for tea" (*na chai*) to nannies. James Heinzen notes that doctors interviewed as part of the Harvard Project on the Soviet Social System Online (HPSSS) acknowledged understanding the differences between fees, bribes, and gifts but viewed them as "part of the age-old relationship between the patient and the caregiver."[140] Those writing on the matter at the time worried about how this kind of practice affected the internal running of the hospital, and in particular the atmosphere it created in wards, as well as the needless pressure on sick and vulnerable patients. As was often the case, blame rested on older workers' shoulders. It was their fault for introducing "old habits," and now Soviet workers would have to work hard to stamp out these "cursed tsarist" ways.[141] But as medical workers might very well have argued, they needed to survive, and their wages alone were not sufficient. If the state could not provide for them, then patients, quite literally, would have to pay the price.

To improve material conditions for medical workers, the state addressed the unequal rate of pay in 1931 and 1932.[142] These increases favored medical workers in industrial centers and in transport, unsurprising in the context of industrialization.[143] Sovnarkom introduced a decree on "measures to improve the material and social status of medical workers" in June 1932. This law had the purpose of regulating medical workers' pay and determining wages according to position, rates, qualifications, and quality of work.[144] Following on from Sovnarkom, Ukrainian authorities issued a resolution on "measures to improve the everyday conditions of medical workers," whereby middle and senior medical personnel and their families could access food at the same level as engineers, teachers, and technical workers. This was to go into effect on July 1, 1932, through the special closed system of distribution or through cooperatives.[145]

But issuing resolutions did not necessarily lead to any improvements, because local authorities did not always implement central directives regarding medical workers' wages. In Tatarstan the public health organ was accused of refusing to implement the new rates for medical workers, repeatedly ignoring union requests to do so.[146] In Krasnodar, a medical worker received only 12 kilograms of flour to a teacher's 18 kilograms of flour per day; in Tatsinskii, Rostov, a teacher received 2 kilograms of flour to a medical worker's 600 grams of bread per day.[147] Medical workers, like those working in industry, felt unfairly treated, especially as teachers were also not particularly revered.

During the 1920s medical workers almost seemed to be at war against the state. They quite justifiably considered their living and working conditions unacceptable and repeatedly called the union and Commissariat of Health to account. These two bodies, to be fair, tried reasonably hard to improve conditions but were hamstrung by wider socioeconomic and political circumstances that were largely beyond their control. The press and the general population, who seemed to be at war with medical workers, complicated the situation. There was a clear disjuncture between the state's endorsement of science and medical research, on the one hand, and public healthcare and the plight of medical workers, on the other. Research institutes promoted the kind of scientific experimentalism and innovation that awakened fascination and awe, but medical workers in hospitals and clinics largely stirred up feelings of fear and hostility among the population.

As the First Five-Year Plan unfolded, a process of entanglement took place that meshed nurses and other medical workers together. Nurses still had a strong presence in the medical institution, but they were on equal footing with other middle medical workers and even junior medical workers as the lines between their daily duties became increasingly blurred over time. A reading of the medical trade union literature is ample of evidence of this. Nurses were never really distinguished in the union file headings, referred to largely as middle medical workers. Medical books and journals also tended to use the more inclusive term "middle medical worker" when discussing nurses. That might have happened on purpose to suppress any lingering sense of bourgeois identity among nurses and show that they were no different from other medical workers. As part of the working class, they would merge with the greater collective whole and fit in with orderlies, schooled feldshers, and other middle medical workers.

The socialist system that was developing in the 1920s and early 1930s appeared to have two faces to those reading some of the general and medical literature at the time. Even though the state took an unequivocally firm line on medical care and ran a propaganda campaign urging workers and peasants to trust the doctor, the message was evidently not getting through to many who still viewed doctors and nurses in white coats with suspicion. The hostility directed toward medical workers marked them out as different, even outsiders. Medical workers were in turn often cynical and hostile toward the hospital administration, the union, and the Commissariat of Health. One historian has characterized labor relations at the start of the First Five-Year Plan as "fundamentally adversarial," and this certainly holds up in healthcare.[148] The various battles that medical workers fought in the 1920s continued into the 1930s, but the overarching political narrative was changing to reflect Stalinist directions by the middle of that decade. What remained unchanged was the desire to innovate public healthcare and produce medical workers who would meet a standard of excellence in patient care.

CHAPTER 5

Stalinist Care

Cadres Decide Everything

Over the course of the 1930s all aspects of the public healthcare experience came under scrutiny to improve the service to patients. Immense changes during the Cultural Revolution of 1928–1931 saw medical education expand and the number of graduates increase. The situation was in need of further attention in the context of the Seventeenth Party Congress on January 26, 1934, the "Congress of Victors," and the emphasis on cadres. Medical cadres were no exception. As the providers of socialist healthcare to Soviet citizens, the state needed qualified and cultured medical workers. The shift in attention to cadres in the mid-1930s reflected an increase in the "clinical gaze."[1] Medical workers' visibility grew steadily as they were gradually recognized as important representatives of the state.

As intermediaries between the state and the people, medical workers acted as conduits of state care and attention. Their behavior and competency held symbolic value. Indeed, the Soviet state's concern with the birth rate and raising good communist children came to define its attitude to women and nursing. If the years of the New Economic Policy (NEP), the First Five-Year Plan, and collectivization saw increasing tensions and disharmony between medical workers and the state, the years leading up to the 1936 Constitution saw medical workers, but especially nurses, capitalize on the narratives of care that came from above. As the Stalinist state sought to provide its citizens with a decent healthcare service in return for their hard work, nurses in particular became the subject of growing rhetoric about cultured care and compassion.

Anybody who had any kind of interaction with Soviet public healthcare, especially patients, realized that the rhetoric was far removed from reality. Despite the many problems afflicting healthcare—and there were many—the state continued its ideological crusade to improve it. Dwelling on Soviet public healthcare's failings misses the fact that optimism periodically prevailed. There was sporadic hope of fixing the broken system, and the authorities, especially in the early Soviet years, seemed to believe they could fix it. Plenty of acolytes, not yet jaded by hardship or disillusionment, supported the cause. And enough ideological skeptics were committed to the underlying ideals of the mission. Speaking about hope and optimism seems misguided in the context of the 1930s. Yet these had their place.[2] This chapter captures some of that elusive hope.

During the political repressions that increased over the course of the 1930s, culminating in the Great Terror of 1937–1938, state calls for greater care and devotion grew louder. Such incongruity was not alien to the Soviet system. Historians have shown how the Gulag, a place of disease, death, and violence, was at the same time a space where medical workers were ostensibly charged with monitoring and improving the physical health of prisoners.[3] Others have asserted that the Soviet government was "engaged in an enormous pronatalist campaign" at the moment it was "killing hundreds of thousands of people."[4] With its focus on the Stalin Constitution and the Great Terror, this chapter casts light on some important issues that came to the fore during this rather short period. These include the creation of very particular narratives of care that were harnessed during the years of the Great Terror, as well as changes in the education and status of nurses that directly connected to questions of professional expertise, authority, and control. The ongoing process of creating new narratives of care and gradually promoting nurses and medical workers more generally helped resolve some of the problems that had characterized the relationship between the state and medical workers during the period of industrialization. That said, the ethics of care that Mikhail Kalinin espoused in 1924 remained undeveloped and would stay so until after the Second World War.

Narratives of Care

In light of doctors and medical personnel continuing to face accusations of incorrect treatment and callous behavior, Sovnarkom put pressure on the

Commissariat of Health to ensure that medical workers were "thoughtful" and "considerate" when it came to the patient.[5] Authors writing in the journal *On the Public Healthcare Front* (*Na fronte zdravookhraneniia*) foregrounded the important role of nurses and believed they should want to dedicate themselves to the welfare of the patient.[6] There were clear echoes of Kalinin's 1920s call for greater humanity in Soviet healthcare. Drawing on the work of a certain K. Kissling, the author M. E. Zhitnitsky argued that the position of nurse was a "vocation," not only an occupation, because nurses "possessed a deep, internal desire" to care for patients.[7] Soviet healthcare, Zhitnitsky believed, might benefit from drawing on some of the Christian ideas that influenced medical practice in western Europe.[8] One such notion was that women were "suited to patient care" and "their female qualities: gentleness, patience and the ability to renounce" made them ideal caregivers.[9] For these reasons, patient care was to be exclusively in the hands of nurses/women.

Care and womanhood were inextricably bound up, even in the supposed socialist utopia where women were apparently free of traditional gender baggage. This view was at odds with revolutionary rhetoric about women considered equal to men in the workplace, though in keeping with the conservative values of the 1930s.[10] While female workers predominated in other workplaces, for example, the textile industry, in the second decade of Soviet power the nursing profession became associated with prerevolutionary concepts of feminine care. Nurses, as women, were to be inherently attuned to and mindful of patients' needs. Yet in a broader context, such debates were not all that unusual. In the 1920s and 1930s the international nursing community and leaders of the International Council of Nurses (ICN) were trying to negotiate the "ideologies of gender, race, and class," which became more problematic as the organization expanded.[11] Nursing leaders and organizations in other countries were having a similar conversation. In France, for example, nursing reformers had "different experiences" as a result of "conflicting beliefs about woman's 'natural calling,' her status as an individual, her duty to the republic, and her place in public institutions."[12] As nursing in Russia developed, Soviet writers on the subject engaged in similar debates about care and gender that had characterized nursing in Europe and elsewhere.

Healthcare writing, but particularly nursing literature, evinced tropes of the kind nurse with increased frequency in the 1930s. The Stalin Constitution reduced many a healthcare discussion to saccharine sloganeering. Nurses and orderlies were "commended for responding to the government call and to the patient."[13] Medical workers noted that patients must be "surrounded with love and attention."[14] The medical press portrayed nursing as a "heroic profession," with tropes of modest, caring, and self-sacrificing nurses deployed.[15] These tropes endured.

In their 1955 publication on nurses, Ia. I. Akodus and A. A. Skoriukova wrote that women's care for patients was "especially significant" and dependent on the "particularities of the female character," where her gentleness and patience could encourage the patient.[16] Indeed, they argued that there was perhaps "no other more 'female' profession than that of nurse." The emphasis placed on the female character indicated the type of moral values that Soviet nurses were increasingly exposed to in the second half of the 1930s and beyond. The case of Soviet nursing reaffirms the philosopher Martha C. Nussbaum's claim that the "moral education of women in many societies cultivates, to a greater extent than does the moral education of men, the high evaluation of personal relationships of love and care that are the basis of most of the other emotions," whereas men are encouraged to seek "separateness and self-sufficiency."[17] Traditional gender stereotypes became intertwined with morality and ideas of educating women and men to adhere to society's cultural standards.

Although the Soviet state initially attempted to tackle and deconstruct gender stereotypes through integrated schools for young people, producing the "first Soviet generation" in 1935, this was frequently challenged when it came to professional training, such as nursing, which both reinforced and challenged gender stereotypes.[18] Efforts to place women on a par with men did not always play out in practice. Conservatism was still entrenched at state and societal levels. There was a "spectrum of models of Soviet womanhood" in the 1930s.[19] The conservative turn that has typically characterized the 1930s, led by the sociologist Nicholas Timasheff's discussion of a "great retreat," was also not so clear-cut. Historians have argued that the conservative changes taking place in the 1930s were not quite as abrupt or straightforward as the "great retreat" theory suggests.[20] Radical or even liberal ideas petered out in the 1920s. Although the state wanted nurses to shed their veils and bourgeois pasts, they remained working in the healthcare system in the 1920s and 1930s. Similarly, a conservative element remained in Soviet attitudes to care and its delivery. In spite of calls to recast medical workers as scientific and revolutionary, it was never entirely clear what this meant in everyday clinical practice. The lines between the 1920s and the 1930s were blurred, and, if anything, a gradual progression in how the state came to understand medical workers defined shifts in public healthcare as much as a wholesale retreat in terms of politics and ideology. Once again, there was no singular vision of the Soviet nurse.

The official view of women and nurses was often at odds with medical workers' experiences. Nurses had their take on narratives of care and the system in which they worked. Idealistic projections of patient, devoted, and loving nurses were all well and good on paper, but in the real world, nurses and other medical workers had to get the job done. They had a heavy workload, and at the end of a long day working on the ward, demonstrating "female kindness" was probably low on their agenda. A senior nurse in Leningrad, E. M. Parkhomenko, complained that experienced nurses left hospitals and patient care for administrative work in polyclinics, where there was less work and responsibility but more pay.[21] Stalin's kind and loving nurses were shown to be more economically savvy than idealistic. This example illustrates further tensions among nurses who favored more high-status administrative work as opposed to those who saw patient care as the primary function of the nurse.

Even in the context of the widespread terror of the later 1930s, there were discussions about care and the value of human life. In *Medical Worker* the professor A. I. Abrikosov wrote about the value medicine placed on human life and the genuine care doctors felt for their patients.[22] The well-being of the patient was paramount in medical discussions of the 1930s, a trend that filtered down from the state level. "Party leaders," as one historian has noted, "embraced a broad concept of social welfare whereby the government would guarantee workers' well-being."[23] Care, humanity, and femininity regained their place in medical and especially nursing vocabulary in the second half of that decade. The message was unmistakable: Stalin cared about everyone, and public healthcare would reflect this.

The Stalin Constitution and Medical Education

Providing good care depends on knowledge, skill, and time, but by the end of the First Five-Year Plan problems remained with the quality of medical training and the quantity of medical workers.[24] There were similar problems in industry, where technical education could not keep pace with the rush to expand the labor force.[25] On June 19, 1930, Sovnarkom issued a decree on the reorganization of doctors' training with the purpose of "furthering integration of training with the needs of the health service."[26] A "second wave" of medical institutes followed in the period 1928–1934.[27] In spite of decrees and changes from the top, patients failed to benefit. Hospital patients often complained about basic neglect, such as "attending nannies not answering their calls or critically ill patients forced to get out of bed for various reasons," while hospital wards and beds were not always clean or tidy.[28] This was a basic lapse in care, with no training required to simply look after the rudimentary needs of patients.

In public healthcare there was constant pressure to train large numbers of nurses and medical workers for medical institutions and to ensure that medical workers already in employment had the requisite skills to competently perform their duties. Reforms in 1936, for example, invited nurses who had not completed middle medical education to attend a retraining course or to pass an exam.[29] As middle-level medical workers, nurses had a range of responsibilities. These included—in brief—turning and lifting patients, reading to patients, feeding weak patients, monitoring patients' condition (physical and moral), as well as preparing and analyzing blood smears, using enemas, applying compresses, *banki* (cupping), dressing wounds, preparing casts, giving intravenous injections, draining fluids, administering drugs, dealing with prescriptions, recording illnesses as directed by the doctor, observing and assisting junior personnel, in addition to being able to perform emergency first aid and cope with trauma and death situations.[30] In short, nurses did a lot. And more was to come.

Some of the changes to middle medical education in 1936 reflected new Stalinist policies. These brought women's rights under greater state control. In a glut of decrees between 1936 and 1940 the Commissariat of Health extended its "care and vigilance over women's reproductive behavior."[31] Kindergarten nurses joined the list of middle medical personnel, as a reflection of the postnatal policies of the Soviet government. A new *kul'turnost'* (culturization) inflection could now be found, as nursing schools had to equip nurses with a "deep knowledge of [their] specialism" and "a wide sociopolitical outlook" and train them as "cultural worker[s]."[32] If Soviet officials had come to see the family as an important transmitter of Soviet values, especially in exercising control in the upbringing of children, then nurses and in particular kindergarten and school nurses were significant instruments of the state.[33] Similarly, social assistance nurses and their role in the dispensaries presented another official route to shape culture and behavior through home visits.[34]

The cultural and political standing of the nurse became an increasingly important factor in producing an ideologically sound Soviet nurse. In the eyes of the state, only cultured and ideologically reliable medical workers could administer care. Nursing curricula were consequently to include thirty hours on the Constitution, alongside other classes totaling twenty-three hours respectively on the Russian language, math, and Latin, and some sixteen hours on modern history.[35] There was a total of forty-six hours of physical culture, in addition to the usual medical and scientific classes. These kinds of subjects were central to shaping a new kind of nurse who would be a true product of the Soviet state. Political and ideological training extended to those in different specializations. For example, nurses training to specialize in surgery over a three-month period were to take eighty hours in political education.[36] Those nurses seeking to advance their training to the senior level would have to take a total of eighty hours in the history and Constitution of the Union of Soviet Socialist Republics (USSR), where they could learn about, inter alia, the economic changes of 1924–1936, the organs of state administration, and the electoral system.[37] Semester 2 had a total of forty-five hours, with nurses not required to take any medical or scientific classes during this period.

The curriculum was also the case in 1939, when nursing courses for students without complete middle medical education included a total of eighty hours in history—more than math, at forty-six hours, and Russian language, at sixty-nine hours. Nursing students took more classes in history than they did in children's illnesses, venereal diseases, and eye, ear, nose, and throat illnesses.[38] And the health authorities wondered why there were problems with the quality of care! The rhetoric of care might have come to dominate nursing literature in the 1930s, but nurse training reflected a greater concern with training ideologically reliable medical workers.

In terms of their proletarian credentials, medical workers more or less ticked all the right boxes. They were largely drawn from the working classes by the 1930s—those proletarians the Commissariat of Health wanted to attract in 1919 when setting out the agenda for Soviet nursing. The First Five-Year Plan and rapid industrialization meant that medical workers, like industrial workers, had become proletarianized.[39] The ethnic and gender makeup of nursing schools was overwhelmingly Russian and female: Moscow's Medsantrud school in 1937 included fifty-four female students, forty-eight of whom were ethnic Russian, five were Jewish, and one was German.[40] None of them were party members, although eleven were in the Communist Youth League (Komsomol). Some forty-nine students had not completed seven years of education. It was a similar case in the Rusakov hospital, where all but two of the sixty-three students were ethnic Russian (two were Jewish). There was one male student.[41] In the Rusakov hospital a majority, just under half, were from working-class backgrounds, four were kolkhozniki, and sixteen were white-collar workers. There were just eight Communist Youth League members.[42] Other Moscow hospitals recorded similar statistics, with ethnic Russians remaining the majority ahead of ethnic Jews, Ukrainians, Belorussians, Poles, Georgians, Tatars, and Armenians. Again, very few of the nursing students were party members (I counted one in the Frunzenskaia school), and Communist Youth League membership was generally in single figures.[43]

But class, at least in principle, ostensibly played a lesser role in the mid- to late 1930s.[44] Attention was now on ensuring that cadres were politically loyal as well as educated and skilled. The latter was harder to achieve. One of many short-lived initiatives, known as the hospital-based medical college, trained people as they worked.[45] It ran in Leningrad's Mechnikov hospital for two years but failed. One doctor, an interview respondent of the Harvard project, described it thus: "They would take an attendant in the hospital and send her to a school in order to become a nurse, and they would take a nurse and send her to the university to become a doctor while working."[46] The respondent was head doctor of the department where this scheme was run. It had been a center of excellence, but after most of the good nurses were shipped off to university "the entire section was destroyed." Luckily, the department had managed to hang on to a couple of nurses.[47] The entire enterprise showed the ongoing struggle to reform medical education, but it ultimately undermined the value of orderlies and nurses. Such initiatives also demonstrated a fundamental lack of understanding about the role and responsibilities of nurses.

The medical institutions were dealing with students who often lacked a complete high school education. It was therefore a tall order to expect lecturers to teach advanced medical subjects to these students in a relatively short space of time. Hospitals and clinics were frequently forced to promote nannies and orderlies with medical experience instead of freshly trained graduates. Although the state wanted greater numbers of medical workers, resources were not in place to ensure that these workers were properly trained. The quota filling that typified Soviet society also had a detrimental effect on the public healthcare system. For example, only about twenty-five thousand nursery nurses had completed middle-level medical education, but they were mainly promoted junior medical personnel without training in infant care.[48] This was a fairly common occurrence across the public healthcare sector, for the state had to meet its targets.

Tensions and frustrations existed in this kind of pressurized climate. One professor, a certain Vengerov, when speaking about plans for middle medical schools in July 1938, recalled nasty comments he had heard made against the medical profession. He wanted medical workers to "rise against" the criticism and feel proud about their profession.[49] He provided an example of the unrealistic expectations placed on medical workers, recalling one head of school saying of a newly qualified medical worker, "Well, he's not only inexperienced, he doesn't know anything and cannot do anything."[50] Vengerov argued that a newly qualified nurse could not possibly have experience and required nurturance and guidance.[51] Vengerov's comments in support of middle medical workers were admirable and to an extent true, but there was a problem with medical graduates who were not well trained.

The statistics were moving in the right direction, though. By 1939 some 85.5 percent of nurses in Leningrad had legal middle medical education, compared to just 53.4 percent in 1934.[52] The number of nurses, and indeed other medical workers with recognized qualifications, was slowly growing, at least in urban centers, in spite of the challenges that students and instructors faced. This trend was broadly in line with developments in Stalinist society, where the push for mass education formed a crucial part of modernization efforts.[53]

Winds of Change: Professional Control and Autonomy

When featured in medical or press discussions in the 1920s, nurses were usually derided and accused of negligence, inexperience, and rudeness. To be sure, much of the criticism was justified, but the negativity was not constructive. For much of the 1920s, nurses in many ways remained subject to discussion, rather than engaging in any discussion themselves. But nurses gradually became active agents in Soviet society. No longer shunned as suspicious medical workers, nurses instead became acceptable and even admirable Soviet figures. The increased state value placed on nurses in the 1930s manifested in a number of ways but particularly in terms of professional recognition and development. They became more assertive as a result, and the number of platforms on which they could participate increased. Indeed, as the public healthcare system and its institutions expanded, medical workers in some ways became agents of social control. As such, they could hold considerable power. But this additional power and control also led to tensions. As nurses gained expertise and asserted their autonomy in the workplace, they often encountered obstacles such as a discord between caregiving and administrative work as well as tensions with physicians who challenged their autonomy.

From the mid-1930s on, nurses had more opportunities to increase their knowledge base and learn more about the profession. They could read about medical matters and contribute to journals such as *Medical Worker*, although this was not exactly a high-quality professional publication. An alternative was *Feldsher*, but this was not directed to the professional interests of nurses (the monthly *Feldsher and Midwife* [*Fel'dsher i akusherka*] was first published in 1936 and *Nurse* [*Meditsinskaia sestra*] in 1942). The quality and standard of the medical literature available to middle medical workers was questioned in 1934 when union members criticized *Medical Worker* and claimed it was out of touch with workers.[54] Critics argued that the journal covered neither the most salient questions of public health nor medical workers' interests. They also claimed that its reach was too broad, trying to connect with everyone "from professors to orderlies" and that it "completely ignored" rural medical workers—

those "most in need of a newspaper's help."[55] Instructors from the provincial committee, together with representatives from *Medical Worker*, criticized the journal for frequently missing its publication deadlines, and they also supposed that nobody read it.[56] The discussion seems to have instigated change in the publication.

In the following year, *Medical Worker* ran a feature article on nurses' experiences. In many ways, nurses' accounts reflected the concerns of those writing about healthcare. Senior nurse Zhuliubina of Medsantrud's gynecological department wrote of a "negative attitude" to senior nurses and complained that she and her colleagues had to carry out housekeeping work.[57] After she became a senior nurse in the gynecological department, she claimed that she spent less time with patients and more time on menial tasks.[58] Nurses from the Botkin hospital seemed to have a better experience, and a nurse, Tolokonnikova, described her working day as being very much connected to caring for critically ill patients.[59] Based on these experiences those nurses who had close interaction with patients found their jobs more personally rewarding.

Burobina, a senior nurse from Moscow's Basmannaia hospital, complained about her lack of contact with patients.[60] She mainly did administrative work from 11:30 a.m. to 4:00 p.m. and saw her patients only after 5:00 p.m., when she could "chat to them quietly and find out how they were."[61] She felt that she was not completely informed about her patients' condition because she did not go on rounds; that task fell to the department's five interns (*ordinatori*) while Burobina did paperwork. She wanted senior nurses to be "free of administrative work" so they could be more involved in medical matters.[62] This, by all accounts, quite frank discussion of nurses' experiences illuminated the differences in how medical institutions in the Soviet Union functioned; the medical workplace was a space shaped by various factors, including location, budget, resources, and personnel. A nurse working in one hospital had a considerably different experience and workload from those working in other hospitals.

These workplace differences coupled with the increasing and varying levels of autonomy that medical workers held were problematic. We have already seen how issues of discipline could influence the ethics of care, but autonomy was also a factor in determining ethical outcomes in the medical workplace. Back in 1924, Kalinin, in his call for greater humanity in the medical profession, also claimed that Russian medical ethics were weak and undeveloped. The absence of clear ethical guidelines became glaringly apparent in cases of medical negligence that occurred in the late 1920s, the 1930s, and beyond. Cases of misdiagnosis were often put down to a lack of self-criticism or discipline, conveniently shifting the blame to individuals rather than the system—cadres decided everything, after all.[63] And although nurses were most definitely viewed as assistants to the physician, they nonetheless could wield a great deal of control when it came to patient care.

But such autonomy, especially when directly related to treatment, was not always welcomed. In a generally positive article about nurses, the eminent surgeon Nikolai Burdenko wrote about not crossing a line when it came to care; he knew of cases where nurses administered laxatives or tranquilizers to patients "on their own initiative" because they wanted to "help the patient." Burdenko called on nurses to instead take "less action and false humanity and show greater discipline and accuracy in performing what is permitted."[64] The incident raises questions about reasoned judgment and humanity or sentiment in the medical workplace, but it also suggests that female agency and autonomy "threatened power relations within medical care."[65]

Nurses elsewhere could exercise their autonomy. A nurse and occupational therapist working in a Kiev sanatorium from 1928 to 1941 (with a two-year break between 1936 and 1939), interviewed as part of the Harvard project, wrote that she had a good deal of autonomy.[66] As an experienced nurse she administered codeine and other medication to patients without the doctor's permission because the doctor trusted her.[67] She emphasized that the chance to earn extra money and retain her nursing position was completely at the discretion of the head doctor in her department. She understood that she was "protected by the doctor" but "could be thrown out at any moment."[68] If her orderlies did not receive their food rations, she could order extra rations for her patients and distribute them to the orderlies, but she understood that "in another place you could be tried for one glass of sour cream."[69] Her account of working life in the sanatorium—the conditions, professional relationships, equipment, labor discipline, and even wages—all depended on the head doctor, even though she experienced degrees of professional autonomy. Power and autonomy worked in subtle ways, and nurses found means to exercise both to secure better conditions for themselves and their colleagues.

These examples are fairly representative of an ambiguity deriving from the lack of organization within Soviet healthcare and a blurring of the boundaries between authority and control. Lack of regulation and organization might not be so telling when competent, highly educated, well-trained personnel had autonomy, but when this was not the case serious problems arose. Patients could die. Medical workers who made mistakes were usually investigated and then censured or dismissed, or both. Hospital bosses were reprimanded or dismissed (or, if it was 1937 or 1938, possibly arrested and executed). But as a system that issued innumerable directives on care or education yet fundamentally lacked the resources and organization necessary to enforce these, it failed medical workers.

From the perspective of those at the head of healthcare, the problem was usually the worker. Inexperienced and unqualified junior personnel rather than the doctor or the nurse frequently cared for patients.[70] As was often the case, and not just in the Soviet Union, it was the "subordinate members of the health care team" who spent the most time with patients.[71] This was not good enough for the Soviet healthcare authorities. As the example of the nurse from the Basmannaia hospital showed, many nurses spent a great deal of their working day on administrative tasks. To the vexation of the medical authorities and pedagogues, it was thus orderlies who cleaned the wards, distributed medicine, made the beds, and even carried out "a few medical procedures [*manipulatsii*]."[72] In rural areas it was more common for orderlies to care for the patient, in addition to doing the "dirty work of cleaning the premises, kitchen, and grounds."[73] For these reasons, those working in and writing about healthcare expressed concern about whether patients received sufficient care. Moreover, there was disquiet at the thought of patients spending time with "uncultured" and "uneducated" junior medical personnel, which was very much at odds with Stalinist calls for *kul'turnost'* and a cultured way of living.

But discussions about patient care also spoke to fears about loss of control within the various public healthcare institutions. One contributor to *On the Public Healthcare Front* went so far as to write, "At present there is almost total lack of control over the treatment of the patient."[74] Although brigades or committees inspected hospitals, their visits were primarily concerned with ward tidiness, patient diet, or the accounts—the nature and quality of treatment "constantly escaped" them.[75] Stalinist public healthcare institutions, and indeed post-Stalinist institutions, remained gray zones in the sense that those bodies within—patients and medical workers—could not be fully regulated.[76]

Anti-egalitarianism

One way of addressing the problem of little-trained medical cadres and a lack of control in the medical workplace was to introduce degrees of stratification. The creation of the role of senior nurse was one example, but others included wage differentiation. Stalin's speech on June 23, 1931, titled "New Conditions— New Tasks in Economic Construction," also known as the "Six Conditions" speech, led to various changes in industry that were also felt in healthcare. These included wage differentiation as well as a rehabilitation of "bourgeois" specialists, bringing about huge changes in the education system. In his speech Stalin declared that wage scales in factories reflected "an almost total disappearance of the difference between skilled and unskilled" and asserted: "We cannot tolerate a situation where a rolling mill worker in the iron and steel industry earns no more than a sweeper."[77] This shift from egalitarianism that began in the factories also made its way into the medical institutions.

Medical workers' wages were set to increase on March 1, 1935. Thereafter worker categories reflected their seniority and experience (the categories were more than ten years, between five and ten years, and up to five years). An urban-based nurse with middle medical education could now expect to receive, depending on the experience category, 200 rubles, 170 rubles, or 150 rubles per month.[78] By now, wages were being explicitly linked to the quality of care, which was still considered below acceptable levels. The head of a surgical department in one medical institution claimed that graduates of the medical college were not cultured people and that they were "not able to provide quality medical service and could not be a valuable assistant to the physician."[79] But, the doctor added, connecting the wage of nurses to their professional experience and education changed matters. The nurses in his department were good, and he had seen "literally in a few days" how work had improved as people began to value their role.[80]

The experience of a senior nurse, Elkina, confirmed his impressions. She had worked in a hospital for fourteen years and under the March 4, 1935, wage revisions received 250 rubles instead of 90 rubles, a staggering increase. She admitted that work was generally "bad" but pledged this would change; nurses would study and work harder to raise their cultural level and provide better care for patients.[81] Nannies with considerable experience also received a pay increase, and, as a result, one promised to frequent the theater more often.[82] In this *Medical Worker* article, a virtual ode to the party and government, medical workers wrote of their joy at having such value placed on their work and how they would try to improve conditions in hospitals.[83] The framing of these happy medical worker vignettes occurred in the context of the party and state increasing their level of care for people, both patient and medical worker.[84]

Despite the press image of the happy, better-remunerated medical worker, complaints mounted. At a city meeting of medical workers in November 1937, a Leningrad worker grumbled that orderlies worked day and night for a meager wage.[85] The worker, Cheremushnikov, wanted to make it known—in the presence of Commissariat of Health representatives—that this demonstrated a "harmful attitude" toward this group of medical workers and required urgent action.[86] Conditions were so bad, he claimed, that workers hired one day were gone the next. Lack of financial security led to junior medical personnel shortages.[87] The situation was reminiscent of that in the United States at around the same time, when absenteeism and high turnover resulted from staff nurses moving to better-paying jobs in larger hospitals.[88] A heavy workload, low wages, and high expectations for standards of care placed hospitals and medical workers everywhere in a precarious position. State reactions to these problems differed enormously.

Back in Leningrad, officials overseeing healthcare came under huge pressure. In 1937 a certain Alekseev from the city health authority noted that he had seen orderlies' pay slips with amounts of 520–580 rubles.[89] He paid 28,000 rubles in overtime and wondered where he was to obtain the money to cover it. He had even been "threatened with Solovki" for such overruns.[90] Medical workers in his hospital needed to eat, he argued, but there was no money to feed them, so they would eat at the expense of patients.[91] Once again, financial and economic conditions, now accompanied by the fear of denunciation and arrest, placed local health authorities and hospital administrations under colossal pressure.

Either the wage increases of 1935/1936 were not enough, especially in light of rising inflation, or they simply were not implemented, because salaries and the general economic situation were still the source of discontent a couple of years later. In the Botkin hospital one nurse, Fridman, had completed a Red Cross course and, after two years working there, was earning a wage of 100 rubles a month.[92] Alongside her worked other nurses with fifteen years' work experience and refresher courses under their belts. They were considered better workers than Fridman but received the same wage.[93] Orderlies were in a similar position. Neither the hospital administration nor the local committee addressed the matter, despite appeals in the local wall newspaper (a type of poster or placard newspaper in schools, workplaces and other sites where people gathered).[94] If this was happening in some of the largest and best-known hospitals in the Soviet Union, then it was most likely occurring elsewhere. In spite of calls for an end to the wage leveling instituted after the revolution and corresponding regulations to realize these calls, medical workers still found that their wage was not commensurate with their professional skills and experience.

Recognition and Resolution

In spite of difficult economic conditions, nurses were advancing professionally by the end of the 1930s, especially in Leningrad. The Leningrad city health authority organized the first conference of hospital nurses on May 11–12, 1939.

At this conference nurses presented thirty papers on patient care and treatment.[95] Medical workers took part in some one hundred presentations at conferences in local hospitals in the run-up to the Leningrad event. Through their participation in conferences and collaboration with other medical workers, nurses developed their expertise and in turn their autonomy and control. Several decades later some regarded the conference on care for newborns held in Leningrad in 1939 as a catalyst in helping to raise the profile of middle medical workers.[96]

As a sign of support, the head of the Leningrad health authority released 25,000 rubles to publish the conference proceedings and urged city hospitals to hold nursing conferences on a regular basis, as well as awarding the title of "Excellent Health Worker" to the best nurses in Leningrad.[97] By the end of May 1939 medical workers of all rank received awards for their work.[98] Across Leningrad Province more than sixty midwives and nurses presented papers and participated in discussions on infant care in fifty hospital and district conferences.[99] The midwife D. A. Kaplan of the Central Scientific-Research Midwifery-Gynecological Institute (TsNIAGI) and the Mechnikov hospital's pediatric nurse I. V. Velitskoi were joint winners of the 500 rubles for first prize.[100] The emphasis on pediatrics was a telling sign of Stalinist pronatalist policies and the themes prioritized at the conferences. While there is no doubting the achievements of medical workers in many institutions, those rewarded were often from the biggest and best hospitals and research institutes in Leningrad and Moscow. Other cities, towns, and provinces might very well have had excellent medical workers, but it is also likely that resources and wages were just not at a comparable level. Consequently, attracting "excellent" health workers and providing a high standard of care would have presented a greater challenge.

As conferences were being held, nurses continued to show their knowledge and experience. At one Leningrad nursing conference in 1940, the medical union "awarded sixteen of the best nurses" with prizes that included resort passes to rest homes and sanatoria.[101] These nurses were akin to Stakhanovite, or hero workers who excelled at their jobs.[102] The Commissariat of Health's Grashchenko was in attendance and made a speech noting the "huge political and practical significance of this first [sic] scientific conference of nurses."[103] Moscow hospitals followed suit, and in 1939 nurses published conference papers on a range of subjects, including pediatrics, trauma, burns, gastric bleeding, and angina.[104] The papers' themes were this time illustrative of the growing militaristic climate.

A Sovnarkom decree of May 1939 raised the wages of junior and middle medical workers so that urban-based nurses with more than ten years' experience who worked in hospitals, polyclinics, or sanatoria earned 245 rubles (185 rubles for rural-based nurses).[105] This pay raise was to include middle and junior workers only. Nursing expertise was now officially rewarded and celebrated. One could cynically argue that this satisfied the state's military agenda, but progress also took place in other professions. Nurses, like teachers, engaged with the system and drew on their professional expertise to elevate their position in society.[106] Indeed, medical workers more broadly, through their engagement with state institutions, gradually improved their professional situation.

Despite some progress, medical workers across the Soviet Union had very different professional experiences and did not all work in the same conditions.[107] Far away from Moscow and Leningrad, visiting doctors in the Primorye Territory often had to stay with acquaintances or sleep on their office desks. Not only were the awful living conditions a source of dissatisfaction and a deterrent to working in the region, but they also contributed to medical workers attempting suicide after arriving from central medical institutes.[108] In July 1940 a medical worker from the Tauride hospital infused arsenic and morphine in a suicide attempt. A nurse sent to work in the same hospital also attempted suicide in July or August that year. Later that year a doctor sent to work in a fish processing plant attempted suicide.[109] The author of a report on the region reached the grim conclusion that "the regional health authority, through its training of middle medical personnel, dentists, and pharmacists, should have addressed the very difficult conditions for medical workers in this part of the Far East," but the matter had been grossly overlooked.[110] Medical workers far from the center did not receive much reward or recognition.

Care amid Denunciation and Violence

Despite ongoing efforts to reform and improve the public healthcare system, hospitals remained chaotic spaces in the 1930s. Not even a major Moscow hospital, such as Medsantrud, seemed organized.[111] In January 1934 a group of shock workers denounced orderlies from the Medsantrud hospital for being rude to staff and patients.[112] Nannies also came under fire for not cleaning around beds and thus "violating the work schedule." Head doctor El'sinovskii wanted the matter addressed immediately.[113] One incident in particular seems to have caused him much anxiety. Although only one nanny was to be on dishwashing duty and the rest were to be in the wards with patients, El'sinovskii discovered three nannies and a senior nurse in the buffet room one January morning while he was on rounds in the therapy department.[114] Two of the nannies washed dishes, while a third, Konova, ate biscuits from a plate destined for a patient. The senior nurse took no action, and El'sinovskii was furious: he considered the behavior of Konova "criminal and completely unacceptable" and condemned the senior nurse for her negligence. He recommended dismissing Konova and the senior nurse and also wanted to deprive Konova of her ration cards.[115]

The actions of the nannies certainly elicited an extreme reaction, and while head doctors were undoubtedly under immense pressure, a reprimand might have seemed more appropriate. El'sinovskii probably wanted to send a message to all medical workers that patient care mattered and every action taken or not taken by medical personnel had an impact on the patient experience. But this incident took place in a culture where doctors were constantly on guard to avoid attracting the attention of the authorities. One former Soviet doctor noted that it was common knowledge that "any dissatisfied patient could write a letter of complaint to the health authorities or to a newspaper," with a commission established to investigate the accusation if deemed necessary.[116] A culture of fear thus prevailed.

Indeed, a high-profile medical investigation took place not long after the Medsantrud incident. In early October 1934 a complaint arrived in the offices of Sovnarkom in the form of a letter from a professor of the Moscow Medical Institute, Przheborovskii. The matter concerned his very ill sister, who was transferred from the Moscow Medical Institute to the Moscow Institute for Oncology.[117] Despite having the appropriate documents, the attending doctor refused to accept the patient, and she was admitted only when the nurse accompanying her requested the refusal in writing. When the patient asked for more regular pain relief injections, the attending nurse "rudely refused," and her pleas were not met until the doctor on duty the next day eventually agreed to increase the frequency of injections.[118] When the patient asked for one of the service personnel to call the patient's brother, Przheborovskii, the doctor refused the request. The professor contacted Sovnarkom asking that it investigate the oncology institute immediately in the "interests of all patients."[119]

On October 14 the minister of public health, Kaminskii, wrote to the head of Sovnarkom, Vyacheslav Molotov, about the results of the investigation—a sign that the state took accusations of rudeness seriously.[120] Responding to the incident, the director of the oncology institute issued an order criticizing the "neglect and rudeness" of his staff and reprimanded them.[121] Similarly, on October 10, the Moscow Health Department circulated an order underlining poor labor discipline, a failure to carry out instructions properly, and poor relations with patients.[122] The incident, which made its way all the way up to the ministerial level, showed how much care mattered to the Soviet government.

Sometimes discipline seemed severe, with workers censured for what they might have considered to be minor offenses. But in the 1930s, and especially after the death of Leningrad party head Sergei Kirov in December 1934, fear and suspicion increased, and so the pattern of strict discipline was not out of place. Calls for greater vigilance and discipline often occurred in the context of the "hunt for terrorists" that consumed industrial enterprises in the fall of 1936 and that also spread to hospitals and clinics.[123] Any threats to patient health, safety, and well-being could now easily assume a dangerously political character. One of Medsantrud's deputy head doctors, Byk, reported work violations in the hospital laboratories in early 1936.[124] Byk found that a nurse from the men's department completely forgot to provide a patient's stool analysis to the laboratory, and this resulted in an "unnecessary race" for the laboratory staff that impeded their work.[125] The nurse at fault received a reprimand, while all department heads were reminded of the importance of sending samples to the laboratory at the appointed time. Nurses were to "personally" oversee the delivery of samples to the laboratory, a further example of placing responsibility—and potentially blame—on those lower down the chain of command.

Another Medsantrud deputy head doctor, P. A. Golonzko, expressed concern about critically ill and dying patients' relatives not receiving notification until it was too late (some relatives arrived in the hospital after the funeral).[126] Head doctors, as those with responsibility for the smooth running of the hospital and patient satisfaction, were keen to improve standards. A few years later, some of these very doctors became caught up in the denunciations and violence of the late 1930s.

Indeed, terror was soon unleashed on Soviet society with the first of three high-profile Moscow show trials beginning in August 1936, as well as the executions of those accused of industrial wrecking, treason, and espionage in the case of the Anti-Soviet Trotskyite Center of 1937. Soviet citizens feared that the country was under siege from internal and external forces.[127] After the Central Committee plenum of February 22–March 7, 1937, in which Stalin highlighted the important role of "little people" and chastised local leaders for failing to promote "criticism and self-criticism," terror engulfed Soviet society. When a nurse in a medical emergency center in Moscow's Dzerzhinsky District found herself in hot water in March 1937 for failing to provide her name over the telephone, it was probably not too surprising that she was charged with gross indiscipline: the head of the center had decided to make an example of the incident to remind employees of their responsibilities while on duty.[128] The process of "unmasking" hidden enemies filtered down from the party and government to industry and medical institutions.

The Great Terror, a term traditionally attributed to the period 1937–1938, when over one and half million arrests and almost seven hundred thousand executions took place, did not spare medical workers, who, like many others, fell into the category of "enemy" and were victim to the mass operations of that period. On March 13, 1938, the People's Commissariat of Internal Affairs (NKVD) arrested and later shot Medsantrud's head doctor, El'sinovskii.[129] Although a brigade from the Basmannaia hospital denounced him, Medsantrud colleagues lost no opportunity in denouncing their former boss after his arrest; the party committee secretary referred to him as "the enemy" in a March 1938 general meeting of Medsantrud employees.[130] Former colleagues leveled a series of dubious charges against El'sinovskii, who now proved the scapegoat for any number of problems experienced in the hospital. One worker even claimed that El'sinovskii called some young nurses one night and "forced them to give him a stomach massage" and that they were "all very happy the bastard was isolated" (etot gag izolirovan).[131]

Love and Duty

Narratives of care were juxtaposed to the vitriolic, coarse language of the Great Terror that some of the Medsantrud hospital workers adopted. While enemies were hounded and often described in derogatory terms to elicit disgust, others were characterized as compassionate.[132] As terror ripped through families, Soviet citizens were told that Stalin and the state loved them. Medical workers were presented with images of hero workers to show the kind of care the Soviet state expected. Older, experienced nurses were often presented as those most capable of providing cultured care. The press described orderlies with twenty to thirty years' experience as real heroes, but also "modest" workers who had remained in their posts in spite of the horrors of the civil war years.[133] These tropes of simple, modest people drew directly on Stalinist language that promoted the idea of everyday heroes.[134]

Natal'ia Mikhailovna Anpilogova was one such hero nurse. She came from humble origins, a "modest worker" who entered Sisters of Mercy courses in 1907. A self-educated peasant, Anpilogova worked as a feldsher in a military hospital during the First World War and in 1918 joined a Moscow polyclinic, where she often performed surgeries with no doctor present.[135] Anpilogova worked as an assistant to the surgeon Nikolai Burdenko for fifteen years, and he invited Anpilogova to work with him in the newly established Institute for Neurosurgery in 1929.[136] She became a lecturer on the courses for surgical nurses established in 1937. The Commissariat of Health awarded her a personal wage of 450 rubles; the director of the institute where she worked gave her a "valuable" present to mark her jubilee; and the medical union's central committee rewarded Anpilogova with a resort pass.[137]

The publication *Noble Sister: N. M. Anpilogova (Znatnaia sestra: N. M. Anpilogova)*, the first issue in the popular series Experience of the Best (Opyt luchshikh) published by the Moscow city health department, celebrated Anpilogova's career.[138] The publication described her "blue eyes radiating faith and happiness," so dedicated to her patients that she often worked after her shift had ended. Drawing on the usual tropes and narratives of care, including that of maternal care, nurses were frequently depicted in medical publications as conscientious workers who loved their patients.[139]

The Value of Care

Such narratives of nurses as the embodiment of care and commitment conveyed that love and duty were high priorities for the Soviet government. Any transgressions were supposed to be taken very seriously. In January 1939 deputy head of Sovnarkom, Bakhrushev, wrote to Molotov and his Sovnarkom colleague, Nikolay Bulganin, describing an incident that had occurred in the maternity department of Moscow's Klimovskii hospital earlier that month. The hospital, located in Podol'sk, was the scene of an unnerving and horrifying incident, though not an unfamiliar one. Rats in the hospital had nibbled the lips and tongue of one infant and the neck of another.[140] Bakhrushev apportioned blame for the incident to infringements in basic medical and sanitary rules, including a breakdown in the labor discipline of medical workers who were "rude to patients," slept on night duty, and did not take proper care of the babies. The building that housed the maternity department was overrun with rats, causing sick women "to run about screaming."[141]

Midwives had to hold the "corpses of babies in their arms" during the night to protect their bodies from the preying vermin, but that was not always successful, and a shelf containing the corpses had fallen victim to the rats.[142] The horrifying conditions were in spite of the fact that the hospital was a model institution, as Bakhrushev claimed. The hospital administration, the district health authority and the Moscow Province health authority "had taken no measures to establish order in the hospital" or destroy the rampaging rodents.[143] Sovnarkom investigated the matter and referred the case to the procuracy. Bakhrushev promised Molotov and Bulganin that he would bring those individuals found guilty of neglecting their duties to justice and restore "normal conditions" in the hospital.[144] The orderly work of medical institutions received much attention by the 1930s, so much so that serious infringements came to the attention of the highest levels of government by the end of that decade. When model institutions were subject to investigation, the outlook for Soviet healthcare was bleak and did not bode well for other, less prestigious medical institutions that did not receive the same level of funding or attention.

In fact, conditions elsewhere were desperate. A maternity hospital in Vladivostok's Egershel'd District had no running water or sewage system, while other hospitals had cockroach, bedbug, and lice infestations.[145] Hospitals also lacked basic resources. Lack of care reached appallingly low levels in this part of the Soviet Union. New mothers at a maternity hospital in Tavrichanka were often left lying in soiled sheets that smelled of blood.[146] Hospitals were dirty and had leaking roofs. One Vladivostok hospital put corpses in a barn because it had no morgue.[147] There were also cases of patients dying as a result of misdiagnosis in medical institutions in the Primorye Territory, which operated with 60–65 percent of the required staff and had young, inexperienced physicians.[148] Doctors had a "criminal attitude" toward some patients, as demonstrated by an incident in the Spasskoi city hospital in September 1940. After a mother had given birth to twins, one of which was unconscious, the doctor, midwife, and orderly diagnosed neonatal death and "threw" the nonresponsive baby into some dirty linen in the corridor, assuring the mother that the child had died. The mother took both babies home, noticing on the way that her supposedly dead infant was still breathing, but it gave up its fight for life later that day.[149] Soviet healthcare had its fair share of "undervalued and overstressed" medical workers who mistreated their patients.[150]

Many Soviet citizens continued to suffer at the hands of medical workers and the healthcare system more generally. And the state continued to investigate and charge those responsible. But the ethics and humanity that Kalinin first drew attention to in the mid-1920s appeared to fall on deaf ears. To discuss ethics and care in the context of late 1930s Soviet Russia seems deeply problematic. But care must be theorized within a social and political context and must be "assessed in its relative importance to other values" in order to "serve as a critical standpoint from which to evaluate public life."[151] My aim is not to provide a moral and political theory of care but to show how the ethics of care that developed in the Soviet Union was directly connected to the broader political context. Altruistic measures shored up support for the regime and entrenched power at the same time that the Soviet state branded medical workers and local officials "enemies of the people" for their attitudes or actions toward patients.[152] In this way, public healthcare came to form an important arena for the demonstration of Soviet state care for the people. The years of "excisionary violence" in the hunt for enemies saw a heightened interest in public narratives of care.[153] Discussions of care thus contribute to dismantling the totalitarian paradigm that posits Soviet citizens as atomized, subjugated, and terrorized. While the Soviet state set about implementing mass violence to eliminate certain categories of perceived political and ideological enemies, at the same time it continued to investigate claims of callous behavior among medical workers and ensure the maintenance of certain standards of care.

During the 1930s there was a specific appeal to sentiment and compassion to mobilize middle medical workers. Often this took the form of a gendered discourse that drew on women's femininity. But the discussions of nursing in the 1920s and 1930s also came to place considerable emphasis on values of trust. This speaks to the philosopher Annette C. Baier's discussion of trust as a value and a mark of respect.[154] When medical workers did not earn the trust of people and the authorities, they struggled to win their respect. Medical workers, especially nurses, as leaders in the economy of care, held a moral responsibility to ensure that patients received treatment that reflected the "humanity" expected of the Soviet state. By the end of the 1930s, healthcare workers were under enormous pressure to fulfill these expectations. This pressure and responsibility came at a time when nurses were professionalizing. As nurses and other middle medical workers progressed through the Soviet healthcare system, they developed complex expertise and skills. As a professional cohort, middle medical workers expanded significantly between the First and Second Five-Year Plans.[155]

While Soviet society became ever more polarized in the late 1930s, and as heroes and enemies dominated the political and ideological landscape, public healthcare captured the complexities of how this played out on the ground. The high-level interest in patient care and the state's very clear stance on providing the best care to Soviet citizens were constantly undermined by several factors, not least lack of resources, insufficient training, and low professional prestige. Although these problems were gradually addressed (but not resolved) in the 1930s, the scale and depth of the problems were immense. The Soviet government was simply not able, and to an extent not wholly willing, to properly invest in healthcare. Public healthcare institutions, even model hospitals, could not overcome the serious deficiencies in the system. Perhaps that is why the appeal to individual healthcare workers—the heroes rewarded for their outstanding care and service—was so important. If Soviet citizens were really to receive good quality healthcare, it would have to be at the hands of individual medical workers and not at an institutional level. The compassion and humanity of medical workers, especially nurses, would have to overcome systemic problems. When poor medical training and lack of resources were so rife, perhaps the commitment and compassion of healthcare workers would comfort patients. But nurses who wanted to effect change to improve the patient experience were, as the chapter 6 shows, competing for attention in a crowded arena.

CHAPTER 6

Fortresses of Sanitary Defense
Preparing for War

When the 1930s dawned across the European continent, people awoke to a decade that brought increased militarization, violence, and war. The Soviet Union had already experienced much of this in the 1920s, and so the following decade continued with emphasis on health, sanitation, and defense serving to promote the interests of the state and boosting the military preparedness of Soviet citizens. Through its commitment to defense, the party-state gradually brought the nursing profession back into greater focus. While of course most often overtly propagandistic, the attention brought to bear on nursing not only highlights the state of the nursing profession during this early Soviet period but also illustrates how the socialist state understood the values, traditions, and status of nursing. By the late 1930s, nursing had become an important career choice. Soviet nurses were to care for patients but also to train in the ways of sanitary defense.

The greater push for sanitary literacy in the second half of the 1920s and the militarization of medicine in the late 1930s were not exceptional in an international context.[1] The Japanese Red Cross had three elements at its core, "the subordination of personnel, organized patriotism, and military authority over Red Cross operations."[2] These elements, grounded in particular ideological and political conditions, gradually came to characterize Soviet nursing to varying degrees in the 1930s. Alongside calls for improvements in standards of healthcare (chapter 5), parallel campaigns were taking place in the Red Cross and Red Crescent that emphasized patriotism and military preparedness. There were many times when these two campaigns—those by the Commissariat of Health and the Red Cross—interacted.

The mobilization campaigns of this decade often touched on gender issues. Women formed the backbone of the healthcare service and Red Cross work. In the early Soviet period the range and type of training for nurses, including paramilitary training, reflected a binary concept of gender.[3] While traditional gender stereotypes existed—the narratives of care that prevailed in the context of civilian healthcare discussed in chapter 5 testify to that—some Soviet women could dismiss these as irrelevant.[4] Women could identify with hero nurses wielding rifles as easily as hero nurses sitting by the patient's side.

Although the focus on family and motherhood in the mid-1930s positioned women back in the home and with a double burden to bear—working in factories in addition to carrying the bulk of responsibility for looking after children and the home—women still maintained degrees of agency and emancipation. The All-Union Society of the Red Cross and Red Crescent USSR (SOKK and KP USSR [hereafter shortened to SOKK]) expansion in nursing in the 1930s, along with the renewed emphasis on the nursing profession in the face of war, provided many women with opportunities for upward mobility. The range and type of course on offer afforded them greater flexibility in shaping their career path. But for all that it offered women and medical workers, the essence of SOKK work and the efforts to improve sanitary defense across the entire nursing profession were not about elevating women in society or expanding training opportunities for medical workers. Rather, SOKK efforts centered on (1) organizing a patriotic workforce with first aid skills; (2) buttressing any weaknesses in the healthcare system; and (3) deploying nurses and sanitary workers to defend the Soviet Union in the event of war. This chapter analyzes the Soviet state effort to build fortresses of sanitary defense through mobilizing Soviet citizens and especially women to become involved in first aid and nursing and how these efforts transpired in practice. Promoting sanitary defense and nursing worked both ways, and while the state benefited from women's involvement in civilian defense, women in the 1930s were able to take advantage of the training on offer in the healthcare professions to advance on the career ladder.

New Representations of the Nurse

Although the Communist Youth League was a Soviet institution, the Red Cross and Red Crescent was not. In order to better appreciate some of the challenges confronting the Red Cross, one needs to understand how people perceived that organization in Soviet Russia. While the SOKK was successful in drawing in Communist Youth League members, it was an ambiguous organization with prerevolutory and international roots—two negative ticks in late 1920s and early 1930s Soviet Russia. Popular understanding of the SOKK in the Soviet Union seemed to be unfavorable, and the organization had to work hard to present itself in a positive light to the public. Press accounts suggested that the SOKK worried that some people harbored doubts about the organization. One anecdote from *Women's Journal* (*Zhenskii zhurnal*) described a discussion on a bus in Tver' that drew contrasts between the prerevolutionary Russian Society of the Red Cross (ROKK) as an organization for the wealthy and the Soviet SOKK as an organization for the Soviet people.[5]

Women reading *Women's Journal* were to understand that the Red Cross played a crucial role in Soviet society and Soviet citizens should lend their support to the organization. The ideologically equivocal position of the SOKK nurse after the First World War, and in particular the nursing profession's links with aristocracy and religion, adversely affected nurse recruitment and prestige in the early Soviet period. The separation between the old, tsarist Red Cross and the new Soviet variant came across in different ways. In 1930, SOKK uniforms, for example, still apparently had "more crosses than the pope," and one writer suggested that it was time to move away from the "old monastic form."[6] Read in this light, it is unsurprising that the SOKK joined forces with the Communist Youth League and youth, the vanguard of the revolution. Attaching itself to this most Soviet of institutions enabled the SOKK to operate with a greater degree of credibility and gain street kudos.

Moves to connect nursing and civil defense were further strengthened in 1930 with the publication of the monthly journal *For Sanitation Defense* (*Za sanitarnuiu oboronu* and, from 1938 on, under its new title, *Sanitary Defense* [*Sanitarnaia oborona*]).[7] The campaign to produce higher numbers of nurses was gaining ground, with various organizations and the media promoting nurse courses and a militarized image of the nurse. The SOKK, which was struggling to consolidate its Soviet identity and win the support of those who still associated the organization with the old regime, devoted many pages of *For Sanitation Defense* to convincing readers that the Red Cross and its nurses were bona fide "Soviet." Readers were informed that the Moscow city committee conducted checks on the sociopolitical credentials of students enrolled in nursing courses and medical colleges, because the training system had been "contaminated" (*zasorennosti*). When a supervisor in Moscow's Zamoskvoretskii District asked about the high dropout rate, he was told it was "a consequence of passport introduction" (*sledstvie pasportizatsii*).[8] A majority of students recruited did not receive passports (internal passports were reintroduced in 1933), and so the "former merchant class deftly wriggled their way into nursing courses and wanted to use the nurse's headscarf as a visor to hide the face of an enemy."[9] Press accounts such as these made it clear to readers that constant vigilance was necessary to unmask the enemy. They could rest assured that the Red Cross was a legitimate and reliable Soviet institution. Readers were also reminded that their moral and physical safety was being monitored through state surveillance mechanisms.[10]

The 1936 film *Girlfriends (Podrugi)* and its press coverage was a Soviet attempt to harness interest in the nurse. Lev Arnshtam's film, with a musical score composed by Dmitry Shostakovich, placed nurses front and center.[11] This was the first time, and one of the few times (at least prior to World War II), that Soviet nurses appeared as screen heroines. The film takes place primarily during the Russian civil war, when Asia, Zoia, and Natasha, three Petrograd friends, decide to become Bolshevik "red nurses."[12] The timing of the film was important, for it marked the point when nurses received increased attention and when national campaigns to train nurses gained momentum. The heroism, compassion, and patriotism these characters displayed served to cast nurses in a new light, depicting them as strong women who could inspire the next generation of red nurses. In the mid-1930s the press heralded nursing as a worthy and respectable profession. Nurses came to be medical workers in their own right, and not as simply one category of middle medical personnel.

In the late 1930s, publications such as *For Sanitation Defense* emphasized the title of "nurse" as honorable and respectable, often drawing on the heroic red nurse of the civil war years to illustrate this point.[13] An article penned by a certain L. Bronshtein noted that the red nurses, as depicted in *Girlfriends* by protagonists Asia, Zoia, and Natasha, were "excellent proletarian fighters in the most patriotic and heroic moment of their lives."[14] The story of the three red nurses apparently had a "huge influence" on Soviet youth.[15] The film was "an opportunity" with educational (*vospitanie*) potential. The campaigns seemed to pay off in rather spectacular fashion: Red Cross membership grew from a modest seventy-five thousand in 1926 to over five million in 1934, an incredibly high increase, while its activities extended to over 1,890 administrative districts.[16] In 1934 almost half a million women completed the Communist Youth League civil defense nursing courses.[17] Such increases were an impressive feat.

The 1941 film *Girlfriends at the Front (Frontovye podrugi)* presents further propaganda efforts to place nurses in the limelight.[18] The film follows the wartime fate of three friends who complete Red Cross training and volunteer after the German invasion and start of war. The opening scenes take place in their

local Red Cross committee center before the three friends go to a field hospital and then to the front itself. Signs of heroism, particularly that of their group
(*druzhin*) leader, Natasha Matveeva, are evident throughout. After planes roar
in the skies above the makeshift military hospital, the cluster of Red Cross volunteer nurses gathered inside become anxious and turn to Natasha for reas-
surance. Natasha, unsure of what to do, walks to the operating room and
observes doctors and nurses quietly getting on with work. When a bomb whis-
tles by and explodes, the nurse assisting the surgeon loses focus and looks up,
but the surgeon, asking repeatedly for forceps, tells her "to pay more attention" and "not to be distracted from work." Now knowing what to do, Natasha swiftly returns to the Red Cross volunteers and tells them to look after
the patients and "not be distracted from work." Natasha is later shown reading to patients, caring for them, distributing letters and presents, and also sing-
ing to patients. She is brave and fearless on the battlefield. Her character was
the kind of Red Cross volunteer the Soviet state required. Bronshtein and his
press colleagues would, no doubt, have been very pleased with the film, which
depicted proletarian fighters equipped to deal with anything that came their
way. The image of the nurse was in the process of changing thanks to media
and press campaigns.

Mass Mobilization: Calling all Youth!

Changing representations of the nurse in the period 1929–1945 fit the charac-
terization that this was "an unbroken time of crisis that provided young people
with opportunities even as it surrounded them with violence."[19] Such a description applied to young people interested in entering the medical profession, where the boundaries between civilian and military nursing, presenting
both opportunity and danger, often overlapped. Much of the opportunity that
came the way of young people arrived at a time of political tension as the NEP
declined and then later through the years of collectivization, industrialization,
and purging. Toward the end of the NEP, the SOKK, the Communist Youth
League, and Pioneer organizations assumed an active role in first aid and sanitary training.[20] These organizations, as well as the Red Army Military-Sanitary
Service and the public health organs, all had a duty of care to the injured and
sick and a responsibility for providing help during times of crisis, such as natural disasters, accidents, or epidemics.[21]

This work was no doubt given further impetus by the war scare of 1927
and buoyed by international recognition of the Soviet Red Cross in 1928.[22]
At this time, between 1926 and 1927, the Red Cross "organized 400 sanitary

detachments and 'courses for reserve nurses.'"[23] The Pioneers organized sanitary detachments, or *sandruzhiny*, to augment the work of institutions and organizations during periods of mobilization and war.[24] Indeed, by July 1927, local Communist Youth League organizers in Kazakhstan, Northern Dvinsk, and Taganrog implemented calls from on high by expanding sanitary groups (*kruzhki*), nursing courses, and programs for youth league members.[25] For example, the secretary of a Taganrog Communist Youth League group wrote to the organization's Central Committee reporting that its members, male and female, participated in local factory-organized sanitary groups.[26] Young girls, often league members, who signed up and completed nursing courses then went on to a central outpatient clinic (ambulatory) for practical training.[27] From the mid- to late 1920s, young people were thus drawn into sanitation and defense work through their involvement in the Pioneers and the Communist Youth League.

In spite of these early organizational efforts, some Communist Youth League reports (*svodki*) at the local level registered a note of concern when it came to youth and wartime mobilization. A correspondent from Irkutsk wrote that "young people underestimated the threat of war, seeing it as something distant, and were consequently not in a position to defend the country."[28] A Communist Youth League member and tannery worker in Irkutsk reportedly said at a cell (*iacheika*) meeting: "We talk so much about military danger, but all the same there will not be war. The Western bourgeoisie cannot fight with us." The report also noted discontent in Martovskii district: "In a construction workers cell a mixed gathering of Communist Youth League members and non-party youth claimed they did not want to hear reports about war danger and shouted: 'Give us dancing.' The war reports were removed."[29] At a meeting in Leningrad's Sverdlovsk District only fifty-one of three hundred people turned up to discuss the "week of defense and Communist Youth League tasks."[30] Still, paramilitary training remained an important part of the Soviet education system, whether in schools or the Communist Youth League. Indeed, integrated paramilitary training was obligatory in Soviet school curricula from 1932 on, and Soviet children were enrolled in a military-political program from the age of eight.[31] The Communist Youth League, born in the crucible of war and revolution, was no stranger to militarizing youth.[32]

Some local league members worried about involving girls, who were apparently not drawn to military or sanitary work because they had to "give birth, not fight."[33] Since its inception, the Communist Youth League had been male dominated, and the gendered discourse it promulgated continued under Stalin.[34] But as the organization turned its attention to making young men into soldiers in the 1930s, it sought to make young women into loyal Stalinists in the domestic sphere.[35] Nursing offered a route to attract more girls and women to the organization. Over the course of the 1930s, millions of Soviet women "came of age at a time when being a good Soviet citizen meant acquiring military skills."[36] Military and defense training was often a key component of nursing courses and an obligatory qualification for those already working in medical institutions.

The SOKK Central Committee ratified and ran various courses in conjunction with other organizations and departments, such as the Communist Youth League. This expansion in civil defense, at least with regard to nursing, coincided with the push to draw more workers into higher education that had begun during the First Five-Year Plan, but also connected to broader efforts to expand membership in a whole host of organizations (the Communist Youth League being a prime example).[37] Through its engagement with the Communist Youth League, the Red Cross reached a much wider audience and campaigns served the needs of both organizations.

Once enrolled on Red Cross courses, students attended two-hour classes that taught them about the structure of the Red Cross, including its work in industry, collective farms, and sociopolitical campaigns and its cooperation with other social organizations such as the Communist Youth League and trade unions.[38] Students also held classes on sanitation with a requirement to pass the Get Ready for Sanitary Defense (GSO), as well as classes on the role of the SOKK in public health.[39] Students learned that factories were to be "fortresses of sanitary defense."[40] Their participation was part of their patriotic duty, helping to strengthen and solidify Soviet military preparations. "Stalinist political language" was after all "awash with campaigns, battles, and fronts," and Soviet society was effectively "organized for war and lacking in clear boundaries between military and civilian life."[41] This language coupled with the war scare of 1927, the Japanese invasion of Manchuria in 1931, and the rise to power of Adolf Hitler in Germany in 1933 lent a degree of credence to rumors of foreign threat. Similar mobilization efforts extended to the countryside, where the Red Cross organized springtime sowing campaigns and helped out in village hospitals and ambulatories.[42] Sanitary defense and nursing had their place alongside some of the other mass mobilization campaigns of the late 1920s and early 1930s, including physical fitness campaigns, industrialization, and collectivization.

Some three years after the introduction of the Communist Youth League–inspired Get Ready for Labor and Defense (GTO) norm in 1931, the SOKK launched the GSO norm. This was to train young women and men in civil defense skills such as nursing. The Communist Youth League played a big role in this scheme. Mass literature about the GSO norms accompanied its launch, and the SOKK printed 500,000 slogans, 75,000 posters, and 35,000 textbooks.[43] Campaigns such as these, while focused on devolving the state's duty of care to ordinary Red Cross–trained citizens, reflected the ideology of the time and an emphasis on building the New Soviet Person. Collective responsibility and duty to one another was at the heart of communist propaganda in the early Soviet years, when citizens could improve themselves "by contributing to the social whole."[44] Both the Communist Youth League and the SOKK were at the forefront of making Soviet society a beacon of sanitary defense.

A Sovnarkom resolution of December 3, 1938, prioritized sanitary defense work in the Communist Youth League and the SOKK.[45] The Red Cross and Red Crescent was to "widen its system" of sanitation work in industries, collective farms, and institutions.[46] It was to ensure that "masses of cadres would become nurses, orderlies, and disinfectant personnel" and that the civilian population would engage in sanitary defense work.[47] Glebov, from the Red Cross Executive Committee, wrote to Shteinbakh of the Communist Youth League Central Committee, advising that the league assist the SOKK through member involvement in reserve nursing courses.[48] Glebov suggested that N. A. Mikhailov, the Communist Youth League secretary, include the following less than catchy slogan in his speech: "The Communist Youth League must train the best girl-patriots in enterprises, state farms, collective farms, and educational institutes in reserve nursing courses."[49] To help students pass the nursing courses, Glebov pressed for there to be no interruption to production work and for regular monitoring of the young women in courses. Mikhailov acknowledged that women wanted to participate in war but argued that they brought "a better advantage as nurses."[50] The increasingly pragmatic emphasis on defense training necessary in the event of war applied to nursing, as well as paramilitary training more generally.[51] As one Red Army representative noted at the Seventeenth Communist Youth League Central Committee Plenum in April 1939, while aviation or production might be attractive to some young women, their "main role was to care for soldiers and work in hospitals."[52] This was the line taken in much of the propaganda around wartime nursing in the late 1930s and was especially clear in films such as *Frontovye podrugi*. Mass youth would mobilize but in different ways and according to gender-prescribed roles.

Courses and Challenges

A growth in the quantity and quality of trained cadres (every second inhabitant in Moscow was studying by the end of the Second Five-Year Plan) might

have characterized the years 1932–1936, but serious problems remained unresolved.[53] Trouble brewed behind the scenes of mass mobilization campaigns
to train nurses. One of the perennial issues with Soviet education—poor studying conditions—also afflicted nursing. Press coverage showed that schools
suffered from frequent changes in staff, flu was rampant owing to the freez-
ing conditions inside the schools, and classrooms lacked textbooks, visual aids,
and even desks.[54] The conditions in classrooms, needless to say, hampered
teaching. One correspondent wrote that an SOKK and KP course was being
conducted in a "room that was only a little warmer than the street."[55] Inadequacies such as these were prevalent in general education in the 1930s as a
result of rapid expansion and urbanization.[56] At that time both urban and
rural schools shared "structural impediments to effective instruction."[57]
Students may very well have enrolled in courses and bolstered statistics, but
whether they attended their courses was another matter. The usual problems
of recruitment and retention plagued nursing.

That seemed to be especially the case for SOKK and KP courses. Many of
the nurse training courses took place in whatever rooms or spaces were available. Courses in Moscow's Kazanskaia District, for example, took place in the
corridor of a chemical-bacteriological lab.[58] Providing enough qualified teachers was also a problem and again one that afflicted the educational sector as a
whole.[59] Elsewhere, half the students dropped out of Red Cross nursing courses
in Ivanovo Province: no wonder, when classes took place in a room adjoining
the physical culture classroom, where those exercising (*fizkul'turniki*) regularly
met and "stamped about, shouting and behaving in a hooligan way."[60] This
"wrecked" the nursing classes. The physical culture organizers were, no doubt,
carrying out the same kind of mobilization campaigns asked of the Red Cross;
on this occasion, they ended up stepping on each other's toes.

In 1935 the Red Cross courses graduated fourteen thousand nurses and had
ten thousand enrolled in postgraduate courses.[61] Red Cross and Red Crescent
personnel cared for more than five and a half million people that year.[62] Nonetheless, recruitment and retention remained a challenge. Moscow's Dzerzhinsky school received almost two hundred applications but accepted only
thirty-five to classes commencing September 1, 1935. By October 15 two had
dropped out, and by January 1, 1936, a further five had dropped out; the numbers were neither "stable nor current."[63] Reasons cited for the dropout rate
were poor literacy levels, illness, relocation from Moscow, and living and working conditions. Further difficulties arose once students managed to pass the
courses. Sometimes SOKK and KP–trained nurses slipped through its net.
One committee report noted that the military and Red Cross service took
only 77 percent of those finishing the nursing courses (perhaps the remaining

23% found better-paying work in industry).[64] To address the problem, the SOKK and KP Executive Committee distributed special nursing booklets for every student to complete. The booklets would contain marks and act as "passports" for those who completed nurse training courses.[65]

In other places, doctors did not want to teach nursing courses. A certain physician, Gomfel'ford, went on the record saying, "Nobody will read lectures for free, including me."[66] As was often the case in the Soviet 1920s and 1930s, the success of schools and courses depended on the enthusiasm and initiative of directors, teachers, and instructors; this was also the case for Red Cross and regular nursing courses. Some instructors were so overburdened with work that they were simply unable to instruct on nursing courses; others went to great lengths to help students and colleagues. Outside of major urban centers doctors received no fee for training nurses, while in cities they could earn "up to five rubles an hour."[67] But money was often not the issue. A doctor interviewed as part of the Harvard project worked several jobs until 1938. He taught in a postgraduate institute, the Second Moscow Medical Institute, and a hospital. He also worked in a closed hospital as a consultant, two maternity hospitals, and a railroad polyclinic eight hundred kilometers from Leningrad. His motivation for working long days was to help his students, who "for every infraction . . . could be brought into court."[68] Professional empathy and compassion worked in different ways. His students qualified as doctors.[69] Where the system failed, individuals often stepped into the void and assumed the burden of training and education.

Upwardly Mobile Patriots

While civil defense was certainly a leading factor behind the organization of Red Cross courses, there was also a vital and immediate need for nurses to work in civilian hospitals and clinics across the Soviet Union, a need the current nursing education system did not meet. The Commissariat of Health and the government were also aware of problems in healthcare. A decree in 1933 had noted the low level of nurse training in the polytechnics and the insufficient numbers of graduates to meet the demand for medical workers.[70] The newly certified Red Cross nurses no doubt helped to stave off problems with short staffing and turnover in hospitals and clinics. After all, not only were courses in first aid and nursing to provide workers and collective farm workers with basic medical skills or train them as "military-sanitation workers," but they were also to give them a taste for medicine and function as a path to further medical education. The SOKK had to look on the short-term nursing courses as a base for higher medical education. Hospitals could boast about the class origins of their workers, celebrating nurses who had left their collective farm to become first orderlies and later nurses.[71] As Henry E. Sigerist, the Swiss-born doctor with a keen interest in socialist healthcare observed, the Red Cross and Red Crescent "adapt[ed] themselves to the government agencies" and contributed to "fulfilling the health program of the nation."[72] And as we have seen, this fulfillment assumed many forms. By working with both the Communist Youth League and the Commissariat of Health, the Red Cross and Red Crescent helped to promote both sanitary defense and nursing.

Working in a range of institutions allowed for various forms of career progression and some degree of flexibility in terms of where nurses decided to work. Young people who did well in courses and participated in the various norms—the GTO; GSO; Society for the Assistance of Defense, Aircraft, and Chemical Construction (Osoaviakhim); and Voroshilov sharpshooter (*Voroshilovskii strelok*[73])—had good credentials and a range of options when it came to medical work.[74] One young woman recalled that local Communist Youth League district and school secretaries had to round up good students and send them to nursing courses or military college.[75] After studying at the six-month SOKK courses, graduates could continue their studies at a medical college for five years, a two-year nursing college, or a three-year feldsher college.[76] Attending courses could thus be in a person's interest, especially those eager to fast-track their career in healthcare.

One could dismiss much of the hullabaloo around propaganda and mobilization as rhetoric, but nursing courses seemed to genuinely appeal to some. A young woman from Yaroslavl' Province who "really loved children" read a notice about courses for medical workers. She "very much wanted to be a medic" and enrolled in a course in the training school of a hospital nearby. After passing the exams, she went on to study in Moscow, where she also worked as a nanny. She studied for two years and qualified as a midwife.[77] A temptation to view the press stories and statistics as bombast does not do justice to those who were interested in working in healthcare. Propaganda played a role in helping to promote nursing, and the SOKK press in particular took a positive stance on the profession.[78] Frequent press references to the "honorable" or "proud" title of nurse suggested that people had hitherto not viewed nursing as a desirable profession. This changed by the mid-1930s as a new wave of workers joined the ranks of nurses, no doubt in hope of a bright future.

The opportunities available to urban-based nurses—who received higher salaries than their rural-based counterparts—were generally far greater than those working outside of the major Soviet cities.[79] In a *Medical Worker* article about orderlies, two authors reported on a conference of nurses in the Leningrad District of Moscow. One Communist Youth League member and participant, Galina Men'shova, when asked if she wanted to be a doctor, replied: "I will be, for sure."[80] The assumption was that orderlies or nurses who were any good would naturally want to become doctors. But it was not always straightforward for medical workers to advance in their specific career. For that reason, it was sometimes easier for them to move specializations and qualify as a doctor or move institutions.

A doctor from Voronezh interviewed about her life and work as part of the Harvard project commented that in the institution where she worked, five of the best *sidelki* were promoted to the laboratory, another three were promoted to nursing courses, and four former orderlies were completing their studies in the *rabfak* (school for workers) so that they would enter the medical institute in the following year.[81] The Red Cross courses effectively provided medical institutions with trained cadres. For those with an interest in medicine but who lacked a full secondary school education, nursing was a means to access further medical education, and many nurses availed of this opportunity. For some, whether SOKK-trained nurses or regular Commissariat of Health–trained nurses, promotion could mean leaving the nursing profession. Soviet policies during the First Five-Year Plan period opened opportunities for the upward mobility of workers and peasants.[82] But these opportunities came with a price in healthcare when some of the most qualified nurses sought to move to medicine by the mid-1930s. Despite propaganda efforts to popularize nursing, medicine remained the preferred career choice. For nurses who had advanced so far in their education, training to become a doctor seemed to be the next logical step up the career ladder.

After working for a period of three years as nurses, some women in their middle to late twenties then decided to make the move to medicine. For example, twenty-four-year-old Aleksandra Aleksandrovna Larionova graduated from a medical institute in Leningrad in 1938, having worked as a nurse in pediatric consultation for three years.[83] She was assigned work as a doctor in Murmansk.[84] Sometimes nurses worked in their chosen profession for ten or even almost twenty years before deciding, as women in their middle to late thirties, to train as doctors.[85] This decision to change profession and move jobs and often location was sometimes made when these women had young families (those with family could request to remain in the same city as their spouse or submit special requests about the health or education of a dependent). Perhaps the prospect of better pay was a deciding factor, although these women would have been close to attaining senior nurse status, if not having done so already. There were also women without children or spouses, or both, who decided to become doctors after working as nurses for a substantial period of time. One unmarried woman, Aleksandra Ivanovna Semenovskaia, born in Novgorod, completed a one-year nursing course in 1916 and worked as a nurse for nineteen years. But in 1935 she opted for change, and in 1938 she graduated from the First Leningrad Medical Institute, at age thirty-nine. She was assigned work as a therapy doctor in the town of Olenets, Karelia.[86]

Besides wages, another reason for a sudden career move, and one that reflects poorly on nursing in the Soviet Union in the 1930s, was motivation. Although the archive record is silent on the matter, it is very possible that these nurses were intellectually or professionally unfulfilled in their role as nurse or senior nurse. Nurses with considerable experience and an interest in further specialization may very well have found that they had reached a dead-end and saw no challenge or future development in their career. Becoming doctors thus allowed them to pursue a deeper or higher level of knowledge, training, and recognition. Of eighty-seven students graduating from the Second Moscow Medical Institute in 1938, more than a quarter were middle medical workers; twelve had worked as nurses, twelve as feldsheritsas, and one as a midwife.[87] One Harvard interview respondent, who studied at the Odessa Medical Institute from 1928 to 1933, noted that many of the students there were nurses and feldshers pursuing a medical degree.[88] They received a small stipend—"just enough to buy bread"—and one nurse worked during the day and studied at night. Many of them fell asleep in class but continued their studies in spite of the circumstances.[89] These middle medical workers were desperate to qualify as doctors. Such a position would result in receiving a higher wage and a greater degree of professional prestige.

Yet training large numbers of nurses was the primary objective of nursing courses, and those with Red Cross certification could enter medical institutes or work as middle medical personnel in hospitals, clinics, and dispensaries. By 1938 and 1939, especially after the battle of Lake Khasan, the press presented nursing as a respected, valued, and responsible profession.[90] Khasan precipitated great interest in paramilitary and nursing courses (see chapter 7), but enrollment numbers were not as high as expected.[91] For those already working in the public healthcare service, the Khasan experience generated mass political enlightenment work in hospitals, with the head doctor of one Odessa hospital noting that it held meetings of doctors and nurses, as well as senior and middle-level personnel, to discuss nurses' role in public healthcare and how to learn from the Khasan experience.[92] These kinds of experiences promulgated romanticized images of war and technology to instill patriotic values in young women.[93] Training young women to become nurses was all very well, but there was no guarantee that nurses would remain in their posts.

Senior medical workers worried about the upward mobility trend and how they would replace valued nurses with twenty to twenty-five years' experience.[94] They expressed concern about young people finishing medical college and nurses considering work in the hospital temporary, "striving to study further." As one senior surgeon observed, the hospital became a "waypoint" between the medical college and the Institute of Higher Education, and while he did not begrudge young people the opportunity to improve themselves, he wondered where hospitals would "get good nurses."[95] Writing about women and career development, Ellen D. Baer concludes that a "continuing societal misconception is that nursing is a sort of junior medicine" and not a discipline in its own right.[96] In the Soviet Union, women often did not aspire to become nurses; they aspired to become doctors. Here the "ladder from nursing to medicine" meant that the highest achievers in nursing moved into medicine (although this applies to middle medical workers more generally, as feldshers might have aspired to become doctors).[97] But it also speaks to the problem that the American Quaker Anna Haines identified at a very early stage—that those in charge of nursing viewed it as a type of medicine in miniature form.

Fears about the blurring of professional boundaries between women doctors and nurses have surfaced in Europe and North America. Some scholars have suggested that women doctors in the West fear nurses encroaching on their territory, particularly in obstetrics, where nurses might "undermine their own diagnostic abilities and counseling skills."[98] Today, gender dynamics and class shape workplace relationships between doctors and nurses, as women doctors and male nurses are now more commonplace in hospitals and clinics. The women's studies scholar Rosemary Pringle argues that women doctors have usurped the caring role of nurses to demarcate their own territory as distinct from that of male doctors.[99] The widespread entry of women doctors has left the nursing profession in an uncertain position, and so "the relationship between nursing and medicine will need to be worked out around an ethos of mutual respect."[100] These kinds of gendered and professional issues already existed in the Soviet Union. Soviet public healthcare was heavily feminized, and nurses frequently made the move to medicine to qualify as doctors.

The absence of a clear, distinct nursing profession proved problematic in many ways. Medicine focuses predominantly on diagnosis, but nursing is about the patient, and as Baer astutely asks, "What good is a brilliant diagnosis and treatment order if the person activating the treatment does not do it correctly, cannot interpret patient responses accurately, and does not have the judgment to intervene if necessary?"[101] In the early Soviet period the dialogue on nursing more or less relegated nurses to the position of assistants to the doctor, with little autonomy in activating any kind of treatment. The lack of professional independence for nurses and the general upward mobility that was so characteristic of Soviet society during this period harmed nursing and made it a halfway point on the career ladder.

Militarizing Medicine

Increasing militarization put upward social mobility for nurses on hold. In the late 1930s the government seemed more interested in producing as many nurses as possible with transferable skills for war. There was no escaping the militarization of these years, and the Commissariat of Health had to balance state needs with institutional needs.[102] Newly qualified and experienced nurses in hospitals, polyclinics, and sanatoria found themselves caught up in military and defense training. One such nurse, interviewed as part of the Harvard project, had received two years training in anatomy, physiology, first aid, and other subjects in a Red Cross military hospital in Arkhangel'sk in 1914–1916.[103] She generally liked her job and wanted to help people. Like other nurses in the second half of the 1930s, she had to pass a military training course of about a month's duration each year that included lectures on planes, gas, bombing, injections, and care for soldiers.[104] Some of the military instructors told the nurses that they would be armed "like any rank-and-file soldier." When she stated that the International Red Cross took care of people and did not fight, instructors told her that these "were the remnants of bourgeois ideology." Of the nineteen to twenty students in her feldsher course, most were older nurses who, like her, "had not yet adjusted to the Soviet pattern" and received the opportunity to raise their qualifications. She and the other tsarist-era trained nurses and doctors could "spot someone's social origin in two words" and "understood each other, almost by sign."[105]

Other nurses with wartime experience, such as Lidiia Ionovna Vtorova, who worked in the Botkin hospital, found new roles in this militarized society.[106] The most senior member of her local Osoaviakhim group, Vtorova had served at the front during the Russo-Japanese War and the First World War. She often shared her experiences of war with senior class pupils in local schools.[107] Women, and nurses, had to participate in a vast array of defense-related activities, whether at work or as part of their collective social and political obligations. Nurses attending full-time, two-year Commissariat of Health courses also undertook defense training. In the 1937 study plan, military-sanitary training totaled sixty-eight hours, which was one hour less than general patient care.[108] By 1938 and 1939 sanitary defense classes had increased to ninety-two hours, and, additionally, physical culture classes in 1939 (also ninety-two hours) included rifle training.[109] Militarization was now a core component of nurse training and education. In a little under two years, many of these nurses had to put these skills to the ultimate test.

Nurses could also become flight nurses (*bortsestry*). The SOKK first conducted training for parachuting nurses and organized training for operation nurses in 1936.[110] Its Executive Committee trained nine nurses, nine medical students, and two doctors to parachute jump.[111] Parachuting seemed to be quite a popular activity among women. Aviation offered women a "symbolic and real" escape from the monotony of everyday life.[112] In spite of positive press portrayals of parachuting or nurses, there was sometimes a dissonance between the picture of mass patriotism and genuine enthusiasm.[113] Some women may not have been so keen to take part in the different sanitation and defense activities but participated as a result of various societal or peer pressures, or, like the nurse who worked in the Kiev sanatorium, they believed that they were serving the greater good.

Press coverage continued to highlight the success of the militarization campaigns and to encourage nurse participation. Although some of these campaigns encountered problems, particularly related to parachuting and aviation accidents, the effort to reach out to women continued unabated. The GSO norm placed emphasis on training nurses for antiair defense.[114] Osoaviakhim, which had responsibility for chemical and defense campaigns, had by 1940 turned its attention to focus more specifically on medical work and antiaircraft defense.[115] But militarization campaigns did not appeal to everyone. In Leningrad the provincial party committee (*obkom*) criticized the work of the provincial Red Cross committee: "huge turnover" occurred on the Red Cross committee, there was no political work, the sanitation brigade program kept changing, and there were no premises for nurse training.[116] Still, orders to mobilize continued to rain down from on high.

Militarization campaigns in nursing and sanitation were often tempered by references to womanly care and compassion. In the Kharkov confectionary factory "October," women wanted to train as nurses because this was a "holy vocation" and would help the Red Army in the event of war.[117] In harking back to the Sisters of Mercy imagery, and presaging the "holy war" to come, women workers deployed symbolic language that echoed the narrative of compassionate and devoted nurses. Wounded soldiers could be miraculously healed by "female care [*zabota*], attention, gentleness, patience, and bravery."[118]

In spite of efforts to attract women to nursing, some authorities in the Commissariat of Health doubted whether those who completed short-term nursing courses were able to work in a military medical capacity. One surgeon,

Prof. N. N. Priorov, when speaking at a plenary meeting of the Hospital Commission in January 1939, asserted that many middle medical personnel wanted to work in military hospitals, but he wondered: "[How could they] send them there if they have not studied the appropriate subjects?"[119] Medical professionals recognized that the standard of nurse training needed vast improvement and that nurses had to assume greater professional responsibilities to ease the pressure on overburdened doctors and surgeons.[120] Much discussion centered on whether nurses should take x-rays and perform blood transfusions (although, as it transpired, some hospitals already allowed their nurses to independently perform blood transfusions). The head doctor of Moscow's Ostroumov hospital argued that nurses should know how to do blood transfusions in a defense context, understand the basic techniques of x-ray, and be able to define the blood groups.[121]

With war breaking out in Europe in September 1939, the Soviet drive for defensive expansion increased in the second half of that year and throughout 1940. On the northwestern edge of the Soviet Union, the Soviet-Finnish War in November 1939–March 1940 necessitated the establishment of short-term medical courses so that sanitary brigade members and reserve nurses could work in military hospitals or the Red Army.[122] By 1940 the Commissariat of Defense was involved in the campaign to train greater numbers of nurses with a very specific skill set, specifically in surgery and blood transfusions.[123] Undertaking this kind of training required "tens of thousands of doctors to assume lecturing roles, a huge quantity of hospitals with surgical departments for use as an academic base, hundreds of thousands of textbooks, and many thousands of different study aids."[124] The SOKK responded by establishing more reserve nurse courses, to begin on February 1, 1940.[125] In 1939 it trained about forty thousand reserve nurses (compared with nine thousand nurses trained between 1933 and 1938).[126] Evgeniia Filippovna Tarasova (Kharchuk) was one of two hundred female students at Kiev University who enrolled in a reserve nurse course for the Red Army in December 1940. She worked in an evacuation hospital four days after the German invasion, in 1941.[127] Less than six months had passed between Tarasova's enrolling in a reserve nursing course and serving in a hospital. Demands for a further increase in the nursing courses were necessary in light of a recently organized system that was still not strong enough—problems remained with student attendance and high dropout rates—and impending war.

A variety of state bodies were now involved in nursing. Next to take part was the People's Commissariat of Internal Affairs (NKVD), which requested reserve nursing courses and ordered training for about twenty-five hundred of its employees.[128] The trade unions were also drawn on to help with the training of wartime nurses and sanitary brigades: central, provincial, factory, and local trade union committees were all required to quickly establish short-term courses to attract women workers and housewives to nursing and sanitary brigade training in a range of workplaces.[129] As war raged in western Europe, the drive for training masses of Soviet medical workers was in full swing. The Soviet Union was not alone in its promotion of nurses—the United States harbored fears about a nursing shortage during war and also undertook recruitment drives in early summer 1941. Army nurses penned articles for the *American Journal of Nursing* to popularize military nursing, and the American Red Cross launched an enrollment campaign for reserve nurses.[130] As the prospect of another world war loomed, nurse recruitment campaigns assumed mounting importance.

The tempo of the Soviet campaign increased further after the German invasion. At the start of the war there were 412,221 middle medical workers in the Commissariat of Health system, and 154,000 of these were nurses.[131] In addition to the Red Army—and NKVD—organized nursing courses, the Red Cross and Red Crescent organized further reserve courses, following a Sovnarkom ratification on February 22, 1941.[132] The reserve nursing courses were to train highly qualified nurses with a focus on surgical skills and first aid, as well as provide military-medical training for the Red Army and the navy.[133] But this was a tall order. Evgenia Tarasova recalled that she had acquired no practical skills and very little by way of theory in the reserve nursing course that she attended in Kiev.[134] Reserve nurse courses ran for five and a half months (without a break from work) and took place in collective farms, military academies, and other military institutions, as well as in medical institutions (general and military hospitals).[135] There were few who were not involved in some kind of military medical training in the months immediately preceding the German invasion and following it. Partisan training was not overlooked, and the partisan brigade nurse (*sestra-druzhinnitsa*) had to know how to treat a range of illnesses and injuries in the absence of immediate medical help.[136]

Another Sovnarkom decree on June 29, 1941, seven days after the German invasion, further mobilized the public healthcare organs to form sixteen hundred evacuation hospitals close to the front.[137] By December 31, 1941, six months into the war on the eastern front, the Red Cross and Red Crescent had trained 216,809 nurses and 355,445 sanitary brigade members.[138] Training middle and junior medical cadres depended on mobilizing patriotic support as well as wartime needs. This was especially important during the initial stages of war, when Soviet losses were heavy. Medical and sanitation work symbolized women's commitment to the cause, with "hundreds and thousands of Soviet girls and women striving to be medical workers."[139] Early in the war, the Red Army could count among its ranks 200,000 doctors, 300,000 nurses, and 500,000 sanitary brigade members.[140] By 1943 the Red Cross and Red Crescent was responsible for training the bulk of Soviet nurses; these nurses could still enroll in a Commissariat of Health course, but during the war the commissariat's focus had shifted to producing feldshers and midwives.[141] A huge network of more than 12,000 doctors and about 30,000 nurses had to supervise practical classes to train .5 million nurses, sanitary brigade members, and orderlies.[142]

In peacetime the commissariat's various healthcare organs had set up evacuation hospitals through organizing premises and medical equipment and training medical personnel. The health organs had also accumulated considerable experience in deploying evacuation hospitals in a range of conflict zones including Khasan (1938) and Khalkhin Gol (1939) and in the Winter War (1939–1940). But the weaknesses of the medical services and especially their lack of preparation had also been glaringly apparent.[143] On July 7, 1941, the government decreed that the public health organs would deploy an additional 750,000 beds (593,000 in the RSFSR) by January 1, 1942.[144] There was only so much last-minute preparation that the authorities could do, and the massive efforts to improve medical training, especially in surgery, were not enough. In September 1941 the head doctor and a military doctor in a regional health department (kraizdravotdel) in Khabarovsk, in the southeastern corner of Russia, claimed that most operating nurses were only in the process of "acquiring surgical skills."[145] In spite of early efforts to bolster sanitary defense, the courses and campaigns of the late 1930s had evidently not been sufficient to produce skilled medical workers. Similarly, the Commissariat of Health—which ran specialist courses for training surgical nurses—had largely failed in its bid to educate mass numbers of nurses competent to assist in surgery.

The final decades of the 1930s saw a coordinated state program of mobilization and militarization that incorporated a range of organizations and agencies. Government concern with war preparation and its eagerness to make the Soviet Union a fortress of sanitary defense had already begun ten years before, precipitated by the 1927 war scare. Red Cross and Red Crescent activities, along with Communist Youth League assistance, were crucial to the country's military preparedness. Nurse training was foremost among these activities. The late 1920s and early 1930s drive to rapidly industrialize and enable the Soviet Union to "catch up and overtake" the West mobilized all Soviet citizens. But it was not only peasant farmers or urban factory workers who had to help construct socialism. Medical workers, especially nurses, were clearly called on to serve the state and engage with the wider militarization campaigns and attend SOKK courses. The Nazi-Soviet Pact in August 1939 did not result in an easing of defense preparations. That said, Stalin "continued to believe that war could and would be delayed until 1942."[146] The war in Europe that started in September 1939 and the Soviet attack on Finland in November that year meant that defense and war preparations gained momentum.

Already by the end of the 1930s there were many training courses for nurses that catered to different specialized areas such as dietary nursing, surgery, blood transfusion, and x-ray, as well as courses for senior nurses. Some of these could be undertaken while the nurse remained in full-time employment in the hospital (the favored approach), but for other courses time off work was necessary. The Commissariat of Health approved all courses. Impending war refocused state interests on the training of its middle strata of medical personnel, especially nurses, who were now urged to improve their skills and knowledge. But unlike in publications such as *Sanitation Defense*, the rhetoric of patriotic duty was largely absent in discussions taking place within the professional medical community. The tenor of medical discussions was serious but shared the general sense of urgency around the need to train nurses who were competent and prepared to perform their duties in the context of war. When war came it tested all medical workers to their limits and had repercussions long after the last battlefield wound was dressed.

CHAPTER 7

A Decade of War and Reconstruction

A children's home teacher, Ekaterina Demina, was on a train to visit her brother in Brest, Belarus, when war broke out on June 22, 1941. She found herself stranded and under German fire in Orsha, Vitebsk, not far from the Russian border. Demina had no medical training, but she and several other women helped the wounded, until Demina herself was injured and ended up in a military hospital. Once recovered, she signed up for a short-term nursing course, joined the navy and "saved more than 150 wounded, killed 50 fascists, and was injured three times."[1]

Vera Ivanovna Ivanova-Shchekina was seventeen when war broke out. She was in Leningrad and wanted to go to the front, but the enlistment office (*voenkomat*) advised her to study and train as a sanitary brigade member. She was already at the front by the time the course finished. Shchekina began work in a military hospital, where her "skill, tenderness, care and attention" eased the suffering of soldiers. In September 1941 she became commander of her sanitary brigade and transferred the sick and weak in her assigned residential district to the hospital. Shchekina received a Florence Nightingale Medal in 1975 for her efforts in the Leningrad Blockade.[2] The narrative of patriotism and sacrifice that had been building over the course of the 1930s was put into full effect by the outbreak of war. Countless women like Demina and Shchekina were eager to contribute to the war effort. The invading German army unleashed a swell of emotions across Soviet territory, and the Soviet government channeled these toward patriotic service to the motherland.[3]

In the Soviet Union and elsewhere, connotations of femininity and family associated with the civilian nurse provided a "powerful cultural affirmation of the nurturing nature that supposedly defined women biologically."[4] But the brutality and scale of a war that saw the loss of some twenty-seven million people ensured that many women became embroiled in the horrors of war, whether in battle or at the home front. Such circumstances tested family and femininity. Violence, deprivation, starvation, and hardship defined the wartime experience for Soviet citizens. The harsh policies of the Soviet government, particularly those during the first year of the conflict, were to steer the Soviet Union through the war and save socialism from the clutches of fascism. Less than two months after the launch of Operation Barbarossa on June 22, 1941, Order No. 270 decreed punishment for Soviet soldiers and their families who surrendered; Order No. 227, known as "Not a step back," issued in July 1942, threatened retreating soldiers with execution. It was in this extreme context that women enrolled and served as nurses across the western front, in besieged cities, as well as in hospitals, factories, and clinics far away from the bombing and fighting. This chapter shows how nurses negotiated the changing political and professional terrain during the 1940s, coping with not only the horrors of war but also the difficulties of the immediate postwar years.

The months preceding and immediately following the war are particularly important in understanding Soviet medical preparedness and strategy. Nurses' struggles did not end in May 1945 and therefore the immediate postwar years serve as a reminder of the short- and medium-term consequences of the war for medical workers and healthcare. How did wartime nurses integrate into the civilian healthcare system? What was the state's stance on nursing following their contribution to the Soviet victory? The nursing and broader medical experience of the war shows that, in spite of the civil defense preparations of the late 1930s and rapid industrialization, the Soviet healthcare system was not in good shape prior to the war and that many of the challenges confronting the country after the war had been present beforehand. In that context, the efforts of medical workers should be appreciated all the more. These wartime efforts, and of course the continuing demand for medical workers during the war, were important in cementing the prestige of the nursing profession. It was in 1942, after all, when a journal dedicated solely to nursing, *Nurse* (*Meditsinskaia sestra*) was first published in the USSR. For that reason, the war was a turning point and helped to accelerate some of the changes already occurring in the profession in the late 1930s.

Nurses and women in war were usually celebrated for the care and attention they showed to the wounded and sick.[5] Professional as well as voluntary nurses, such as Demina and Shchekina, felt duty-bound to contribute to the war effort in some way. Some 41 percent of frontline doctors were women, of which 43 percent were surgeons.[6] The number of female military feldshers stood at 43 percent and female sanitary instructors at 40 percent, and 100 percent of nurses were women.[7] All these women made real and significant contributions to the war. But they played a role in the rear too. While many medical personnel raced to the front, the sick and injured at the home front also required care. This chapter brings some degree of balance to the wartime nursing story in the Soviet Union by analyzing the range of caring activities that medical workers performed. It also places the war years in a slightly longer chronological context, with a focus on the 1940s rather than the war years per se.

The Nurse Experience of Frontline War

Communist Youth League women were often the first to volunteer for nursing at the front. One such nurse, Valia Savenkova, was celebrated for her wartime heroism. In the heat of battle, and with the help of a girl from a neighboring village, she evacuated 325 injured behind the front lines and received a medal for bravery.[8] The twenty-two-year-old worker Antonina Alekseevna Lebedeva, who completed a sanitary brigade course in August 1941, went to the military hospital after her day's work.[9] During the war Lebedeva put her skills to good use by evacuating hundreds of injured and earned the praise of her superiors. Another twenty-two-year-old, Communist Youth League member Varvara Emel'ianovna Khomenko, worked as a nurse in a military hospital beginning in February 1942. According to the head doctor, she had "quite mastered medical techniques" and was one of the "best workers" in the hospital.[10]

Much of this rhetoric of praise was already familiar to Soviet youth from previous industrialization or militarization campaigns, but this time it was different: the Soviet Union was actually at war. During and after the Great Patriotic War, as World War II is known in Russia, thousands of medical workers, many of whom were women, received praise for their wartime endeavors.[11] Some had already cut their teeth during the Winter War. Twenty-five-year-old Anna Efimova Ostrovskaia, a Communist Youth League member and student at Leningrad State University, had no nurse training but was celebrated for her brilliance as a surgical nurse in a military hospital, where she looked after patients with "love and maternal care."[12] Much of the Great Patriotic War rhetoric about heroes and sacrifice was present during the Winter War, with Communist Youth League members often at the forefront.[13] The militarization of the late 1930s and war with Finland had raised awareness of the importance of wartime nursing, although nothing could have prepared Soviet youth for the experience of the Great Patriotic War.

Often those who decided to work as nurses at the front when war started had no idea what awaited them. A young teacher, who trained as a nurse and went to the front with her husband, described the horrors of caring for wounded soldiers. When nursing a sergeant with a leg wound, blood spattered all over her face and she initially "lost herself," thinking she could not go on, but then composed herself, fixed up her patient, and sent him to the hospital.[14] She was not prepared for what she faced at the front. As she told her Harvard interviewer: "There is such a difference in the theory and practice of military nursing. Everything seems so nice and neat and orderly when you're learning, but when you are actually involved in treating wounded, your arms are covered with blood up to your elbows."[15] The rivers of blood, especially during amputations, overwhelmed another nurse, Maria Selivestrovna Bozhok. She said, "I was always bloody. . . . Blood is dark red. . . . Very dark."[16] Another woman, who completed her nurse training in a hospital at the beginning of the war and received some military training in a polyclinic before being sent to the front, recalled bandaging so many wounded patients that it seemed to her that "her hands smelled like blood."[17]

Sometimes eager volunteers barely out of school went to the front but soon found they were out of their depth. One recalled bringing a bedpan to a man with no arms, and it took her a few minutes to figure things out. In her words: "I had to help him. . . . And I didn't know what to do, I'd never seen it. They didn't even teach it in the courses."[18] Even though many of these nurses had only the most basic medical training and were ill equipped to deal with the wounds and injuries that confronted them at the front, they nevertheless managed to take care of soldiers with serious and life-threatening injuries. They also had to deal with constant threat of danger and injury to themselves.

Anna Grigor'evna Menzorova, from Novosibirsk, completed a nursing course without a break from work and went to the front when war broke out. She was "injured four times but each time she recovered and returned to her battalion." According to her senior commanding lieutenant, Menzorova had "iron nerves." During one battle a mine exploded near her, and they "all thought that was the end of their 'Siberichka,' but she got up." She continued her work after somebody bandaged her head wound.[19] Not all were so lucky.

A group of three medics remembered their friend Polina. She died after throwing herself on a patient during a bombardment.[20] Such tales of courage and sacrifice became part of the foundation myth of the war. The harrowing and heroic experiences shared among comrades defined the memory of the Great Patriotic War. These memories still endure.

Private memories often differed from official, public narratives. When Xenia Sergeevna Osadcheva returned home after nursing in a frontline hospital on the Trans- and North Caucasian fronts, her mother did not recognize her. Even though she later moved to Crimea and lived by the sea, she admitted: "I'm worn out with pain, I still don't have a womanly face. I cry often, I moan all day. It's my memories."[21] Nurses and medical workers at the front experienced trauma and posttraumatic stress disorder. The sights, sounds, smells, and thoughts of war were horrific, and memories of war lived on long afterward; nurses in war often remember the smell of burning or blood, the sounds of bombs and screaming, and the sight of mangled bodies.[22] Soviet nurses, like those in other war zones, felt the stress of war to be great. One American Medical Corps nurse working in a field hospital in Germany wrote that she was "desperately tired, hungry, and sick of the misery and futility of war." After losing one young patient, she "wept uncontrollably," her tears falling on her patient's "bandaged remains."[23] In a 1946 article American Mary Walker Randolph, an army nurse and lieutenant, wrote that army nurses would need time to "recuperate from the stress and hectic schedules of field duty and nursing wounded young men" and, in her words, to recover from the "nervous tension and fatigue built up by life in a foxhole and under shellfire."[24] They needed to get reacquainted with "American life" and enjoy missed luxuries such as a "silk night-gown, a bathroom."[25] In the Soviet context nurses could not admit to some of the issues that nurses elsewhere might have discussed openly, such as compassion fatigue and emotional stress owing to having to care for mass casualties or the severely wounded.[26] This was a group of women whose wartime experience became subsumed to the Great Patriotic War narrative of sacrifice and glory. To publicly tell of their personal horrors, fears, doubts, and lasting pain was to undermine the myth of the war. Rather, their stories had to "suit the stereotype" and be a "conversation for the public."[27]

The everyday heroism of medical workers lay not only in saving lives or dramatic rescue efforts but also in their commitment to the more mundane task of organizing courses, instructing others, and just helping out. After the Red Army liberated Kharkov, nurses and sanitary brigade members home from the front taught classes for two months before returning to duty.[28] Nurses in evening classes who studied for seven months without a break from work were all exhausted after "putting in a twelve-hour day and then showing up to classes."[29] The memoirs of medical workers attest to the sense of camaraderie and friendship that existed. One nurse told her I Remember / Ia pomniu interviewer, "We looked out for one another."[30]

The dedication of nurses during the war was amply demonstrated in the statistics. Medical workers returned 72 percent of the injured and 91 percent of sick Red Army troops to the front. During and after the Great Patriotic War, thousands of medical workers received official praise.[31] Some 116,000 medical workers—40,000 of them women—received honors. Of the 52 medics awarded Hero of the Soviet Union, 15 were women.[32] But praise did not extend to all female medical workers. The nurse Anna Vasilevna Bogacheva, when asked in an interview if she was awarded a medal for "fighting merit" and how often medical personnel received this medal, replied that she received this award but that very few medical workers enjoyed these particular honors.[33] Another nurse interviewed had a similar view and attested that few medical workers received awards, except those who died and posthumously received the Red Star.[34]

When women received recognition for their feats, their efforts were often framed within a gendered discourse that placed women in a caring rather than combative role. As one historian has argued, although the central press was to place women at the front in "caring, sacrificing, and noncombatant" roles, journalists were not always consistent in doing that, nor could they "form a coherent perspective on women's desire to fight."[35] To use the words of the writer and historian Svetlana Alexievich again, stories about women and nurses had to "suit the stereotype."[36] This was the case during but especially after the war. In literature and the press, representations of Soviet medical workers conformed to ideals of heroism and self-sacrifice and feminine, maternal care.

Public tales of heroism often overshadowed accounts of despair during the Great Patriotic War. This despair also applied to women's private lives, where loss, uncertainty, and trauma shaped their relationships. Female medical workers at the front, or *frontovichki*, often fell in love with soldiers, lost their husbands, had sexual relations with soldiers, or were victims of sexual assault.[37] As some historians of Soviet women in war contend, "Women in the Red Army not only had to confront a lethally misogynist enemy but also at times a sexually predatory environment among their own male comrades-in-arms."[38] The 1957 film *The Cranes Are Flying* (*Letiat zhuravli*) depicts the impact of war on those at the home front through the experience of the main protagonist, Veronika. After her fiancé leaves for the front, his family takes her in and they head for the rear, along with her fiancé's cousin, Mark. When Mark rapes and marries Veronika, viewers gain insight into both the vulnerability and betrayal of women.[39] Women and medical workers had to wrestle with not only the hardship of their work but also preying men and the judgment of others.

Women in war who became romantically involved with soldiers were often derided as war-field campaign wives (*polevye pokhodnye zheny*, or *PPZhe*). As one medical assistant remarked: "There were only men around, so it's better to live with one than to be afraid of them all. . . . But after the battle each of them lies in wait for you. . . . You can't get out of the dugout at night."[40] The nurse Ester Man'kova (Fain) wrote in her memoirs that soldiers were more blunt than officers, asking girls they met if they would "do it or not."[41] Senior army personnel were often presented with "trophy" wives; female feldshers became the field campaign wives of decorated military men, including Marshalls G. K. Zhukov, I. S. Konev, and A. I. Eremenko.[42] Oleg Budnitskii's work has shown how many women returned from the front with reputations as "ruined" women. Malicious rumors that began in the army followed them into civilian life: many of these women consequently preferred to conceal or downplay their wartime past.[43]

The Soviet press and propaganda presented nurses and other medical workers as caring sisters and mothers, but some of the deeper personal traumas were not given voice. War would be won at any cost. One historian of British nursing argues that notions of sacrifice during the First World War formed part of nurses' "healing work" as opposed to a reflection of their "subordination" to the establishment.[44] In this way, nurses "subordinated their own emotional and physical needs to those of their patients" because that was how they contained trauma and promoted a patient's well-being.[45] In the Soviet Union, nurses also contained various forms of suffering and trauma from the Second World War. While much of this was a direct result of their role as nurses and medical workers, sometimes the hardship they experienced was due to the fact that they were women.

Healthcare on the Home Front

For nurses and other medical workers, the situation was just as difficult away from the front. In conditions of total war, the state directed the vast majority of resources to defense. Yet medical workers populating military hospitals or evacuation hospitals struggled to cope. Medical workers, who already had a multitude of grievances about their living and working conditions as well as their financial situation, endured extremely harsh labor conditions during the war years. The Labor Law of 1940, which was instituted in workplaces including hospitals and clinics across the country, made already difficult working conditions much worse. This draconian law meant that basic infringements, such as being late to work, became criminal offenses.[46] Workers could be incarcerated for two to four months if found guilty of leaving their job without permission from management.[47] The June law met with widespread resistance in various workplaces across the Soviet Union.[48] The former head doctor of a village hospital in Yakovlevna District, Primorye, was not pleased with the law on the eight-hour working day and seven-day week, which he found to be "unclear" and "unacceptable," because "the work was very difficult and the pay was so little."[49] Nor did the law seem to ease problems with labor discipline. In the central maternity hospital in Vladivostok, 50 percent of medical workers received convictions for violating work discipline and two workers received sentences for two months' imprisonment.[50] In another district of the Primorye Territory, a worker was sentenced to four months in prison for repeated truancy.[51] The outbreak of war put an already stretched healthcare system to the test and placed frustrated medical workers under even more pressure.

One of the reasons provided for worker dissatisfaction was the low salary and the high cost of living, a problem discussed in previous chapters. Doctors worked part-time in several places. Medical personnel at all levels were seriously unhappy with their standard of living in the Far East and "simply refused" to work in the public health system.[52] This was a far cry from the medical training and military preparation—the so-called fortresses of sanitary defense—being undertaken elsewhere in the Soviet Union. These medical workers in the far eastern corner of the Soviet Union were speaking out against conditions at a time when the state was trying to stir up patriotism and just seven months before the German invasion almost ten thousand kilometers to the west.

The civilian public healthcare system had to get by on the scraps, making do with the least-experienced doctors and nurses. Medical workers far from the front also had to deal with the most vulnerable in Soviet society—the old, the infirm, infants, and those ineligible for action. They also treated exhausted workers.[53] Rationing meant that many were often near the starvation point.[54] One sixteen-year-old nurse recalled that she always had food when she was at the front, but that was not the case when she later worked at a military hospital behind the front lines in Baku.[55]

Staffing evacuation hospitals proved challenging too.[56] Medical personnel in the evacuation hospitals consisted of different medical specialties, and most were SOKK nurses. In the city of Gorky, now Nizhni Novgorod, 30 percent of hospitals had one doctor for every one hundred patients; surgeons were in even shorter supply.[57] Doctors, nurses, and other personnel were needed at the front in field hospitals, behind the lines in evacuation and military hospitals, as well as in civilian hospitals and clinics. In spite of the immense challenges, a "majority" of evacuation hospitals returned 96–98 percent of the discharged to action in the first five months of the war.[58] Medical workers in Yaroslavl' and Vologda had to cope with makeshift and awful conditions when treating vast numbers of malnourished and diseased evacuees from Leningrad in March–June 1942.[59] Many nurses, despite their inexperience, quickly mastered the basics of care. Their role was more than just medical; they "read newspapers to the patients, wrote letters to relatives, gave talks, and taught patients first aid."[60] When performing their medical duties, nurses and feldshers were to do so "with loving care."[61] One medical commentator reminded readers that Commissar of Health G. A. Miterev believed medical workers had a "huge responsibility" to the "motherland and humanity."[62] He cited the commissar, noting that infectious diseases and epidemics were "considered anti-state business" that weakened and undermined the country's defense.[63] In this way caregiving became subsumed to the Soviet Union's patriotic rhetoric. Betraying their responsibility was akin to betraying the country.

In spite of the mass training in sanitary defense before the war, the spread of disease remained a constant threat. A report on the conditions of work in November 1940 showed that tuberculosis was a prime contributory factor to this rate, and early forms of the disease were often not detected.[64] There were "hundreds of patients who should have been isolated [but] were instead living in dormitories and apartments, infecting healthy people around them." As a result, the number of deaths from tuberculosis in the Primorye Territory had risen from 336 in 1938 to a staggering 864 in 1939.[65] There were already 467 deaths for the first half of 1940.[66] These were the awful conditions that existed before the privations and increased threat of epidemics associated with war descended on the region. Once war was under way medical workers had to cope with the rapid deterioration of the public's health.[67] By late 1941 and 1942, measles, typhus, and other diseases spread eastward along evacuation routes, taking the lives of infants, children, the old and the infirm; by 1943 and 1944, medical workers had to cope with vast numbers suffering from starvation and tuberculosis.[68] The authorities took the threat of disease "extremely seriously," and local officials put various sanitation measures in place to control the spread of infectious diseases.[69] The State Defense Committee became involved in all anti-epidemic work, with Miterev made a plenipotentiary.[70] But once again, Soviet efforts seemed to be a step behind, responding only after disaster threatened.

A massive health crisis confronted medical workers on the front lines of care. In addition to caring for patients, healthcare workers also had to conduct sanitary-enlightenment work with patients and their relatives. At an interprovincial meeting of workers from infectious disease hospitals in the Urals-Siberian provinces, head doctors acknowledged that it was hard to find people as "devoted" as some of their medical workers, who sometimes worked in almost impossible conditions. The doctors believed that it was "wrong" to ask so much of them and "give them so little."[71] While some doctors felt this way, the state had no qualms about asking citizens to go above and beyond the call of duty.

Duty of Care: State and Citizens

Like medical workers elsewhere in the civilian system, healthcare workers in factories and plants were also under enormous pressure. They had a duty of care to their patients but also to the state. Workplaces had to meet their employees' healthcare needs and ensure they were fit to work. When the Stalin Chemical Plant in Stalinogorsk received orders from the Tula provincial health department to ensure that middle medical personnel worked in the plant's health center round the clock, the plant had five days to make that happen.[72] The plant was also ordered to appoint one doctor and five nurses to the center, and an infirmary for daytime shift work was to be set up in another factory shop.[73] Of the civilian population, it was these workers in defense industries, a total of about four million in 1943–1944, on whom "the Soviet regime concentrated its medical efforts."[74] Workdays lost due to illness cost the defense industry, and therefore medical services for industrial workers expanded during the war through the establishment of medical-sanitary sections to oversee the shop-based and factory-based health centers such as those in Stalinogorsk.[75] Efforts to set up health centers for workers in defense were rolled out across the country, with more medical workers expected to fill these positions.

The state extended the arm of care to people for economic and defense reasons rather than individual or collective well-being. Concerned with typhus outbreaks in 1939 and 1940, the Commissariat of Health sent a series of recommendations to a long list of local and republican health authorities in the RSFSR.[76] One of the suggested recommendations was for directors of schools and children's homes to assume "personal responsibility for the sanitary condition of the institution."[77] The health authorities also wanted to ensure "compulsory sanitary supervision of rural schools, including nursing schools and schools for other medical workers."[78] The Commissariat of Health urged local health authorities to make doctors and feldshers "strictly liable for refusing any patients with typhus, and for the sanitary condition of the hospital, as well as for dispensing any items not disinfected for typhus."[79] The state placed the blame for mistakes and shortcomings on individuals within the system rather than the system itself.

War conditions meant that doctors unfamiliar with the structure and methods of Soviet public healthcare arrived in military hospitals. Head doctors considered many of the doctors medically qualified but "completely unfamiliar with the structure and methods of public health."[80] They were equally worried about nurses. Doctors felt that many nurses who completed only the "shortest of courses" basically "did not know anything, could do nothing" and yet had responsibility for a whole host of critically ill patients. Consequently, the doctors had to constantly work with nurses and feldshers.[81] Doctors, nurses, and other medical personnel had to work overtime to compensate for inadequate training and resources.

The exigencies of war tested those working in Soviet hospitals and clinics in different ways. This was all the more so because medical workers did not work on a level playing field. In Novosibirsk Province the evacuation hospitals relocated from other Russian cities were "fully provided with an administrative apparatus, political personnel, doctors, and nurses."[82] But not all the hospitals were so well staffed.[83] During the war, military hospital No. 1017 (the location was not provided, but the hospital seems to have been in Molotov, now Perm') experienced considerable difficulties presented by the retraining of middle medical personnel. This was partly because of the diverse nature of their qualifications, which included nurses who had graduated from feldsher schools, nurses with a legal middle medical education, wartime nurses, and those trained in short-term SOKK courses—in sum, people with different medical training and "with different cultural levels."[84] Some hospitals and clinics ended up addressing training and quality issues in a variety of ways, including through holding conferences.

Medical conferences, which had started to drive the nursing profession forward from the mid-1930s on, continued over the course of the war. Some 97 interdepartmental conferences of nurses, including 131 talks, took place in 1941.[85] During the war, conferences were a forum for discussion and an important means of bringing newly qualified medical workers up to speed. But they were not quite the professional showcases of the late 1930s. Conferences functioned as important spaces to share knowledge and work experience. The state mobilized medical workers to overcome deficiencies in the system, and they had to figure out ways of dealing with problems in training and education themselves. The Wehrmacht advance on Soviet territory heightened medical workers' sense of duty.

Contours of Care

Medical workers, as we have seen, wanted to provide the best care that they could under very trying circumstances. They had responsibilities to the state and patients and had to meet the expectations of both. In 1942 several patients in a local hospital wrote to the editors of the newspaper *Cheliabinsk Worker* (*Cheliabinskii rabochii*) expressing their gratitude for the careful and attentive treatment they received.[86] They thanked the head physician, Il'ia Naumovich Fridman, who was "ready to give everything to his patients," as well as a group of nurses and a nanny, Anastasiia Sineglazova. Patients wrote that personnel were always "good and gentle," and they felt that the medical workers cared about them. The patients had all arrived in the hospital with high fevers, and some of them had even lost consciousness, but they hoped that "within 15–20 days" they would return to full health after their stay. They were already feeling "much better" after six to eight days and put their recovery down to the care they received from the "hospital collective."[87]

These patients depicted an orderly picture of life in a Soviet hospital during the war. Their positive experience was portrayed as a direct consequence of medical workers' careful attention. Memoirs of nurses based in military and evacuation hospitals interviewed as part of the I Remember / Ia pomniu project also attest to the care afforded to wounded soldiers. There were certainly devoted nurses who held fond memories of their time caring for patients during the war.[88] The extremities of war and the struggle for victory seemed to bond medical workers and patients all the more.

The All-Union Committee for the investigation of sick and wounded Red Army soldiers and commandants received letters and reports with examples of care and love for soldiers and officers. In Moscow's Dzerzhinsky District, the head of hospital No. 1072 wrote about the patronage work it was doing with local industry in the area.[89] The hospital head wrote that the community provided huge assistance to the hospital and was so rooted in hospital life that it was hard to imagine the staff's work without these "modest, motherly, caring and affectionate" women and girls who gave their free time to care for the wounded, "day and night." They assumed the role of *sidelki*, cleaned and decorated wards with flowers, and helped the injured write to their relatives and friends.[90] Local women took on roles that fulfilled a more general caregiving function and provided patients with spiritual and emotional comfort. During the war, women assumed all manner of work to help the cause.[91]

Nursing work and the general healthcare situation was closely monitored during the war, especially in military hospitals. In November 1941, when the German Wehrmacht was attempting to take Moscow, a Communist Youth League secretary in Stalingrad, O. Mishakov, wrote to A. A. Andreev, secretary of the Party Central Committee, detailing the work in the military hospitals in Stalingrad.[92] Despite good work, Mishakov admitted that there were some difficulties. Hospitals and clinics, he noted, struggled when it came to caring for Red Army soldiers—even maintaining basic sanitation proved difficult. There were similar problems with shortages and lack of resources elsewhere. In Stalingrad, for example, medical workers had to wash linen in a communal city laundry facility.[93] Conditions across the front varied considerably. Further north, in battle-ravaged Kalinin, Rzhev, and Vyaz'ma, doctors, nurses, and orderlies cared for patients in a way that "only a mother could give." Only the Rzhev District received complaints, but it dealt with them swiftly—it moved to dismiss a "rude" nurse as an example to other hospitals.[94]

Another report to Andreev, this one written by the deputy head of the Red Army's main military-sanitation administration, highlighted a lack of care toward the mood of patients. In some Commissariat of Health hospitals, medical workers' "careless monitoring" of patients' mood and actions led to wounded soldiers committing suicide by jumping out of windows or using razors to inflict wounds (the latter in Kazan, Ulyanovsk, and Kirov). This was a "consequence of the completely inadequate political-educational work among the wounded and permanent hospital staff."[95]

Mishakov reported that in Stalingrad wounded soldiers walked across town in their hospital gowns to stand in queues for beer.[96] Drunkenness and misbehavior among the patients and some staff were problems, with anti-Soviet behavior noted in the case of one patient who had a fascist flyer that he showed to other patients in his ward.[97] To the northeast of Stalingrad and further up the Volga, in Kuibyshev Province, complaints about discipline and sanitation filed in. With no designated smoking area, patients "smoked everywhere," but "medical workers failed to take any action."[98] There was a shortage of surgeons, and 30 percent of the middle medical personnel were nurses from short-term courses.[99] Given medical workers' workload and the pressure they were under, disciplining patients for smoking on hospital grounds was probably the least of their concerns. Patients and the Red Army had different expectations of care. For the former, cleanliness, comfort, and food (in some cases, alcohol) mattered, but for the latter, discipline and political-education ranked highly. Medical workers had to meet the expectations of both.

Nurses after the War

In spite of Soviet military successes, planning and preparation remained defense-oriented until the very end of the war. In fact, the narrative of praise for hero nurses became even more pervasive after the war. In 1945 more than 250 nurses received the title "Excellent Student of Healthcare" (*Otlichniku zdravookhraneniia*).[100] The medical press often described nurses in the Soviet Union as a "modest army" whose kind word could sometimes be more effective than medicine.[101] While nurses were generally praised for their love, modesty, and devotion, there was perceptible concern about the lack of education and training, especially among demobilized nurses. What would happen to all the nurses after the war, especially those trained in hastily set-up courses in the immediate years preceding and during the war?

The SOKK had trained more than 310,000 nurses in short-term courses over the course of the war, and these largely entered civilian medical institutions after the war.[102] A Sovnarkom decree of 1918 declared the Red Cross and Red Crescent "autonomous and independent in questions about its organization and its participation in state events," but it was under the ultimate control of the Commissariat of Health: Red Cross personnel and institutions were thus subject to instruction from the commissariat (from 1946 on, the Ministry of Health, or Minzdrav).[103] The civilian healthcare sector could reclaim Red Cross and Red Crescent personnel for its needs. Soon after the war ended, SOKK workers taught in nursing courses for collective farmers to prepare them for work in nursing medical stations based on collective farms.[104] Community workers (*obshchestvenniki*) keen to get involved in social activities, sanitary-defense, and prophylactic work could become involved in SOKK nursing.[105] Indeed, between 1944 and 1950, the SOKK trained 15,300 reserve nurses and 8,438 collective farm nurses.[106] But not all nurses remained in medicine: one woman who had trained in a hospital in the early 1940s found that, when she returned to her hometown in Saratov Province after the war, there was already a surplus of nurses, and so she found work in a car depot.[107] The opposite was the case elsewhere. A woman from Yaroslavl' worked as a sanitary worker in a military hospital and enrolled in a nursing course only after the war.[108]

Given that the quality of wartime training was at best patchy and focused on defense needs, those who had trained in short-term courses needed to now enroll in good quality courses to complete their education. This applied to doctors and nurses who took abridged courses after war broke out.[109] The SOKK received the support of the Soviet government; as an Executive Committee representative remarked in a report, Miterev gave "special attention to the work of the Red Cross courses" and promised that "premises, hospitals, and teachers would be provided to ensure their quality."[110] Such a plan assumed that the instructors were well trained, but in fact many teaching staff were not suitably qualified or committed.[111] Courses were also dependent on premises, and in the postwar Soviet context hospitals suffered from dreadful overcrowding. At the Kiev October hospital, the head of the neurological department requested more beds for patients: there had been two hundred beds before the war, but in the summer of 1948 there were just forty.[112] Growing numbers of patients made matters worse, with up to 150 people waiting to register for a bed on any given day.[113] The end of the war brought little respite for medical workers, or patients for that matter.

Those nurses who had completed short-term nursing courses before or during the war and continued in the medical profession afterward created a sense of stability in some medical institutions. Anna Vasilevna Bogacheva, for example, who studied nursing in Moscow and worked as a sanitary worker and nurse as an eighteen-year-old in Stalingrad in 1942, continued her nursing work after demobilization in 1946. She became a senior nurse in 1948 in Moscow's Burdenko military hospital, where she remained for thirty-five years.[114] Another demobilized medical worker found nursing work in the Kiev October hospital after the war, but conditions there were very difficult, and she often worked day and night and sometimes as a *sidelka*. Still, she was thankful to have basic dormitory accommodation and food. She then moved to a railway hospital, where her work with a young, inexperienced doctor was just as difficult, but she remained working there for thirty-eight years.[115] In a field where labor turnover was generally rife, these cases show that some medical workers were content to remain in their post until they retired. Such workers were no doubt valuable to the institutions in which they worked, passing their knowledge and experience on to younger medical workers.

The end of the war did not signal a lack of interest in nursing or the medical services. Indeed, the number of middle medical personnel increased more than threefold in the period 1950–1974.[116] The character of nursing gradually changed, with a refocus on civilian needs. Large numbers of nurses were still required for the army, hospitals, polyclinics and ambulatories. The postwar environment also created a need for specialist nurses in children's institutions, physiotherapy, massage, and therapeutic physical culture.[117] Polyclinics and hospital departments thus came to focus on providing nurses to cater to these areas, as well as caring for millions of citizens with war-related diseases and injuries. Even though there were 325,000 nurses (and 719,400 middle medical personnel) by 1950, this was still not enough to care for the two million war invalids, let alone the rest of the civilian population.[118] Within this context, the healthcare system accepted medical workers with varying levels of training, including Red Cross–trained nurses.

The end of the war also marked further changes in international relations that did not, despite the best efforts of US nurses, bring Russian nurses closer to their international colleagues. As the nurse and social activist, Lavinia L. Dock, wrote in 1947: "How could we expect the Russians to overlook the daily insults, the malice, the ingratitude, the cold blooded threats of unfriendliness that are daily to be read in our papers, in the talk of Bullitt and Earle over the radio. . . . We nurses have no enemies. . . . We consider it an undeserved grievance that our Russian sisters have been alienated by the American government's attitude."[119] Dock was corresponding with Anna Schwarzenberg, executive secretary of the International Council of Nurses (ICN), about the latter's efforts to draw Russian nurses closer to the ICN. Schwarzenberg had sent several requested publications to a Russian contact, the professor Vladimir V. Lebedenko, and, she wrote, "He in turn promised to let me have the nursing laws, journals (they have medical journals including pages edited by nurses) and any material I ask for. Professor Lebedenko said he did not see why after the war the nurses in Russia should not have their own professional association and be allowed to join the ICN."[120] But a livid Dock blamed the US government for kiboshing the nurses' efforts, leaving her with a "bitter and justifiable grievance against the so-called Truman Doctrine."[121] The absence of Russian nurses at the ICN meeting in Atlantic City, New Jersey, in 1947, left her crestfallen: "[They who] served through the War, who suffered everything—devastation, ruin, even imprisonment—starvation, torture and outrage, are to be left out, as if Russia had been an enemy instead of our strongest ally."[122] The immediate postwar efforts of Dock, Schwarzenberg, and others were to no avail, and Soviet nurses remained on the margins internationally.

Where Care Begins

In the late 1940s many nurses had been through several years of war. They worked day and night in terrible conditions and saw those around them suffer and die. After a war in which about twenty-seven million people died (the higher numbers were not fully disclosed until the late 1980s), nurses had to adjust to daily life in a hospital or clinic. "The true Soviet way of coping with emotion," notes one historian, "was to keep working and salute the flag."[123] Still, the disjuncture between war and peacetime work was noticeable. In its first issue of 1947, *Nurse*'s editors ran a cover story expressing concern about the level of devotion of some nurses who did not see their job as a vocation and did not enjoy spending time at the patient's bedside. Nurses were reminded that "yesterday's soldiers are today's workers, servicemen, and war invalids" and they should be respectful, caring, and loving toward those who had sacrificed so much for the country.[124] Another article later that year also reminded nurses that nursing work was not crude but often "consisted of crude work" that could not be avoided when caring for very ill patients. Nursing was a "humane profession" that every "cultured" Soviet nurse undertook with honor.[125] If nurses wanted to become doctors that was fine, but they were not to "belittle" the nursing profession.[126] The barrage of messages about the important and noble work of nurses suggested that an element of compassion fatigue might have set in after the war and that this, alongside inadequate training, harmed the quality of care.

Often these concerns became criticisms when cases of medical negligence and incompetence arose. It transpired that some nurses did not even adhere to the basic rules of hand hygiene, did not sterilize needles, or did not know how to take a pulse.[127] In a *Medical Worker* article, the correspondent and candidate of medical science I. Trop wrote that nurses in a Sverdlovsk physiotherapy institution made many mistakes, including increasing dosages at the patient's request.[128] Although nurse conferences took place at the institution, Trop believed nurses would be better off "discussing their experiences" rather than presenting "abstract speeches."[129] Commentators tended to blame nursing inadequacies on poor training, general carelessness, and lack of organization and leadership in the hospital. Economic issues and the difficulties of the war were cited as reasons too, but the overwhelming argument forwarded for the shortcomings of nurses was a lack of interest in patient care.

The medical press presented hospital workers as indifferent to insanitary conditions in wards, patient needs, and their duties.[130] One Moscow hospital encouraged nurses to spend more time with patients to improve care.[131] In an ideal world all hospitals would have enough staff to facilitate better patient care, but, as it was, there were simply too many patients and too few nurses. Mistakes were inevitable. If nurses were inadequately trained and overworked, it was the fault of state institutions. If they were suffering from compassion fatigue and exhaustion, then it was the responsibility of the state to take better care of its nurses. War veterans and invalids in need of physical and mental attention could seek help, but what about nurses? As Christie Watson writes, the mental health impact of war focuses on men, not the many women alongside them.[132] How did nurses process the brutality of war and cope with the traumatic injuries, violence, and death that they encountered? Experienced nurses have often written about numbing themselves to pain and suffering to do their jobs. Self-care and self-preservation are important for nurses; compassion starts with the individual, with the self. Those nurses who struggled to provide compassionate care after the war were perhaps in need of care themselves.

Watson recalls that in her job as a nurse in the United Kingdom she worked with many kind, compassionate nurses, but she recognizes that a good nurse can have a bad day and that "it is hard to be kind when you are undervalued by society, by your employers and by the media." Exhaustion and burnout, she argues, are common and serious. Compassion fatigue, first diagnosed in 1950, could have a "terrible impact" on a nurse's "ability to provide the quality care, kindness and compassion that patients need and deserve."[133] Nurses in a trauma situation, in Watson's eloquent words, "repeatedly swallow a fragment of the trauma—like a nurse who is looking after an infectious patient, putting herself at risk of infection." There is no doubt that there were thousands of Soviet nurses and medical workers suffering from compassion fatigue or posttraumatic stress disorder, or both. Expecting these broken-down nurses to be respectful and caring toward their patients was asking too much of them. No matter how good or committed some Soviet nurses were, there were undoubtedly those who felt undervalued. One nurse devoted to the well-being of her patients noted that "if a doctor shouts at a nurse, especially in front of their patient," she then "loses confidence and begins to make little mistakes."[134] It also made patients nervous. This was a nurse who had worked in a field hospital in Stalingrad and had written to *Nurse* for information about nursing patients with gangrene. She was "lucky" to receive the support of the head surgeon, Tamara Genrikhovna Bruk, in the hospital for war invalids where she worked, but this was support offered on an individual rather than an institutional basis.[135] After the war, the Soviet government did not want to be "associated with trauma, ambiguity, and societal division."[136] The troublesome features of a violent war were papered over. The transcendent power of ideology would heal broken bodies and minds.

A Culture of Care

In the late 1940s the state placed a huge emphasis on nurses providing patients with a cultured experience. As a series of campaigns against the intelligentsia, the West, and Jews got under way, systematic commitment to cultural and ideological education pervaded medical institutions.[137] Stalinist modes of operation from the 1930s returned: narratives of care functioned as a useful counterpoint to political campaigns and a culture of fear. Propaganda and press campaigns assured citizens that the Soviet state would see to their every need and ensure their good health and well-being. Once again, nurses became important ambassadors of care.

Care was to be cultured. Cleanliness, order, and patient comfort were important.[138] As the author of one *Nurse* article wrote, "[Wards] should have one or two armchairs and a writing desk as well as games, newspapers, books, flowers and plants." Medical workers were to provide moral support to patients by chatting to them, discussing politics, books, or films. Distracting patients would help them to focus on their recovery rather than "their suffering."[139] Medical institutes and schools were to educate students in the "spirit of Soviet patriotism."[140] This move toward a cultured care fit in with the postwar generation's sense of patriotism and belief in socialist values.[141] The government's modus operandi was to raise the ideological level of medical workers, especially junior medical workers and service personnel, who were not all literate.[142] One medical club organized "Nurse Tuesdays" featuring nursing talks on different themes, such as "caring for the sick with brain trauma." The "Nurse Tuesdays" were apparently very popular among medical workers.[143]

Similar efforts were under way in Kiev's October hospital. The head of the clinical department for neurological illnesses, Dr. Kushnir, had struggled to find information about organizing cultural work in hospitals and so had drawn on examples from industry.[144] He believed that improving the service to patients would help them medically but also ideologically. To this end, Kushnir organized lectures, film screenings, and concerts. Patients could also avail of a library stocked with over three hundred books and journals that many staff and patients' relatives had donated.[145] Nurses were to be "humane" and the closest person to the patient.[146] In the October hospital, plans to raise the cultural level of both staff and patients got under way in 1947. That year, to improve their qualifications, doctors attended lessons on Mondays, nurses on Tuesdays (evidently a convenient day for nurses), and orderlies on Wednesdays.[147] On Thursdays all department staff worked with newspaper material to enhance their political and cultural level, while on Saturdays they attended talks about Lenin and Stalin. A conference dedicated to learning about the party took place every other Friday.[148] In Soviet hospitals cultured care also extended to the appearance of the nurse, with new uniforms introduced to distinguish senior, middle, and junior personnel.[149]

Politics and ideology returned with a vengeance as part of the effort to improve the cultural service to patients. In Moscow's Botkin hospital the biography of Stalin and a short course on the history of the party formed part of the program to raise the educational and cultural levels of nurses.[150] The political-ideological classes held there were "checked twice a month," and the nurse bureau would report the results to the deputy head doctor. The nurse bureau also had to oversee the improvement of nurse qualifications and cultural standards.[151] But not all hospitals were on top of raising these matters. The head doctor of the Vasilevskaia hospital in Moscow's Noginskii District was "morally corrupt and drunk," while the medical service to patients there was "bad."[152] At the medical union's Central Committee plenum in December 1949, the representative of the Moscow Province trade union committee, Shaulin, was critical of the medical union. He claimed that medical workers (some 70%) did not have Marxist-Leninist education, and it was "up to the trade union" to provide this knowledge.[153] As the Soviet Union recovered from war, its exhausted medical workforce had to engage with politics and ideology as part of their training and education. For the Stalinist state, cultural and ideological education would be the antidote to the trauma of war.

As Soviet society hurtled full throttle into war in 1941, medical workers joined in a widespread effort to defend socialism. But the war left the Soviet Union economically devastated, leaving infrastructure, factories, and farms in the western and most industrially and agriculturally developed part of its territory in ruins. Families were torn apart and spent the postwar years coming to terms with death, destruction, and the trauma of war. Invalids, demobilized soldiers, and medical workers at the front returned to a victorious but shattered land. They had to adapt to a new world. Those who had ventured beyond Soviet borders during the war realized that socialism was not the paradise propaganda would have them believe (if they ever believed that). The postwar Soviet space had considerably altered; physically it was in need of total reconstruction, but the new Soviet men and women that the state attempted to forge in the 1920s and 1930s were now sick, maimed, homeless, malnourished, traumatized, or dead.

Four years of brutal war and violence produced a population desperately in need of care, yet medical workers had little time to recover from their own battle scars. The state called on the doctors, nurses, orderlies, and other workers who had cared for comrades at the home front or on the front lines not only to continue this work but also to provide a cultured service. In the late Stalinist period, the needs of nurses were secondary to those of patients. There was no significant discussion of the nursing profession or the trauma that medical workers experienced during the war. Rather than reflect on the wartime experience and come to terms with it, the Soviet state instead drove forward. This was the case for medical workers in all aspects of healthcare, including those working in the area of mental health and psychiatry—the focus of chapter 8.

CHAPTER 8

Caring for the Mind

Soviet psychiatric care has come to our attention in previous chapters, but not to a significant degree. Focusing on a specialization, such as psychiatry, provides us with a discrete case study of nursing. By turning our attention to psychiatry now, we can see echoes from some of the debates that characterized nursing before the war and how this had changed by the 1950s. This chapter allows us to take a broader chronological and thematic approach to nursing, a pattern followed in chapter 9. We also broaden our scope further to understand how nurses working in psychiatry interacted with doctors and orderlies.

Psychiatry was under the wider remit of the Commissariat of Health, later renamed the Ministry of Health, and had to compete with vying interests from other sections in public healthcare, be that the focus on epidemiology, venereal disease, mother and child health, or surgical nursing. But by the end of the 1930s there was growing interest in psychiatry, partly owing to changes in its practice. The custodial approach to care that had characterized psychiatry before the revolution was already changing in the 1920s. The end of that decade saw developments in the field of psychiatry that reflected interest in different methods of treatment as opposed to just custodial care. Working in a psychiatric hospital was consequently physically, mentally, and emotionally exhausting. Conditions were difficult and the work was hard. Medical workers,

largely through the heads of psychiatric institutions and societies, were consequently engaged in an ongoing battle with the state to improve working
conditions.

Like medical workers in other branches of healthcare, those in psychiatry
were also confronted with questions about their skills, training, and qualifications. Much of the discussion about qualifications was reflective of wider debates in public healthcare. As a broader range of therapeutic treatments
developed, medical workers had to train to be able to administer these. By mid-
century, psychiatric care included somatic therapies, insulin treatment, elec-
tric shock therapy, and a number of other therapies. Mental health hospitals
across Europe and North America, as well as the Soviet Union, adopted these.[1]
The treatments did not replace other established therapies such as, for example, hydrotherapy or occupational therapy, but rather provided the psychiatrist with a wider repertoire of treatments from which to choose. New
treatments also presented medical workers with the need to keep their knowledge current.

The Soviet approach to psychiatry, at least in terms of caring for psychiatric patients, bore some similarities to caring for psychiatric patients in the
United States or Western Europe. While standards of care in psychiatric hospitals abroad were not high, conditions in Russian psychiatric hospitals were
particularly deplorable.[2] Both patients and medical workers had to endure very
difficult conditions. Some psychiatric hospitals suffered from terrible overcrowding, with patients sleeping on floors and in corridors. One psychiatrist,
observing a Moscow city hospital in the 1920s, depicted a chaotic and disturb-
ing scene where noisy, screaming patients generally ran amuck and assaulted
personnel.[3] A mixture of agitated patients alongside helpless and dying patients
painted a pitiful picture.[4] But the Soviet state engaged in ongoing efforts to
improve these conditions, and this chapter assesses whether these steps resulted in higher standards of care or better working conditions.

As we saw in other chapters, the state took complaints about medical care
seriously and investigated these to improve conditions for patients. Many of the
changes instituted were a response to advancements in medicine, the changing
ideological inclinations of the Soviet state, and a need to improve working conditions for medical workers. The periods under the leadership of Nikita
Khrushchev, Leonid Brezhnev, and Mikhail Gorbachev each had their own hall-
marks in the healthcare sphere, but this chapter assesses psychiatric care from a
temporally fluid perspective, and chapter 9 examines periodization more
closely. The focus here is on middle and junior medical workers in psychiatric
hospitals and their engagement with the state or state actors. How much control did junior and middle medical workers wield in the psychiatric institute?

Were they atomized and de-professionalized, and, if they were, was this connected to Soviet policy and ideology? Although psychiatry in late socialism is perhaps best known for forensic psychiatry and the incarceration of dissidents on bogus claims of mental illness, the focus of this chapter is on nurses and orderlies working in nonpolitical psychiatric institutes.[5]

Reading Psychiatry

Skilled and educated middle and junior medical workers were central to the everyday functioning of psychiatric institutes. When interviewed as part of the Harvard project, one psychiatrist who worked in a Kiev psychiatric hospital between 1927 and 1940 said, "Our lower staff was excellent, and sometimes a young doctor could learn a lot from this low staff." Medical workers, according to this respondent, "were very close to one another," and their work brought them together.[6] Given that junior medical workers spent so much time with patients, it is not surprising that some had accrued valuable experience, knowledge, and skills. In the United States, "pariah clients" such as mental hospitals usually did not attract elite professionals.[7] The functioning of a psychiatric institution depended on medical aides who, because they spent so much time in wards, could hold a large degree of control over a patient's medication.[8] This was also the case in the Soviet Union, where psychiatric hospitals relied on middle and junior medical personnel.

The body of instructional literature for medical workers in psychiatric institutes came at a time when Soviet psychiatry was undergoing change. Treatments such as insulin therapy (introduced in 1936) and shock therapies finally offered Soviet psychiatrists the opportunity to prove their worth as "scientists" and medical experts who could actively treat mentally ill patients. The handbooks were especially helpful in drawing attention to the "fight against agitation" (*bor'ba s vozbuzhdeniem*), so well described by the historian Benjamin Zajicek in his work on Soviet psychiatry.[9] Maintaining order in overcrowded psychiatric hospitals was essential, and the sound training of junior medical workers formed a vital aspect of winning the fight against disorder and improving medical care. This was particularly important because orderlies and nannies often had to help nurses hold agitated patients and were equally vulnerable to injury and attack.[10] Often viewed as "jailers" by medicated patients who considered themselves imprisoned rather than hospitalized, medical workers bore the brunt of patient fear and vengeance.[11] Arming medical workers with knowledge and skills was thus for their personal safety as well as the health and safety of their patients.

To this end, psychiatric doctors began conducting research on medical workers in psychiatric institutions and compiling and publishing handbooks for middle and junior medical workers. The work of I. A. Berger and other psychiatrists in the late 1920s demonstrated a concern for the well-being of medical workers. By analyzing nurses' notes and talking to them, researchers learned, for example, how tired nurses made mistakes and were most susceptible to attacks toward the end of their shifts.[12] Interest in medical workers and their interactions with psychiatric patients grew in the following decades with the publication of various handbooks. Of particular interest is the unpublished manuscript titled "Guidelines in Caring for Mentally Ill Patients for Junior Medical Personnel in a Psychiatric Hospital," which psychiatrists from the Odessa Psycho-Neurological Institute compiled.[13] The photographs featured in this manuscript are illuminating for the visual contribution they make to our understanding of medical workers and psychiatry. Produced in 1937, the manuscript had the purpose of educating and informing medical personnel faced with particularly challenging conditions during the period of the "reconstruction of psychiatric hospitals."[14]

The large, illustrated volume produced by the Odessa Psycho-Neurological Institute included references to psychiatric practice abroad (as well as the international history of psychiatry) and was important in outlining early Soviet attitudes to psychiatric care. The Odessa Psycho-Neurological Institute existed from about 1930 to 1953 and was a teaching clinic for the local medical institute, although many of its staff perished or fled during the war.[15] Significantly, the manuscript's editors—doctors working at an Odessa psychiatric institute prior to the war—considered it necessary to compile such a guide for the orderlies with whom they worked. The work of auxiliary medical personnel was not of a high standard; the doctors consequently wanted a disciplined and competent staff trained to cope with the demands of modern psychiatry. It was written not only for the junior medical workers in the Odessa psychiatric institute though—the editors wanted the volume brought to the attention of those working in all psychiatric institutions. That did not happen on a wider scale until the manuscript was published in 1947, ten years after it was first produced. The models of care in psychiatric institutions before the war were thus promulgated in the postwar period.

In addition to the Odessa manuscript, a handbook for nurses working with nervous and psychiatric illnesses, under the editorship of V. V. Mikheev and A. V. Neiman, was published in 1939.[16] It varied little from another handbook published in 1937—Semen Konstorum's third-edition handbook for feldshers.[17] Indeed, many of the passages were identical. Mikheev and Neiman reminded medical workers to be "smart and tactful" when dealing with patients.[18] They considered tone important and a key factor in maintaining order and calm.[19] The editors underlined the significance of tact, understanding, and patience in dealing with patients in psychiatric hospitals. In Konstorum's book, medical workers were to know how to handle different types of situations and when to call the doctor (the only figure permitted to use an aggressive tone).[20] Handbook editors were mindful of medical workers misbehaving and were at pains to suggest that the slightest lack of vigilance could have serious repercussions for patients, including their escape or death. Mikheev and Neiman's handbook for middle medical workers and nurses was necessary and important, with later iterations published in 1946 and 1962.[21] Indeed, nurses and feldshers lacked enough literature in the mid-1960s, with some hospitals publishing conference proceedings as instructional tools.[22] In the tradition of the Odessa psychiatric hospital, some medical institutions produced their own literature and training programs to instruct and inform nurses.[23]

The medical press sometimes augmented the work of the guidebooks by publicly celebrating medical workers who were good at their job. Maria Mikhailovna Toporkova, a fifty-four-year-old medical worker, graduated from a feldsher school in 1914 and worked in various psychiatric hospitals in Moscow Province. In 1948 a *Nurse* editorial praised her for her "highly developed sense of duty, and for showing discipline, love, sensitivity, and warm relations to the sick."[24] Much of the discussions in nursing journals on psychiatric nursing echoed those of the handbooks. Nurses working in psychiatric hospitals were to establish a "quiet atmosphere" for patients, but they were also expected to be firm and tactful with both patients and colleagues.[25] At the same time, they were not to whisper or walk too quietly for fear that this might arouse alarm or suspicion. They were also to be thoughtful, composed, and gentle, but "not familiar or sentimental."[26] Nurses were to constantly keep their behavior, actions, mannerisms, and gestures in check around patients. All actions had to maintain a relationship of trust. The medical press reinforced the message of the handbooks so that medical workers would have a better understanding of their role and responsibilities.

Other factors were also at work here. The emphasis on behavior in textbooks for middle medical workers, even if mixed with science, affirmed the psychiatrist's ownership of science and thus authority and power.[27] In the history of nursing, there are links between power relations and gender and class. This is more complicated in the Soviet case, where many doctors were women. By the 1970s some 72 percent of Soviet physicians were women, compared to 7 percent in the United States.[28] As Rosemary Pringle and others have argued, "Medical men wanted to limit nurses' knowledge but at the same time to take advantage of their expertise."[29] As those closest to the patient, nurses and, in the case of psychiatry, orderlies, often knew more about a patient's condition than a doctor did but might not have possessed the scientific language or the qualifications to establish their authority. Junior and middle medical personnel's close relationship with the patient, as well as the fact that many doctors were women, complicated power relations in psychiatric institutions. Young or inexperienced doctors (male or female) might have felt threatened by an experienced nurse or orderly. Unfortunately, it is difficult to discern the complicated nature of power relations in the hospital or clinic, as few doctors, let alone nurses or orderlies, wrote about their experiences.[30]

Although most of the handbooks are very similar in scope and content, there is one exception. Konstorum's 1937 handbook followed type by discussing the care of mentally ill patients and the important role of medical workers.[31] But the handbook presented nurses in a more negative light than other publications. It informed feldshers that nurses working in psychiatric hospitals for many years "considered themselves more competent in diagnosing illness than the doctor." Konstorum's handbook explained that this was because they spent so much time in the wards in direct contact with patients. Lack of understanding led to "mistakes and problems," and there was "no substitute for scientific knowledge."[32] While nurses may or may not have been guilty of such accusations, Konstorum's handbook was hardly helping their case by criticizing them so openly in a handbook for feldshers. Such assertions had the potential to poison relations between middle medical personnel as opposed to creating a calm, collegial atmosphere. The handbook also undermined the trust central to nurses and feldshers successfully working together.

Indeed, the handbook was unusually critical of nurses, claiming they often had a simplistic understanding of psychiatric illnesses, misreading troublesome behavior as "hooliganism" and treating well-behaved patients as "good." Ten years of working in a psychiatric hospital, spending eight hours a day with patients, Konstorum maintained, had led some nurses to think that they knew patients better than the doctor.[33] Konstorum provided no concrete evidence to back up his criticisms. Instead, he just continued to denigrate nurses before his feldsher readers. As a result, the uncritical feldsher might not trust experienced nurses. Nurses reading the handbook would have had good reason to feel aggrieved. Some scholars have viewed the greater need for nursing over medical skills in psychiatric hospitals and the infrequent presence of the doctor as a positive development for nurses. Because doctors had a "less interventionist role," nurses could "gain greater confidence in their own abilities and behave less deferentially to doctors."[34] But confident nurses might also pose a threat to some doctors.

The handbook's editors also claimed that ignorance and misunderstanding of scientific methods led to "incorrect and mechanical approaches to patients and mistakes."[35] Nurses were in a difficult situation. On the one hand, they were to show initiative and authority, but, on the other, they risked criticism for overconfidence and lacking sufficient knowledge. Nurses were after all the key link in the chain, particularly in the Soviet healthcare system, where the three-tiered structure of care—doctor/psychiatrist, nurse, orderly—placed pressure on the nurse to act on instructions from the doctor, manage orderlies, and care for patients.

Fears that nurses in psychiatric institutions were becoming overly confident and complacent remained into the 1950s and 1960s. In 1959 nurses in Moscow's Gannushkin hospital came in for criticism because they had "too much self-assurance." This was to the detriment of psychiatric patients' health and safety.[36] Meanwhile, the Soviet concern with nurses working in a "mechanical" fashion was a long-standing one, present since the 1920s and reflective of wider international concerns about the role of the nurse. At around the same time, the American nurse Hildegard Peplau published texts in the United States that strongly advocated therapeutic rather than custodial care. Peplau's *Interpersonal Relations in Nursing*, written in 1948 and published four years later, emphasized the importance of the nurse-patient relationship and the need for nurses to move away from passively fulfilling doctor's orders. According to Peplau's theories, the relationship between the nurse and the patient was in and of itself therapeutic. Her interpersonal theory affirmed the symbiosis between nurse and patient—both worked together to enhance knowledge.[37] While Soviet medical handbooks indicated a similar interest in moving away from the "passive" nurse, this was yet to be fully articulated when it came to bestowing more power and authority on nurses in practice. Their therapeutic role was certainly acknowledged and valued, but that did not always result in raised professional status or prestige.

Visual Encounters with Medical Workers

The images of medical workers caring for patients in the Odessa Psycho-Neurological Institute illustrate the importance of orderlies as well as nurses. Presumably staged to be instructive, the photographs show how middle and junior medical workers operated within a psychiatric institution. The photographs in the manuscript were not reproduced in the published volume, perhaps because of cost or relevance. Even though the number of those who saw the photographs was perhaps small, they still tell us a great deal about the representation of medical workers. Above all, they provide a visual record of how medical workers restrained agitated patients. The photos show that Soviet doctors took what was then a modern, progressive approach to psychiatric care and frowned on restraining patients with straps or chains. They also suggest that Soviet psychiatric care, or at least custodial care, was not so different from that in other countries. For example, in their work on medical photography, Daniel M. Fox and Christopher Lawrence discuss a striking close-up image of a patient in a padded cell in the Constance Road Institution, London, in 1936.[38] We see medical personnel caring for the patient in a way that is similar to the Odessa photographs in terms of its simplicity and focus on patients and personnel. The similarity indicates that the style of the Odessa photographs is largely in keeping with the late 1930s trend for close-ups, with a focus on patients and on medical personnel at work. When compared with instructive images from the United States produced some time later, in 1960, where nurses from Skidmore College lifted patients in the New York Psychiatric Institute, the photos again do not seem all that unusual.[39] The safety of both patient and medical worker was foremost in the literature, with procedures for lifting and walking patients explained in full.

Unlike Franco Basaglia's *Morire di classe* [Dying because of class], the famous photographic account of asylums in Italy published in 1969, the Odessa manuscript photographs were not purposefully radical or designed to shock; their purpose was instead instructional. But like Basaglia's collection, they are stark, providing glimpses of the institutionalization and suffering portrayed in *Morire di classe: La condizione manicomiale fotografata da Carla Cerati e Gianni Berengo Gardin* [Dying because of your class: The asylum conditions photographed by Carla Cerati and Gianni Berengo Gardin].[40] The photographs help us learn about "people's way of seeing" how medical workers and patients were to behave.[41] They also offer a *"signifying system* through which . . . a social order is communicated, reproduced, experienced and explored."[42] Maintaining order and following guidelines allowed junior medical workers to take control of their environment. The photographs suggest that orderlies were not supervised, thereby confirming that junior medical workers in psychiatric institutions seemed to experience a good deal of autonomy (a positive perspective) or lack of supervision (a negative perspective).

The photographs also allow us to see Foucauldian ways of disciplining and controlling the physical body through images of restraint.[43] We can examine the techniques deployed by orderlies and the importance of knowing how to physically carry, hold, and calm patients. These include holding a patient in a position with the patient's arms crossed (figure 2) and using physical strength

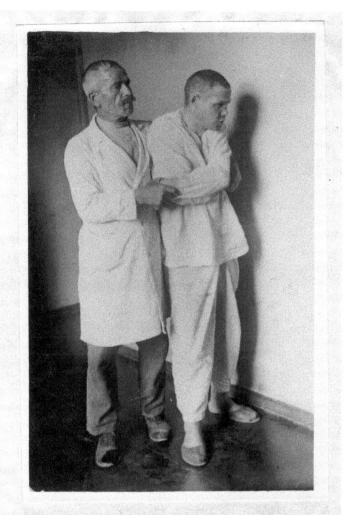

Рис. 15. Удерживание возбужденного больного
одним санитаром в стоячем положении. /Из альбома
Одесской Психиатрической Больницы/.

FIGURE 2. An orderly holds an agitated patient in a standing position. From the Odessa psychiatric hospital album. Source: GARF, f. 8009, op. 5, d. 9, l. 82. Used with permission.

to restrain an "agitated patient" on a bed (figure 3). All the images show that physicality and technique were clearly important in the daily duties of orderlies in psychiatric hospitals. They also highlight the different aspects of custodial care, which included restraint, protection, cleanliness, and order.[44] Custodial and noncustodial tasks were necessary for therapy to be effective.

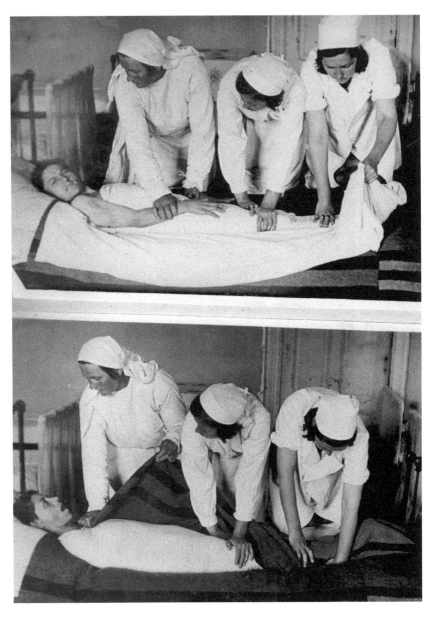

FIGURE 3. Wet-wrapping an agitated patient. From the Odessa psychiatric hospital album. These are two photos from a series. In the third photograph (not shown here), the patient is calm and sleeping, with a medical worker sitting beside her. Source: GARF, f. 8009, op. 5, d. 9, l. 200. Used with permission.

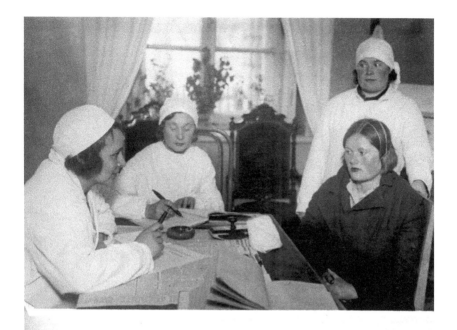

Рис. 44. Прием вновь поступающей больной. На
снимке первая комната приемного покоя, где оформляется
первичная документация поступающих больных. /Из альбома
Одесской Психиатрической Больницы/.

FIGURE 4. Receiving a newly admitted patient. Shown is the room where new patients are registered. From the Odessa psychiatric hospital album. Source: GARF, f. 8009, op. 5, d. 9, l. 179. Used with permission.

In a way, as Peplau had claimed, they were part of the therapeutic process. This was especially so when physicians and nurses assumed more of the administrative work (see figure 4), reducing the amount of time they spent with patients in wards.

The photographs also highlight the emphasis placed on observation and supervision in the handbooks. We see a nurse or orderly observing patients in a "bed rest" ward (figure 5). The image indicates the level of strict control over patients, even when they were sleeping or unconscious. In a bed rest ward one nurse or two orderlies were to supervise some ten to fifteen patients.[45] It was up to these workers to maintain order, calm, and discipline. Silence and "quiet" time were after all central to the therapeutic process, and the Odessa manuscript certainly privileged silence as critical to the patient's well-being. Indeed, this was not restricted to psychiatry, for junior and middle medical workers in

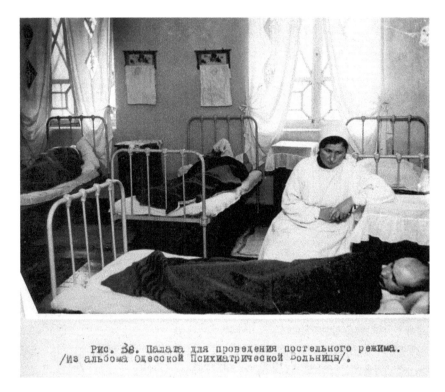

Рис. 38. Палата для проведения постельного режима.
/Из альбома Одесской Психиатрической больницы/.

FIGURE 5. Ward for bed rest. From the Odessa psychiatric hospital album. Source: GARF, f. 8009, op. 5, d. 9, l. 134. Used with permission.

general medicine were regularly urged to speak in a low voice and wear footwear that kept noise to a minimum. The patient's well-being was paramount.

The handbooks for middle- and junior-level medical workers highlight issues around the question of care that also speak to Soviet healthcare more generally. Who were mentally ill patients, especially those undergoing traumatic shock treatments, entrusted to during their time in a psychiatric hospital? The evidence suggests that those with the most medical training and qualifications—the nurses and doctors—spent little time with patients. Junior medical workers often filled their place. Given that orderlies were responsible for custodial care, and that they spent so much time with patients, it was imperative that they knew how to conduct themselves in the psychiatric hospital environment. This was especially the case when handling "agitated" patients, with whom they were to be particularly vigilant, polite, and sensitive and "able to correct a mistake" to maintain the patient's well-being.[46] In practice custodial care and treatment were tightly connected. Yet in theory, the borders between the two were to be sharply delineated by the role of medical personnel. Orderlies oversaw custodial care, and nurses and physicians were responsible for treatment.

Improving standards of training for orderlies and providing better care was not always possible given the poor conditions in which many psychiatric institutions operated. While some junior and middle medical workers were knowledgeable and provided excellent care, others were not. When the custodial care they undertook had an immediate bearing on therapy, treatment, and the general well-being of patients, the significance of these handbooks becomes ever more apparent. The handbooks were published into the 1950s and 1960s, as standards of care remained problematic. Both the handbooks and the Odessa photographs show that junior and middle medical workers were integral to the life of the psychiatric institution and that custodial work and therapy were all part of the same process of caring for the patient.

Psychiatric Training (or Lack Thereof)

Nurses and orderlies who trained in a general hospital school or medical college were perhaps not fully prepared for the psychiatric hospital environment. In the 1937 nursing school curriculum, psychiatric care came to a fairly modest eighty-eight hours, slightly less than care for patients with skin and venereal disease and slightly more than general patient care in the hospital.[47] The lack of specialized theoretical training was likely matched by a lack of practical training in a psychiatric clinic or environment. Many nursing students might have rotated only in the psychiatric wards of general hospitals, if the hospitals had such wards. In 1937 one psychiatric hospital received eighty-seven middle medical workers "specially trained" for the psychiatric hospital, but after just two weeks twenty-five left because they could not stand the conditions there.[48] Medical personnel in psychiatric institutions considered nurses inadequately prepared to cope with their work and needing "to undergo corresponding training."[49] Problems with training and turnover were inextricably connected when it came to psychiatric nursing, posing a constant challenge to healthcare institutions.

Just before the war, a group of psychiatrists (V. M. Banshchikov, I. A. Berger, and M. I. Gurevich from the First Moscow Medical Institute) discussed Commissariat of Health recommendations on raising the qualification of middle and junior medical personnel in psychiatric institutions. Some of the rationale behind these upper-level moves to reform psychiatric training spoke to the "complicated nature of care" for active methods of treatment.[50] Education could not keep pace with developments in Soviet psychiatry. Similar to other medical workers, middle and junior medical workers in psychiatric wards, hospitals, and institutions were to attend courses to improve their qualifications and progress their career. The proposed recommendation failed to quell doubts about the curriculum and the hours per subject, as well as concerns about financing courses.[51] The more common problems of wage scale and experience, discussed in chapter 4, also applied to medical workers in psychiatric institutions.

Middle and junior medical workers had to learn quickly, and they often did. The former British National Health Service nurse Christie Watson admitted that, after three years of training, her understanding of how to be a nurse began only on the first day after she qualified.[52] Theory and knowledge are of course essential in nursing, but experience and mentorship are also crucial. Sometimes junior and medical workers who lacked formal medical education nonetheless became very good at their jobs. As the psychiatrist working in a Kiev psychiatric hospital observed, orderlies there were "very intelligent," often able to understand more about a patient's condition (or perceived condition) than a doctor.[53] This psychiatrist recalled that they had "some very experienced nurses and wonderful attendants."[54] Medical workers were not a monolithic group; some enjoyed their job and were good at it, while for others their job was a means to an end. Whatever training or disposition orderlies and nurses possessed, they performed a vital function in the hospital. And hospitals and clinics could ill afford to be too selective when it came to hiring them. The de facto position was that nurses and orderlies would receive additional training in the clinical setting so that they could properly care for psychiatric patients.

Yet there were limits to progress. Unlike other medical specialists, nurses had not undergone the state attestation (*attestatsiia*) program that had started after the war. Attestations were initiated to check the professional credentials of doctors and improve the healthcare system by recognizing and incentivizing medical specialization.[55] The attestation program for medical professionals was to raise their prestige and authority by rewarding "specialization, length of service and merit."[56] The process of attestation revealed that many medical specialists were not particularly competent.[57] It also led to a purge of the healthcare administration, as well as offering cover for dismissing Jewish doctors in the anti-Semitic campaigns during 1950–1952.[58] The attestation exercise inadvertently drew attention to the issue of training and qualifications. As a result of the attestation campaign, the healthcare professions struggled to shake off doubts about the quality of training and care. Despite the unanticipated consequences of the attestation program, it still, in principle, conferred prestige and respect on doctors and other medical workers—but not nurses. Nursing was evidently not considered a sufficiently prestigious medical profession at that time.

Improving the standards of care was more or less left in the hands of individual institutions, a by now familiar story. In Ukraine, the Zhitomir psychiatric hospital ran monthly educational events to improve medical worker training. This included scientific-medical conferences for doctors and conferences on patient care for middle medical workers.[59] Similar efforts were under way in the 250-bed Romenskaia psychiatric hospital for children, also in Ukraine, where medical workers could take annual courses in psychiatry and neurology.[60] It was not only newly qualified medical personnel who were to attend classes, courses, or talks. In the Karelo-Finnish psychiatric hospital doctors subscribed to the major medical and neurological journals and experienced workers took classes in politics and ideology.[61]

In some cases, the extra training paid off and nurses proved that they could provide quality treatment if given the opportunity. Trained and educated nurses working with and observing epileptic or schizophrenic patients in Moscow's Kashchenko psychiatric hospital became familiar with their patients' diagnosis and treatment and were able to share their knowledge with colleagues in other psychiatric institutions.[62] Given a chance, nurses committed to their career could advance professionally and deliver better standards of care. By the 1950s and 1960s, the path from senior nurse, to head nurse, to administrative positions in the local healthcare sector was open to nurses who were interested in developing their nursing career.[63] The status of orderlies was less clear.

Orderly Care

Discussions about the role of the orderly or attendant were also evident in US literature in the 1940s. During the Second World War almost eighteen hundred conscientious objectors worked in mental hospitals and "schools for defectives," where they tried to improve the system as well as the education and status of attendants.[64] Private groups, attendants, and doctors were key actors in the United States.[65] Such a scenario could never play out in the Soviet context. Although specialist literature catered to orderlies and showed their importance, it was doctors who maintained positions of power and authority when it came to negotiating conditions and making decisions. At high-level meetings it was primarily the head doctors of psychiatric institutions or the heads of professional societies who advocated on behalf of middle and junior medical personnel; the latter did not yet have a high-level platform through which they could voice concerns themselves.

When the Odessa manuscript was published in 1947 it included revisions to reflect the impact of the Second World War on psychiatric care and treatment. Some of the treatments and attitudes to psychiatric care that were popular before the war had become "outmoded."[66] New methods in psychiatry required better-trained feldshers and nurses. The editors of the published handbook, L. I. Aikhenval'd and Ia. M. Kogan, noted that the prewar Odessa guide instructing middle medical workers in how to care for mentally ill patients had proved to be beneficial. Indeed, they claimed there had been a great demand for the guide on the part of psychiatric institutions, whose staff likely encountered the guide at conferences or through professional networks before its publication.[67] The number of copies printed for circulation in 1947 was thirty-five hundred.[68] Besides the editors (Aikhenval'd and Kogan), the 1947 publication did not feature any of the earlier contributors. The later publication shared the same objectives as the 1937 manuscript, but its focus was on new active therapies. The editors again highlighted the important role of medical workers and recognized them as fundamental to the successful treatment of mentally ill patients. Similar to Konstorum ten years before, they criticized the "mindless, disinterested, and mechanical work" in psychiatric institutions. Instead, they wanted medical workers to be well trained and knowledgeable, which would in turn make them "more interested" in their work.[69]

Medical orderlies had to be engaged in the life of the psychiatric hospital, but their voice is virtually nonexistent. Those writing handbooks for middle and junior medical workers made it clear that orderlies (and, to an extent, nurses) existed to assist the psychiatrist, but, at the same time, there was no getting around the fact that they were instrumental to patient care. They were there not only to lift and carry patients, clean, or fulfill menial tasks (although lifting, carrying, and cleaning required some training and expertise too.) For example, in the event of an epileptic patient having an attack, the attending orderly had to call the nurse.[70] But while waiting for the nurse to arrive, the orderly was to help the patient and not stand around waiting for the nurse.[71] In this sense, the later publication granted orderlies additional autonomy and clarified their role.

Orderlies continued to spend the most time with patients. It was presumably the orderly who provided most of the information about a patient's condition prior to any attack or incidents. Time spent in wards meant that their patient observations were evidently crucial to how nurses and doctors formed their opinions about correct diagnosis and treatment. Orderlies might not have had much verbal interaction with patients, but their role as observers was important. In spite of their lowly status within the medical hierarchy, orderlies' contribution to medical care was crucial. Indeed, as the psychiatrist who contributed to the Harvard interview project acknowledged, a "good relationship" between doctors and middle and junior medical personnel was vital to doing "the work they did," and everybody liked these "little people with a warm and generous heart."[72]

Junior medical workers, as is probably clear, were often reminded of their place. They were not to overstep the boundary between custodial work and treatment. Middle medical personnel had to be cautious when medicating patients; they were not to trust junior medical personnel with these duties, and certainly not the patient.[73] The rules were strict and to be followed (although, in reality, all sorts of infringements took place). Examples were often provided to warn workers of the dangers of not being vigilant. One inexperienced nurse made the mistake of handing a vial of medicine to a patient, who claimed they usually took the medicine themselves; the patient overdosed and almost died.[74] By the 1960s some junior and middle medical workers regularly made mistakes and even forgot medical terminology.[75]

Hard Work for Little Pay

As scientists and psychiatrists grappled with Stalin's postwar interventions in psychiatry and science more generally, medical workers got on with the business of caring for Soviet citizens.[76] Working in a psychiatric institution was more challenging than working in other healthcare institutions. Middle and junior medical personnel undertook strenuous and unattractive work, as the Odessa photographs show. Indeed, orderlies working in psychiatric institutions had legal rights that recognized their difficult work.[77] One hour of their work was the equivalent of one hour and twelve minutes of regular work.[78] They were also entitled to higher rates of pay. For example, those working in departments with "quiet" patients received an additional 15 percent to their basic salary, while seven years' experience counted as ten. Those working in wards for "agitated" patients received an extra 30 percent to their basic salary, and for them two years' experience counted as five, while four years' experience was the equivalent of ten. In addition, all employees had forty-two days' leave.[79] The combination of physical strain, shift work, supervisory responsibility, and threat of danger was an important factor warranting higher salaries and additional vacation time. The state recognized the difficult nature of their work (at least in theory). Introducing better working and living conditions for orderlies in psychiatric hospitals was one way of stemming high turnover rates.[80]

Many of the discussions on living and working conditions for psychiatric workers took place in the 1940s and 1950s, a time when political and cultural repression continued to define Soviet society. Purges of the cultural intelligent-sia (Zhdanovshchina), party members (Leningrad Affair), and Jews (Doctors' Plot) signaled the government's intent to rely on coercive methods of main-taining power and control. The late Stalinist years were still dangerous times, and medical workers were often caught in some of the above campaigns. Along with other citizens, nurses and middle medical workers were accused of anti-Soviet behavior, considered an offense under Article 58-10 of the Soviet crim-inal code. State organs arrested middle medical workers for engaging in religious activities, criticizing the Red Army during the war, or criticizing the state more generally.[81] One midwife in Yerevan, repatriated from France in 1947, received a seven-year sentence in the Gulag in 1951. Her crime was criti-cizing the government: after the death of a new mother at age twenty-five, one witness claimed the midwife told workers who had gathered around the deceased that she "seemed to be forty-five years old" and then said, "You live worse than dogs—that's Soviet power for you."[82] Many of the accusations dated to the war, and therefore retrospective "justice" was applied. In the midst of this turbulence, medical workers continued to fight for better living and working conditions.

Those who no longer had the will to fight left their jobs. High worker turn-over, as we have repeatedly seen, seriously undermined the healthcare sector in the late 1930s and 1940s. The situation did not change in the late socialist years. Psychiatric hospitals did not have a full complement of cadres in all cat-egories of medical worker but especially junior medical personnel, which was only at about 10–20 percent capacity and mainly consisted of male work-ers.[83] The turnover of this group and other groups of auxiliary and domestic workers was "colossal."[84] Those concerned about the situation wanted to know what they could do to address the issue. One doctor asked, "Do we cur-tail the number of posts and leave the patients unsupervised?" But they did not want to undermine the quality of their work and "had to permit overtime hours." As a result, psychiatric institutions sometimes ended up paying order-lies "twice their wage." As this doctor noted, an orderly might therefore "earn more money than a doctor, receiving 500–600 rubles with overtime, whereas a young doctor fresh in post received 350 rubles (without overtime)."[85] Another, by now familiar, problem with worker turnover was accommodation. Unsat-isfactory or out-of-town accommodation made the psychiatric hospital unat-tractive to workers. Especially unappealing were hospitals located on the outskirts of town—the last thing nurses or orderlies wanted after a long, dif-ficult day's work was a tiring trek home. Hospitals and clinics were in compe-tition against one another and industry when it came to securing medical workers.

The situation with turnover, conditions, and workload worsened after the war. The destruction of and damage to hospitals and institutions as well as increased workload caused problems for medical workers and the government. The swell of invalids and traumatized citizens after the war placed huge demands on psychiatric hospitals and their staff in the late 1940s. In 1948 the Zhitomir psychiatric hospital in northwestern Ukraine was lucky to have an increase in the number of beds, from 125 to 150, but there was no corresponding rise in the number of personnel.[86] Medical workers consequently had a 36 percent higher workload than the previous year and had to deal with more first-time patients rather than repeat patients—a time-consuming burden.[87] Overcrowding also put additional pressure on psychiatric hospitals that were still recovering from the war.

The situation for medical workers was quite desperate. In November 1950 the head doctor of Moscow's Kashchenko psychiatric hospital, A. L. Andreev, felt that orderlies were in "a bad way."[88] Some female orderlies had limited or no family support and earned so little that it was "impossible" to get by. When an orderly came to him in tears one day, he called the head doctor of another Moscow psychiatric hospital to say that his orderly was "in a difficult situation" and could they find her some work.[89] Those doing menial jobs in psychiatric hospitals were usually unable to find better-paying jobs.[90]

There was at least progress for some medical workers on other fronts. Stalin's death on March 5, 1953, ushered in a period of uncertainty and a leadership battle that was not resolved until Khrushchev emerged as leader in 1956. The purging and violence of the Stalin period and Khrushchev's subsequent condemnation of it as part of de-Stalinization promised no return to the terror of the past. For medical workers, these changes made no major material difference to their professional lives—they were just as badly off as before. But hope was on the horizon when the state addressed the pension issue in December 1953 and outlined plans to improve working conditions in the RSFSR.[91]

Similar to the 1920s, the medical workers' burden extended to violence and assault. There were 17,500 registered attacks against medical workers in seventy-nine psychiatric hospitals in the RSFSR in 1953. Doctors, nurses, and orderlies often became ill and even invalids as a result of their work.[92] In 1954 "alcoholic patients, psychopaths, and the traumatized" lurked in dispensary waiting rooms, which were often scenes of "scandals and debauchery."[93] A lack of orderlies and high patient numbers made establishing order difficult at the best of times. Research on trauma suffered by psychiatric workers identified incorrect distribution of patients, overwork, and insufficient staff as the three main causes of attacks against medical workers.[94] This was a serious problem, but not one specific to the Soviet past. In England, hospital trusts reported 56,500 assaults in 2016–2017, and nurses, paramedics, and mental health workers were the most vulnerable.[95] Understaffing and delays in patients accessing care were the primary reasons for the attacks.[96] Mental health workers in the United Kingdom are seven and a half times more likely to face assault than other medical workers; 33,820 mental health workers were attacked in 2016–2017.[97] Soviet psychiatrists were just as concerned about the health and safety of their workers as those working in healthcare in Britain and elsewhere are today. Governments seem unable to protect the most vulnerable in society, and sometimes that includes professionals such as nurses and orderlies.

Health and safety threats assumed various forms. Dispensary doctors and nurses, for example, were often called as court witnesses and could be victims of aggressive behavior afterward.[98] The police, meanwhile, were reluctant to intervene when incidents occurred on the territory of the dispensary.[99] Everyday work also presented its fair share of health and safety threats to workers. The Gannushkin hospital—one the best in the Soviet Union—provides an interesting study in health and safety. Its 94 doctors, 391 middle medical personnel, 645 junior medical workers, and 126 administrative staff felt the strain of their work every day.[100] The vast majority of medical workers were women (1,111, against 118 men), and 294 of the workers were persons of retirement age—almost a quarter of the hospital's personnel. Most of these older workers were junior medical personnel (35%), followed by doctors (14%) and middle medical workers (7%). Some of these, almost 50, worked in what were typically considered harmful conditions, such as exposure to x-ray, while about 50 nurses worked with treatment that exposed them to allergic reactions.[101]

Over a period of nine months in 1970 there were 818 instances of illness, amounting to 11,108 sick days (almost thirty years!). Just under half of these were a result of flu and associated bronchitis, pneumonia, and pleurisy in the first months of the year. Workers were also struck down with hypertension and cardiovascular illnesses, as well as rheumatism, work injuries, and gastrointestinal and ulcer-related illnesses.[102] The hospital's administration and local committee planned to reduce the problems by addressing workers' well-being and providing regular health checkups.[103] The hospital also vowed to improve workers' living and working conditions, including access to cultured leisure and physical culture classes.[104] Hospital administrations often drew up plans to improve conditions for workers, but one wonders how these translated from paper to practice.

Concepts of Care

A more liberal period, or what scholars of Soviet history have typically called the "thaw," marked Khrushchev's time in power as one of repeated attempts to recast the Soviet Union in a more positive light. Concepts of care were evolving in the late 1940s and mid-1950s, and the range of extracurricular activities for medical workers often reflected that. Some of those present at the Korsakov congress (a congress named after the Russian psychiatrist S. S. Korsakov) in 1954 noted that Soviet medicine, and especially psychiatry, was characterized by a "gentle, humane approach to the patient." Treatment choice demonstrated that.[105] For example, leucotomy, a prefrontal lobotomy, was banned in 1950.[106] Instead of aggressive treatments, attention shifted to somatic methods of treating mentally ill patients.[107] But the shift was not solely grounded in the psychiatric profession. High-level political and ideological anti-Westernness required psychiatrists to validate their therapies and situate them in a patriotic, pro-Soviet approach to practice.[108] For this reason, the work of Ivan Pavlov and his endorsement of sleep therapy gained prominence in Soviet medicine and science.[109] Soviet psychiatrists' concern with humane treatment and therapies extended to care more generally and reflected a broader embrace of ideology and socialist values. This filtered down to nurses, who cited Korsakov and Pavlov as advocates of humane care.[110] Medical workers were also expected to deliver care that reflected a gentle and humane approach to the patient. This coexisted alongside the long-running narrative of providing a cultured service to patients.

The drive to improve the patient experience and make it more humane continued into the mid-1960s, when medical workers were to "raise their cultural service" to patients.[111] Although cultured service was a feature of the late Stalinist period, it became even more pronounced under Khrushchev. Reforms in the 1960s signaled a renewed interest in morality and humanity. These became cornerstones of Soviet politics and ideology. As the deputy head doctor of the Gannushkin hospital noted in his speech at a conference of doctors and nurses, care would improve only when medical workers paid more attention to patients.[112] Some of the reasoning behind his calls for improved labor discipline and patient service related to higher rates of attempted suicides among patients at the Gannushkin hospital in 1964 compared to the previous year (fifty-one in 1964 against thirty in 1962), as well as an increase in numbers of patients attacking other patients, medical personnel, and attempted escapes.[113] The well-being of the individual and the collective depended on the moral health of the medical worker. Brigades and raids undertaken across industry took place in hospitals and polyclinics as workers everywhere responded to the party call to be upstanding members of the socialist community.

Investigations in the Gannushkin hospital revealed that in some cases medical workers were at fault: they slept on duty, chatted, or left patients unsupervised.[114] Concerns about various disciplinary problems and mistakes were also voiced in the Kashchenko psychiatric hospital.[115] A Gannushkin nurse council "raid" in July 1965 revealed several work violations, including a lack of vigilance in "toilet observation" that led to one patient injuring another. Care and attention touched on matters of behavior and attitude too. Medical workers were not to be rude to patients, and, to be fair to the Gannushkin staff, not many complaints of staff being rude to patients were officially reported in 1965.[116] One worker reprimanded for being rude was transferred to another department.[117] The deputy head doctor of the Gannushkin expected medical personnel to perform better after they received a salary increase and even though he acknowledged that they continued to work in very difficult conditions, he still wanted them to "fight for genuine communist relations."[118]

The notion of genuine communist relations also shaped patient responses to their hospital experience. This concern with ideology and culture did not end with the removal of Khrushchev in 1964; the Brezhnev period was as noteworthy in this regard, in spite of its "stagnation" label.[119] By this time, the Soviet Union presented itself as a world leader in healthcare. This was a narrative that some, but not all, Soviet citizens believed. In the late 1960s and early 1970s, the Gannushkin hospital received letters of gratitude from current and former patients. In January 1968 one N. A. Frolova thanked the head of ward No. 14 and its workers for the attention she received.[120] The fiftieth anniversary of the revolution and the day of the medical worker also presented patients with an opportunity to officially express their gratitude to Soviet medical workers. One mother wrote to the Gannushkin staff thanking the doctors as well as middle and junior medical workers for caring for her seventeen-year-old son during his time there.[121] Some patients were grateful for the little things that others might take for granted, such as "sensitive" care and three meals a day.[122] Others were grateful for care and expertise that fully restored their health; after a workplace accident, one woman languished in a Voronezh hospital for five years with injuries that left her paralyzed, but after two months in the Gannushkin she was walking again.[123] Emphasis on the person received greater attention. As the Gannushkin's head doctor noted in a speech given in 1970, the party and government legally enshrined "care for the person, Soviet people, and their health."[124] That fit with the Brezhnev-era policy of injecting humanism into ideology and politics.

Social Rehabilitation and Labor Therapy

As Soviet healthcare standards slipped in the late 1970s and 1980s, the mental health system was one of the few areas that functioned well.[125] Rehabilitating psychiatric patients was an example of innovative thinking that was in line with international standards.[126] But labor therapy also held particular meaning in the Soviet context, where the ability to work defined an individual's contribution to the socialist project. The maxim "He who does not work shall not eat" neatly summarized the importance attached to labor in the Soviet Union. Those not able to work grappled with the question of how to negotiate their standing and rights in Soviet society.[127] Offering disabled, old, or mentally unwell people the opportunity to participate in labor therapy was a logical and long-standing part of the Soviet ideological and economic project. Rehabilitation through labor therapy was one way in which the Soviet medical profession helped the patient "adapt" to normal life in a socialist state.[128] From the patient's perspective, the opportunity to become involved in labor could provide a path to the Soviet way of life as well as "individual and group autonomy" and even "self-transformation."[129]

The agreement drawn up between the Gannushkin hospital and Moscow's electro-mechanical factory No. 1, whereby patients could complete their rehabilitation through labor, was hardly a surprise in light of the ideological emphasis on labor.[130] This 1976 initiative between the psychiatric hospital and the factory offered patients a chance to engage with labor therapy in "difficult and unusual conditions" outside of the medical environment. Factory workers were apparently distrustful and wary at first, while patients were unsure of how they would cope with "serious" work, suspecting that the factory workers were actually "workers" from the psychiatric hospital. But the initiative went ahead, and everyday a brigade of thirty to fifty patients from four hospital departments accompanied by two labor instructors and a nurse showed up at the factory. Sometimes the patients dropped out because the work was too difficult, they lacked discipline, or they became "prejudiced" against some factory workers, but reports suggested that patients encountered no major difficulties.[131]

The initiative seemed to enjoy some success, and by 1978 the scheme had expanded to include patients from eighteen departments.[132] Patients could show a degree of autonomy. In 1977 all the factory brigades had a council of patients to oversee safety and to help weaker patients. Meanwhile, the factory administration and workers acknowledged the patients' good work. The factory paid the hospital patients a salary of almost 20,000 rubles in 1977, and they received this money directly from the factory.[133] Unfortunately, we have only the nurse's perspective of this initiative; we do not really know how factory workers and patients found the experience. But it is unlikely that nurses would have promoted the scheme as a success if they believed otherwise.

We also know that these kinds of employment schemes are beneficial to mentally ill patients. Helping people succeed in paid employment is the "only effective thing in a psychiatrist's toolkit," according to Robert Drake, a psychiatrist and professor of community and family medicine at Dartmouth School of Medicine.[134] In Canada, employees with mental health illness worked as part of a reintegrative group program analogous to that undertaken in the Gannushkin hospital. Up to twelve individuals could join a twelve-week program that combined group intervention with an individual action plan.[135] It was to enable the individual to regain power. The scheme entailed involvement on the part of the employee, vocational consultant, and employer at the job scene; this gave confidence to the employee and "sensitized" other workers. Monitoring took place after the twelve-week period to avoid the employee relapsing. The scheme was a success, with 85 percent of the employees in the program retaining jobs after two years.[136]

Implementing the social rehabilitation program for psychiatric patients was key to successful treatment, according to the Gannushkin nurse Anna Denisova.[137] She noted that more attention was given to patient self-management through the work of the patient council, the relatives' council, and the creative activities of patients.[138] The Soviet interest in social rehabilitation follows a broader trend of giving power back to the patient, an important part of nursing work with mentally ill people. But Denisova was critical of a professor at a conference in Tomsk in 1986; while speaking on the subject of psychiatric patients' rehabilitation, he never mentioned the work of nurses.[139] Even if others forgot about them, nurses such as Denisova knew that all forms of social rehabilitation went through them. Even if gender and professional barriers prevented nurses from getting the recognition they deserved, some such as Denisova had the confidence to realize that nurses propelled social rehabilitation work.

Social rehabilitation was closely connected to labor instruction and labor therapy. In the late 1960s, two senior doctors from the Gannushkin hospital developed a program for labor instruction.[140] The Ministry of Health approved labor instruction in 1972, and as a result anyone with middle medical education could be a labor instructor.[141] But that had already been the case unofficially, as nurses and orderlies had led different forms of labor therapy since the early Soviet period.[142] Denisova lamented that nothing had really changed in the 1970s save for the title and the demands. She wanted change.[143]

In Denisova's view, it was the nurse and not the doctor who treated the patient. Nurses talked to the patients and could comment on their mental health. For Denisova, the "science and art of nursing was understood only in the process of work," and that could take years to master.[144] She felt that the time had come to establish a special college in Moscow for psychiatric nurse training.[145] She also wanted to include social rehabilitation training on curricula. Denisova was prescient in her comments and anticipated the need for the kind of specific psychosocial training that is common in universities today.[146]

There were signs of some progress in different aspects of mental health training. Nurses in the Gannushkin hospital had been experimenting with voluntary art therapy classes with patients from one department since 1984. One nurse found that patients reacted differently, but mostly in a positive way.[147] A former architecture student and current patient diagnosed with schizophrenia produced paintings that were "dark," but the nurse explained that the patient gradually used brighter colors.[148] The art therapy process included analysis so patients could openly discuss problems connected to their illness or mood.[149] Patients also discussed the classical music that they listened to while painting.[150] Medical workers found that creative activities provided patients with a distraction from their illnesses.[151] These were not exactly new developments. Music therapy had been the subject of international research since the 1930s. Music and leisure were also a part of a patient's therapy at the Odessa psychiatric hospital (see figure 6).[152] But these therapies and social rehabilitation efforts in the 1980s illustrated a commitment to empowering the patient, as well as frustration on the part of some nurses who sought greater professional recognition for their work in this area.

Between Fiction and Fantasy

Brezhnev's failing health had been an ongoing concern in the 1970s, and a series of older leaders assumed power after he died in 1982. But a young and energetic Gorbachev sought to reform the Soviet system after he assumed power in 1985. The final decade of Soviet power was one that also signaled a turn toward reform and greater openness (glasnost). By 1987 and 1988 the Soviet Union was changing rapidly, as previously censored material became freely available and the circulation figures for newspapers and literary journals "jumped astronomically."[153] It seemed possible that the socialist system might not be around forever.[154] Although glasnost and perestroika did not lead to doctors voicing their grievances wholesale, the 1989 appearance of a *Medical*

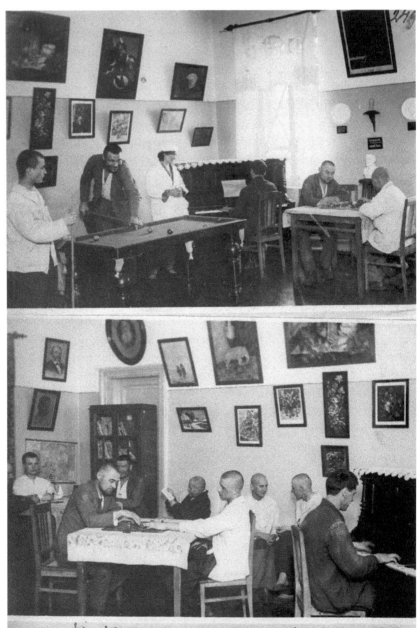

Рис. *X* и *X*. Различные моменты культработы и самодеятельности больных в красном уголке спокойного мужского отделения. /Из альбома Одесской Психиатрической больницы/.

FIGURE 6. Different types of cultural work and activities in the "red corner" of the quiet men's ward. From the Odessa psychiatric hospital album. Source: GARF, f. 8009, op. 5, d. 9, l. 249. Used with permission.

Gazette column titled "What Are Doctors Complaining About?" presented them with an open forum.[155]

Nurses in psychiatric hospitals who had read current publications were also eager to have a frank discussion about the problems confronting Soviet psychiatry. At a 1987 conference at the Gannushkin a nurse, Ivan Vinokourov, delivered an honest and critical paper on the theme of foreign literature, psychiatry, and social rehabilitation. Psychiatry and medical ethics seemed to be almost taboo, he claimed, and, consequently, the majority of the population had a "distorted" view of that part of the profession.[156] But Vinokourov believed there was some literature that broke the public silence on psychiatry and illuminated life in the psychiatric hospital. He took the example of N. I. Lyrchikova's "Splinters" ("Shchepki"), published in *Our Contemporary* (*Nash sovremennik*) in 1987, which highlighted the "contradictions of social realities, when indifference and inequality could bring a person to the psychiatric hospital."[157] Vinokourov asserted that medical workers unable to deal with rehabilitative work failed the mentally ill.[158]

Vinokourov also discussed the late 1980s short story "Goodbye, Green Buckle" ("Proshai, zelenaia priazhka"), by M. M. Chulak, and the serialized publication of Ken Kesey's *One Flew over the Cuckoo's Nest* in the journal *New World* (*Novyi mir*). Kesey's book, published in 1962, and director Milos Forman's film version drew attention to the role of medical personnel and their relationship with patients. Vinokourov also referenced and discussed American John Patrick's 1950 play *The Curious Savage* (*Strannaia missis Sevidzh*). The play, a comedy, depicted the life of institutionalized psychiatric patients. It appeared on Soviet stages in the late 1970s, but, as Vinokourov noted, it ignored problems in the psychiatric profession and instead focused on the flaws of bourgeois society.[159] But in his view, the book was more informative for readers because it afforded them the opportunity to understand the opinion of psychiatric patients and medical workers could "see themselves through the eyes of patients and relatives."[160] Vinokourov did not hold back in its criticism of the psychiatric profession or socialist representations of psychiatry to the public. In his words, he wanted to avoid "stereotypes" and learn about experiences at home and abroad.

From his reading of Soviet and US literature on psychiatry, Vinokourov concluded that patients in US psychiatric institutions saw themselves largely as part of the "medical business." Russian and Soviet psychiatry, he added, was built not only "on professional duty, but also on compassion and empathy with patients," but he worried that a psychiatric hospital's success was not measured in these human terms.[161] Vinokourov was presenting his thoughts at a time when the healthcare system had become chaotic and disorganized, as chapter 9 shows. He yearned for the kind of humanity and compassion called for under Khrushchev and then Brezhnev, but these seemed lost in time.

This nurse told his audience that it had been twenty-five years since the publication of *One Flew over the Cuckoo's Nest* and fifteen years since Chulak's "Goodbye, Green Buckle"; he now sought comparative literature for the late 1980s. He felt that nothing had changed since Chulak's book; time was still wasted on useless activities instead of treating patients.[162] "The fear of responsibility" Vinokourov said, "had left many unwilling to make decisions."[163] Paul de Kruif's *A Man against Insanity*, published in 1958, was another book that this well-read nurse highlighted. The nonfiction account of a doctor and a team of nurses intent on healing patients through a combination of "chemistry and love" impressed him.[164]

Vinokourov bemoaned the loss of the "personal" factor in the work of contemporary medical workers.[165] While generally critical, he also argued that there were plenty of good examples of psychiatric care, but these were not captured in books or plays.[166] Finally, he stated, medical workers had to read this literature and understand it, applying it in practice to "bring out the best in their work."[167] Vinokourov's criticisms of Soviet psychiatry, coming at the end of the 1980s, spoke volumes about socialism. It was all very well to instruct nurses and orderlies on how to care for patients, but if poor living and working conditions, a lack of agency, and bureaucracy marginalized these workers, then how could they be expected to provide cultured care, or even just basic care, for that matter.

The handbooks and guidebooks for middle and junior medical workers leave no doubt that medical personnel undertook a significant amount of patient care in psychiatric hospitals. Indeed, these workers had a good deal of autonomy. But autonomy is not the same as power, and nurses and orderlies did not have much of the latter. This lack of power had more to do with limits on professionalization rather than atomization per se. Nor did the roots of the problem lie in the Soviet system—the prerevolutionary psychiatric hospital was hardly idyllic. The problem was that the socialist revolution did not privilege middle and junior medical workers because they were not sufficiently "proletarian." Socialism in its Soviet guise did not help advance the cause of middle and junior medical workers. Their workload increased, and their living conditions were no better than before the war (they were arguably worse), but they were nonetheless supposed to provide cultured care. Claiming that the Soviet system struggled to provide good working and living conditions for its citizens is hardly news to most readers. Of more interest is the fact that medical workers in psychiatric hospitals such as Moscow's Gannushkin managed to push the profession forward, despite lack of state support.

Middle and junior medical workers certainly seemed committed to their job, pursuing new treatments and championing a "humane" and cultured approach to patient care. To be sure, these terms were ideologically loaded, but that is not to say they were not taken seriously. Many medical workers, in particular junior medical workers, ended up working in psychiatric hospitals because they could not find any other work. But conditions were so challenging that for others, especially nurses, the work was meaningful. To go to work knowing that you have to care for someone who might be physically well but mentally ill, or to face the risk of assault, is hardly something that anyone would take lightly. Many of those who chose to work in psychiatric hospitals, such as Denisova or Vinokourov, believed in the cause. Unfortunately for them, and their patients, their voices were often lost in the bureaucratic, hierarchical, and patriarchal world of Soviet socialism. As chapter 9 shows, medical workers—no matter how hard they tried—could not always extract themselves from their political and ideological habitat.

CHAPTER 9

Communist Morality, Activism, and Ethics

Although an increase in state spending on housing, education, public healthcare, and leisure showed that general economic conditions and standards of living improved under Khrushchev and Brezhnev, hopes of achieving a communist society seemed elusive. The military-command economy, rise of the nomenclature—that is, the privileged party elite—and the growing black market, as well Cold War "hot" flashpoints in Hungary in 1956, Czechoslovakia in 1968, and Afghanistan in 1979, all underlined the fact that the Soviet Union was far from a communist utopia. The problems of the late Soviet economy were also made visible through corruption and a lack of accountability in the medical sphere. The only party dictate that seemed to penetrate this world was discussion of communist morality and ethics. That chimes with the postwar shift in the nursing narrative that began in the final years under Stalin and lasted through to the end of the Soviet Union.

Nurses and medical workers were to show "humanity." Traditional tropes associated with the late-imperial Sisters of Mercy gained currency, and so nurses were to show empathy and compassion. Several reasons explain this shift in the narrative and especially the consistency across the late socialist period, from the 1950s to the 1980s. The Great Patriotic War undoubtedly played a role, and, as previous chapters have discussed, fears of widespread compassion fatigue in its aftermath served as an impetus to reach out to medical workers, encouraging them to care for invalids and veterans. Also, discussion of traditional nursing values found a place in the context of communist morality and the increasing turn toward a more conservative society. Finally, the emphasis on love, compassion, and empathy was likely a reaction to ongoing complaints about inadequate care.

After the war, the demographic imbalance saw women come to dominate healthcare, which became more feminized. In the Soviet Union, as elsewhere, caring, nursing, and womanhood were intertwined. In nursing discourse, discussion of nurses' rights and duties is central and touches on questions of autonomy, altruism, and nurturance.[1] For Soviet nurses, the "order to care" came cloaked in an ideological meaning that placed care in the category of communist morality. Soviet patients, especially those in much vaunted sanatoria, expected good medical service and cultured care.

Middle medical workers, sometimes living in substandard accommodation and working long, hard days, were to smile and provide a cultured, high-quality service. Nurses, through their work, represented the caring face of socialism, and they were regularly reminded of this symbolic role. Medical workers performing emotional labor received different forms of acknowledgment and recognition, whether through patient gratitude or awards.[2] But that did not put food on the table or compensate for work-related illnesses. Although in a better position than they had been during the Stalinist years, nurses and medical workers more generally continued to struggle with difficult living and working conditions. The Soviet healthcare system frequently left both medical worker and patient exasperated.

As a professional group, nurses began to single themselves out from other middle medical workers. Key to this was the establishment of the journal *Nurse* in 1942 and the widespread formation of nurse councils—groups of senior nurses established in hospitals, clinics, and healthcare departments to ensure, inter alia, the smooth operation of patient services, medical training, and the organization of conferences and events.[3] Consequently, in this chapter, more than in any of the others, I can listen to what nurses had to say. And they had a good deal to say. In medical journals, conferences, or hospital meetings there were usually at least a few nurses who were vocal in their criticisms of the healthcare system. They thought about ways to improve the training process, hospital organization, or the patient experience. They were eager to find out more about other hospitals and to compare their professional experiences with colleagues from other parts of their city, town, or the country. Even the so-called stagnant 1970s did not witness a decline in their activities. On the contrary, the stability that the first half of that decade brought allowed nurses some respite. Unlike in previous decades, when nursing was caught up in meeting industrialization, collectivization, and wartime needs, or struggling to achieve basic educational and training levels, by the late socialist period the pace of reform was no longer as frenetic, with the push toward collectivism and communism assuming a more horizontal than vertical form. Nurses drove change from below as the profession and its humanist spirit came to embody communist morality and ethics.

In nursing, the drive for a communist society built on collective action emerges as one of the more positive outcomes of late socialism. But the optimism of the late 1950s, 1960s, and early 1970s had begun to wane toward the end of Brezhnev's tenure, in spite of efforts to reinvigorate ideology through developed socialism. The economic and political crises unfolding in the last fifteen years of Soviet power devastated healthcare and nursing in particular. The medical and national press became engaged in an ongoing attempt to resuscitate the image of the nurse and the socialist project by recalling the past achievements of Soviet nurses in the Great Patriotic War and their kindness and self-sacrifice. The flurry of questions asked about healthcare and nursing were indicative of a wider crisis in politics and fears of a deepening moral malaise in Soviet society.

Gaining Confidence

The moves toward nurses acquiring more professional autonomy and control began under Stalin in the late 1930s and gradually increased thereafter, as previous chapters showed. In February 1952, a year before the death of Stalin, more than ninety nurses from Moscow's Botkin hospital met with the editors of the journal *Nurse* to discuss its work.[4] Although a small step, the meeting was important and a sign that change was afoot—nurses themselves would regularly contribute scientific articles to the journal.[5] Botkin nurses were some of the most experienced and educated in the country—their opinions mattered. *Nurse* editors seeking to improve the content and style of the 1952 issues during the ten-year anniversary of the publication had gone to the right place. The *Nurse* editors explained that they had been struggling to find contributors to the journal.[6] They had a good understanding of their readership— one that was growing each year—and knew that nurses wrote the most popular articles.[7] The problem was that Soviet nurses "wrote very little" for the journal.[8] One of the editors, F. I. Zborovskaia, observed that "readers would not like it" if they published only articles penned by doctors. The editors and, no doubt, readers wanted to know what nurses had to say. Even though many nurses were "very literate people," the editors had come to realize that they were too "shy" to write.[9] Perhaps they were too busy or lacked confidence? In any case, the editors hoped that the conversation with the Botkin nurses would engage them and establish a repository of nurses who would contribute articles to their journal.

Nurses were finding their professional feet, so to speak. Emboldened by the establishment of their own nursing journal ten years before, as well as widespread recognition of their heroic efforts during the Great Patriotic War, nurses—at least those in Moscow's Botkin—were quickly gaining confidence. This confidence only grew after Stalin's death and the broader social changes that followed. Between 1953 and 1955 in the Soviet Union there was a sense of "renewed hope" and energy about Russian culture, science, and education.[10] Nurses shared this sense of optimism and enthusiasm for learning. Discussions such as those that took place in the Botkin in 1952 indicated a growing interest in articulating the professional views and experiences of nurses.

As the Soviet Union shifted course after Stalin's death in 1953, nurses continued to improve their knowledge and expertise through reading academic work and furthering their education. In Sochi's Primorye sanatorium in 1959–1960, nurses read scientific articles in the journals *Nurse* and *Feldsher and Midwife*.[11] Conferences took place regularly in the sanatorium, with both doctors and middle medical workers in attendance. There was an emphasis on acquiring and improving knowledge and skills, with nurses expected to specialize in two to three areas of expertise.[12] Holding internal conferences and seminars for workers helped improve the quality of service.[13] When I spoke to Valentina Sarkisova, president of the Russian Nurses Association, she confirmed that, when she was a nurse in Stavropol' in 1961–1971, she and her colleagues attended such courses and wanted to improve their qualifications.[14]

Medical workers also had access to foreign ideas about healthcare in the late 1950s and 1960s. Khrushchev's doctrine of peaceful coexistence facilitated Soviet participation in the first Asian Congress of Midwives and Gynecologists in Tokyo in 1957, where delegates joined four hundred participants from twenty-two countries.[15] Soviet medical workers were also able to acquire knowledge of foreign medicine through their work in other countries, including Ethiopia, India, and Iran. Female SOKK workers in these countries offered examples of "selfless work" and "helped them in their fight for culture and a healthy way of life."[16] The Soviet Union continued to export medical literature, and in 1959 *Nurse* was the top-ranked exported medical journal, numbering 4,237 copies.[17] It was distributed in China, Czechoslovakia, Bulgaria, and elsewhere in the socialist camp, as well as in England, France, the United States, and Iran.[18] Promulgating ideas of Soviet public healthcare abroad and covering Soviet outreach or missionary efforts in the medical press were important propaganda work that signified international acceptance. Efforts to build professional confidence and prestige were further aided by the fact that education and interest in the sciences grew considerably. By 1959 *Nurse* reached a readership of over 700,000 nurses, and its circulation figures increased annually, standing at 109,000 in 1959, occupying second place among medical journals (behind *Feldsher and Midwife*).[19] With science elevated to new levels under Khrushchev, the Soviet Union's 684,100 nurses took opportunities to develop professionally.[20] But these opportunities were the carrot; the stick was a renewed emphasis on ideology to reboot the Soviet project.

Nurses with Heart

Even though the scientific-technical revolution was reaching its peak in these decades, the state also emphasized the importance of "humanity." The Soviet Union was undergoing a process of being "rehumanized" under Khrushchev, and nurses were constantly reminded of their role in helping to accomplish this weighty task. Future Soviet nurses were to embody love, conscientiousness, and patriotism.[21] A representative of the Moscow Council of Nurses, N. G. Lin'kova, noted at a 1950 conference on Ministry of Health nursing schools that students lacked grounding in historical examples of patriotism and the moral character of the nurse.[22] Lin'kova felt that instructors in nursing schools had a responsibility to inform students that nursing was a "rewarding and wonderful" career but required a "big heart" and was difficult. Nurses were to love their profession—it was a vocation.[23] She argued that this devotion would help to guarantee better care for patients. When allocating roles in the hospital, she noted how she had seen nurses who requested administrative jobs because they could not endure the sound of patients groaning or their "smell"—a far cry from the ideal and compassionate nurse.[24] Lin'kova's message seems to have had some success. The narrative of "communist morality," perhaps most commonly associated with Khrushchev's Moral Code of the Builder of Communism in 1961, was already present in 1955, when socialist patriotism and humanity fused together to provide a powerful narrative. Medical workers were often presented as hardworking women with "big hearts"; no work was too difficult if it was for the benefit of the patient.[25] It was sometimes these diligent and kind orderlies who tactfully showed young, inexperienced nurses how to approach patients.[26] Under Khrushchev, people rather than the state became active agents of social change.

Those involved in SOKK nursing courses in Zaporozh'ye, Ukrainian SSR, for example, were reminded in 1956 that their chosen profession was the "most humane" in the USSR.[27] As those charged with care under communism, Red

Cross nurses there were to show their humanity working in wards and show-case Soviet achievements in science. They also possessed "high moral quali-ties, were educated in ideology, history, science, and politics, and were cultured Soviet citizens."[28] Papers on deontology and patient care appeared on student conference programs.[29] Politics and ideology continued to inform nursing cur-ricula, ensuring that graduates would be properly "Soviet." Nurses in two-year and eight-month SOKK courses in Poltava watched and discussed educa-tional documentaries such as *Take Care of the Heart* (*Beregi serdts*), *Health and Diet* (*Zdorov'e i pitanie*), *Radiation Sickness* (*Luchevaia bolezn'*), and *Ivan Petrovich Pavlov* as part of their program.[30]

During the academic year 1957, nursing students in Poltava (such as in the auditorium photographed in figure 7) heard two lectures on the international situation (just a few months after the Soviet military intervention in Hungary) and various lectures on a range of themes including the moral character of the Soviet nurse and new achievements in domestic (*otechestvennaia*) medi-cine.[31] The school's wall newspaper, "Krasnokrestovets (Red Cross person)" was important in helping to inform and organize students.[32] This was a time of political uncertainty and some confusion following the denunciation of

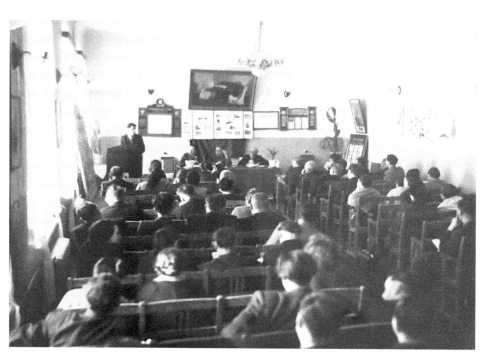

FIGURE 7.   A meeting of heads of two-year and eight-month courses for Red Cross nurses, seminar auditorium, Poltava, 1957. TsDAVO, f. R-4616, op.1, d. 109, l. 136. Courtesy of TsDAVO.

Stalin and the Soviet invasion of Hungary. The authorities worried about the mood of students. The appearance of the RSFSR November 1956 resolution "On Measures to Improve Ideological Work in Institutions of Higher Education" thus came as little surprise.[33] Khrushchev's government attempted to steady the Soviet ship, and students, including future medical professionals, had to be set on the correct course. Nursing students, consequently, continued to learn about Marxism-Leninism as they studied biology and other subjects while also learning about the humanity of their profession. "Optimistic scientists, journalists, and thinkers inside and outside the party," writes one historian, "believed in progress, culture, human reason, and moral revival."[34] Nursing also had these optimistic thinkers.

A nurse from Zaporozh'ye spoke about medical culture and patient care at a conference of SOKK leaders in Ukraine in December 1956. The importance of displaying humane characteristics was again evident. Her comments drew on socially constructed ideas of gender to describe the ideal nurse as having the brain of a man and the heart of a woman. Even though the Soviet Union needed its supposedly emancipated women in the workforce, nineteenth-century views on gender sometimes informed nursing discussions in the 1950s. The nurse drew on the physician Nikolai Pirogov's words in her speech, noting that nurses were "women with a man's education . . . who remained feminine and never neglected the development of the best gifts of their feminine nature."[35] Nurses ended up endorsing official views of women that increasingly promoted traditional notions of femininity, part of the mounting conservatism in late Soviet culture. Doctors and nurses presented a version of the nurse that was often rooted in the past or in ideas of maternal care in order to inspire other nurses to embody not only all the ideals of the Soviet nurse but also the collectivist society of the Khrushchev era.[36] Similar representations of the "wholesome" and "altruistic" nurse dominated US television and film in the 1950s, but that changed in the 1960s and 1970s, when there was "a subtle erosion of the nurse's good moral character" and nurse characters "became the focus of sexual titillation."[37] In the Soviet Union, the image of the wholesome nurse remained. After all, the press interest in the Soviet person and society was to "accomplish both pragmatic goals and socialist ideals" and directed through its propaganda and agitation campaigns.[38] Nurses embodied the ideals of the Soviet person because their profession meshed with the state's ideological agenda of building a humane, compassionate, and virtuous society.

The Third Party Program adopted at the Twenty-Second Party Congress in 1961 and later the Moral Code promised that communism would be achieved in twenty years' time. Even if the Soviet leader vacillated on the world stage

Red Cross Zaporozhe provincial committee exhibition on nursing courses

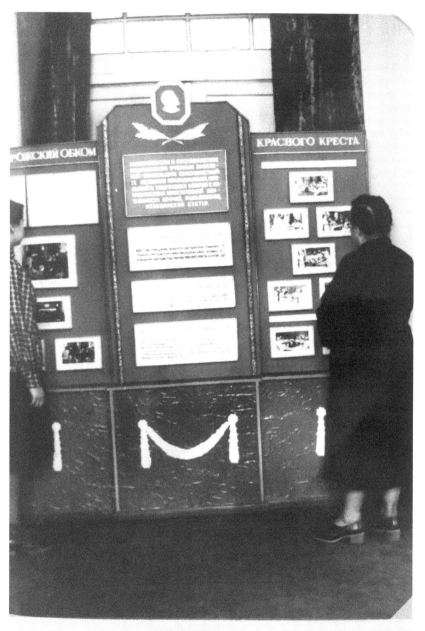

Стенд
Запорожского обкома Красного Креста.

FIGURE 8. Zaporozh'ye Red Cross provincial committee stand. TsDAVO, f. R-4616, op. 1, d. 97, l. 118. Used with permission.

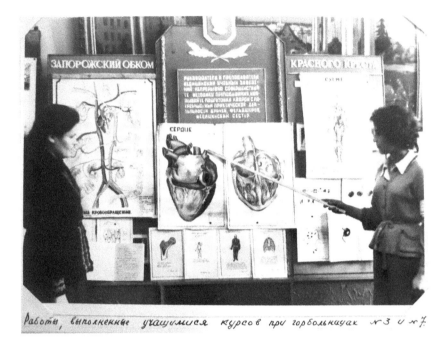

FIGURE 9. Work from students in city hospitals No. 3 and No. 7. TsDAVO, f. R-4616, op. 1, d. 97, l. 119. Used with permission.

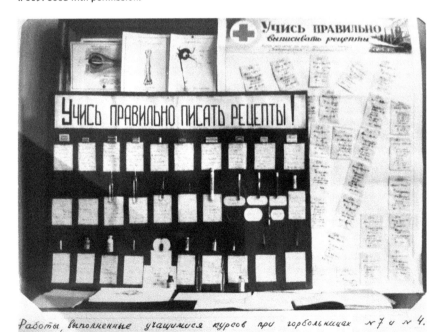

FIGURE 10. Work from students in city hospitals No. 4 and No. 7. TsDAVO, f. R-4616, op. 1, d. 97, l. 120. Used with permission.

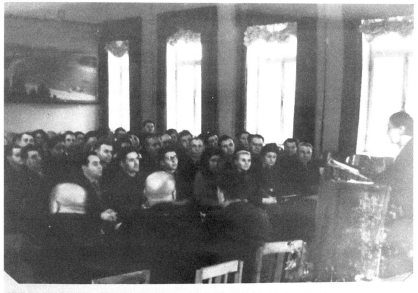

Зал проведения семинара.

FIGURE 11. Seminar auditorium. TsDAVO, f. R-4616, op.1, d. 97, l. 123. Used with permission.

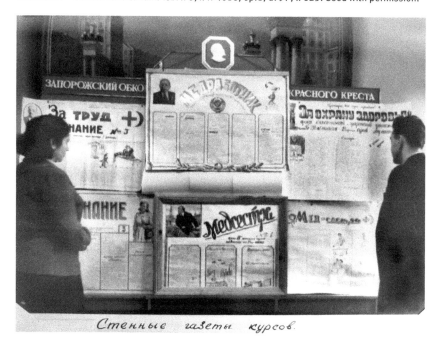

Стенные газеты курсов.

FIGURE 12. Wall newspapers for courses. TsDAVO, f. R-4616, op. 1, d. 97, l. 122. Used with permission.

between 1960 and 1962, culminating with the Cuban Missile Crisis in May 1962, uncertainty did not manifest itself in the working lives of nurses and their colleagues. They busied themselves with building communism. At a 1962 Botkin hospital conference of nurses on the topic of exchanging work experience in the fight for communist labor, nurses' discussions reinforced gender stereotypes.[39] They agreed that the nurse was the "first assistant to the doctor and the good hand of the surgeon" and that the nurse had "to go about wards with a bright smile, with a sympathetic word, and maternal care."[40] People studying medicine in the Botkin, nurses noted, "did so by vocation, that is, for the love of the person."[41] In medical college, instructors imparted students with a "love for the sick person, to care for them."[42] Some nurses did not seem to be able or willing to distinguish between gender and care; care and compassion in their view were extensions of their feminine selves. In the Botkin hospital "modest work by every person and caring for the sick to ease their suffering" was one of the ways to build communism.[43] Women were to fulfill a number of socially constructed roles, both public and private, according to their gender.[44] They worked outside the home and were professional career women. But they were also homemakers. For those working in feminized professions, such as nursing, the role of professional, mother, and homemaker often overlapped. The boundaries between professional and domestic, public and private, were thus fluid.

Conservatism worked in different ways. Questions of values, humanity, and morality led to some interesting, occasionally awkward, discussions. Perhaps buoyed by the political relaxation on censorship at home—1961 saw the publication of Yevgeny Yevtushenko's commemorative World War II poem "Babi Yar," and 1962 saw the publication of Aleksandr Solzhenitsyn's *One Day in the Life of Ivan Denisovich*, a novella about camp life—medical workers felt they could express themselves freely. For example, some regretted the change of title from Sister of Mercy to nurse in the 1920s but supposed reintroducing the former would have a "psycho-therapeutic" effect.[45] The religious question remained unresolved in the 1960s, and ideological activists under Khrushchev thus embraced "positive atheism" to connect with spiritual and emotional aspects of people's lives.[46] In an *Izvestiia* article in 1964 the author was quick to point out that mercy, when separated from its religious associations, meant "mercy of the heart" (*milost' serdtsa*).[47] Although reinstating the title of Sisters of Mercy was not mooted, the debate about whether mercy had disappeared in the age of science and technology, and if it indeed had a place, rumbled on over several years. As one doctor argued in 1971, technology and humanity were both crucial to a patient's recovery.[48] Whenever patients thanked nurses and orderlies, it was for their human qualities of patience and kindness.[49]

Although considered "old-fashioned" (*staromodnoe*), the term "mercy" had made a comeback by the 1970s.[50] Mercy and compassion were the "spiritual basis for the everyday feats of nurses."[51] Nurses were to establish an atmosphere of care and comfort for the patient. Like Pirogov's Sisters of Mercy, they were to preserve their "sensitive heart."[52] These kinds of gendered portrayals of medical workers applied to doctors, too. The 1974 film *Did You Call for a Doctor?* [*Vracha vyzyvali?*] depicts Katia Luzina, the protagonist and a newly qualified doctor, as someone who cares for patients and goes above and beyond the call of duty to ensure their well-being.[53] Her humanity, morality, and "sensitive heart" shine through. The film is a good illustration of the continued struggle to balance medicine and caregiving in practice. Male doctors represent the former, while Katia's actions exemplify the latter.

Niggling doubts about the prestige and character of the nurse, and medical workers more generally, persisted. It was not acceptable for nurses, for example, to inform surgical patients that, rather than the head of the department, under the supervision of a leading surgeon, operating on them, an intern (*praktikant*) had in fact performed the surgery.[54] This kind of information made patients "anxious." Or the nurse was not to tell patients inquiring about how their operation went that she "saw them remove a huge tumor" or "they took away half the stomach."[55] This was not compassionate care. And although efforts were made to provide a public image of the nurse that was positive and in line with communist morality, there was still a prevailing sense both inside and outside of the healthcare profession that good nurses should become doctors. One woman receiving Red Cross nurse support was so impressed by her "gentle" nurse that she advised her to become a doctor.[56] Colleagues suspected that nurses studying medical literature during their free time in hospitals and clinics and taking evening classes in the medical institute were planning to qualify as doctors.[57] Nursing, it seemed, was still not a highly esteemed profession. Still, the state persevered in its attempt to valorize and popularize nursing.

Soviet success in the international Florence Nightingale Medal competition (an award the International Red Cross Committee established) was a testament to increasing Soviet pride in nursing and growing foreign contact.[58] The International Committee of the Red Cross and the Soviet Red Cross and Red Crescent had "significantly widened their contact" in the early 1960s, and, as a response, the Soviets forwarded candidates to the Nightingale Medal competition.[59] Irina Levchenko and Lidiia Savchenko were the first Soviet recipients of the medal, in 1961.[60] The medal, a recognition of exemplary service or sacrifice during war or peace, was awarded to these two nurses who had served during the Great Patriotic War. One of the Soviet winners of the

Nightingale Medal in 1965, Faina Khusainovna, was a nurse with fifteen years' professional nursing experience in Kazan. The medal was a reward for her contribution to the Second World War.[61] The press article portrayed Khusainovna and her colleague, the orderly "Aunt Nastia," both widows caring for elderly parents, as two strong women who understood the importance of human kindness. They were perhaps seen as an inspiration to the seven hundred thousand nurses working in the Soviet healthcare system.[62] To be sure, the Soviet Union's involvement with the international Red Cross and Red Crescent societies heralded its desire to be a real force on the international stage, but it was also in line with broader efforts to frame nursing as a Soviet and noble vocation for domestic audiences.

Activism, Collectivism, and Heroism

When it came to positive portrayals of nursing, the Red Cross and Red Crescent often appeared on the scene. That was the case in the 1950s when the Red Cross and Red Crescent proved itself an important player in the broader Soviet healthcare system, which continued to expand during the Five-Year Plan of 1950–1955.[63] SOKK nursing students and workers were sometimes paid but were more often voluntary workers.[64] An impressive 55,500 students graduated from Red Cross courses in 1955.[65] The SOKK mission to mobilize volunteer nurses also fit nicely with the Khrushchev era's ideological program of civic action and collective responsibility. During the years 1959–1961, the most "talented and energetic" of the postwar generation "sought not only to express themselves professionally," writes one historian, but also "to create a new language of civic culture—a framework of social and moral responsibility, truth and sincerity."[66] This found expression when "ten of the largest Soviet largest cities—Moscow, Leningrad, Gorky, Kiev, Kharkov, Dnepropetrovsk, Minsk, Baku, Tbilisi, and Tashkent—based on experience," became sites of a SOKK initiative that saw the formation of two hundred "nurse bureaus," with a target of one thousand set for January 1961.[67] Bureau nurses were "activists" who had completed SOKK courses and provided care free of charge to the sick at home and those living alone.[68] While Soviet nursing had followed Britain, the United States, and Australia in moving away from "a morally inflected philanthropic model" to a more professional, secular system that privileged science, that position changed after the war.[69] Ideological and political shifts toward scientific success and communist morality required nurses to exercise moral authority in addition to mastering scientific knowledge.

The bureau nurses had different types of medical education and work experience. According to the former minister for health and representative of the Soviet Red Cross Executive Committee, G. A. Miterev, the nurse bureaus helped the state and healthcare system by addressing nursing shortfalls in hospitals and clinics.[70] The SOKK nurses, a mixture of young women, medical students, housewives, and the retired, targeted patients without family or caregivers. Beginning January 1, 1960, bureau nurses had to care for 3,221 people and visit 70,706 people.[71] The Red Cross and Red Crescent received letters from patients in various Soviet cities expressing their gratitude to nurses for their good care and attention.[72]

Mobilizing women was not new to the Red Cross and was part of a second wave of female activism under Khrushchev. Established in 1957, women's councils, or *zhensovety*, were very much involved in this kind of social and welfare work, also mirroring an earlier era of female activism.[73] The movement toward mobilizing women took place at an intraprofessional level too, as nurse councils sprouted in hospitals and clinics across the country. In January 1960 the Ministry of Health issued a decree outlining measures to improve public health, and it spurred on further initiatives, including meetings of senior nurses and representatives from nurse councils.[74] The Moscow city council of nurses, established in 1960, had fifty thousand members two years later.[75] The council organized "raids" in a number of Moscow hospitals and polyclinics.

Indeed, a section on the nurse councils and their activities became a feature in *Nurse*. Although initially established in the late 1930s, the councils became part of the Khrushchev era's "collective mechanisms," engaged in various methods of collective shaming to enforce labor discipline.[76] The nurse councils, medical journals and other platforms now allowed nurses to articulate their needs and interests, as well as offering an important vehicle for specialists to advise on ethics and deontology and report infringements of these. Devolving power, to some extent, fostered a new sense of professional confidence and autonomy among nurses. The greater democratization that came with Khrushchev's de-Stalinization encouraged workers to "become active participants in the management of their own enterprises," or, in the case of nurses, in their departments, hospitals, and polyclinics or in people's homes.[77]

The SOKK also helped train housewives and pensioners in special groups to care for sick people in their homes.[78] These newly trained SOKK bureau nurses talked to patients and their relatives about the Red Cross and Red Crescent and discussed medical and sanitary-hygiene issues with them. They also participated in nurse conferences to improve their qualifications.[79] On an average day the nurse visited four to five patients.[80] Each visit typically took an hour or an hour and a half, depending on the "nature of the illness, the condition of the patient, and the doctor's instructions."[81] The nurses undertook a range of tasks that included giving injections and bandaging patients, taking patients' temperature, helping wash and feed patients, changing bedclothes, and ventilating the premises.[82] On the face of it, echoes of the 1930s prevailed: the state again mobilized SOKK to support the shaky civilian healthcare system, especially for pensioners. But these volunteers differed from the young recruits of the 1930s and were not primarily seeking promotion or adventure; rather, they seemed genuinely interested in helping people.

The cross-generational initiative encapsulated a shared language of civic culture that showed no sign of abating. Over ten years later, in 1974, there were 3,295 visiting nurses attached to SOKK.[83] The Brezhnev-era concern with veterans and patriotism was evident in nursing: more than 72 percent of patients served by SOKK visiting nurses were invalids of the Great Patriotic War, and 1,263 of these were Group I invalids.[84] And, unsurprisingly, SOKK nursing work was described as coming "from the heart."[85] Letters of gratitude to the nurses expressed the heartfelt nature of the work. In 1974 a letter sent to the Georgian SOKK committee from a first-category invalid and participant of the Great Patriotic War, one Z. I. Kritskaia, praised the visiting nurse Tsiala Miridzhaneshvili: "Nurse Tsiala is not only a medical worker, but also a person with a humane spirit [*chelovecheskoi dushoi*]. She warmly participates in the personal life of the patient[s], helps when they are in difficulty, and happily cares for them. She has a warm soul so accessible to all patients that when she comes, all the sores are hidden because of her. Thank you, for educating such good nurses: I want to call your sisters by this ancient name, sisters of mercy!"[86] Such letters make it easy to understand why there was a degree of nostalgia for the 1970s under Brezhnev. People enjoyed not only the relative stability but also a sense of being part of a wider community that cared about people. The volunteers who undertook SOKK nursing work and those they helped both benefited from the experience. Red Cross nursing in the late socialist period tells a generally positive story, but not the whole story. While conditions were much improved, nurses and medical workers were still confronted with a myriad of challenges.

The Milk of Human Kindness Turns Sour

Medical workers as a group were aggrieved on a number of levels. At trade union conferences in Moscow, workers complained about overwork, incorrect organization of personnel, and health and safety infringements in the workplace.[87] Even though the Ministry of Health issued a decree on the protection of medical workers in 1956, workers claimed that local health authorities ignored it. In one Moscow hospital, attending doctors worked for twenty-five to thirty hours straight.[88] Medical workers complained that they were often unable to take their annual holidays.[89] And yet, as one anonymous *Medical Worker* author pointed out the following year, "experience showed that head doctors and trade union local committees that looked after their staff's health and well-being reaped the rewards of fewer sick days."[90] Senior nurses with considerable experience earned fractionally more than their junior colleagues, a repeat of the leveling out of salaries that had occurred in the 1920s. The rise of the nomenclature in the postwar period calcified hierarchies in Soviet society, and, once again, middle and junior medical workers seemed destined to have to make do with generally miserable working and living conditions. One of the worst signs of a lack of concern for medical workers was the low priority assigned to health and safety. Many medical institutions did not have ventilation in x-ray laboratories or instructions for new equipment.[91] Such oversights led to workplace accidents and illness.[92] A *Medical Worker* author lamented that a 1957 trade union resolution to improve conditions in medical institutions had not been acted on six months later.[93] Decrees and resolutions on health and safety continued well beyond the 1950s.[94] The problems afflicting Soviet healthcare in the late Stalinist period seemed just as great as in the 1920s and 1930s. One of the main differences was that nurses at least had their own journal to articulate their grievances.

Half-trained medical workers still stalked hospital and clinic corridors. In 1955 a "significant number" of students failed the state exams: in one Moscow medical college only two students made a plaster cast and the remaining twenty students simply "observed."[95] Doctors who taught in medical colleges had other jobs and were overworked (a familiar story). An editorial in *Medical Worker* a few years later accused the republican and local health authorities of not being sufficiently firm with regard to those in charge of the health departments.[96] Younger doctors were not very well equipped to teach, and there were few courses for training medical college instructors: indeed, instructors were in such short supply that some considered recruiting retired doctors.[97]

Medical workers continued to make mistakes, which some commentators put down to carelessness and a lack of responsibility for their work.[98] In 1965 the Ostroumova hospital penalized orderlies for missing work without a valid reason, being drunk at work, and being rude to colleagues, while the following year a number of nurses were called out for violations of labor discipline, including carelessness in carrying out doctors' instructions, being rude to visitors, and leaving work early.[99] Patients complained about standards of care.

Even sanatoria, supposed havens of communist rest, did not escape criticism. Back in February 1921, Nikolai Semashko had envisaged resorts as "repair shops" for the toiling masses, an opportunity for Soviet people to strengthen their health.[100] But workers convalescing in Sochi's Dendrarii sanatorium in the 1950s claimed: "Everything is far from wonderful here, starting with the admission of patients."[101] Medical personnel complained about patients and patients complained about medical personnel.[102] Patients pilfered and broke cutlery and "ruined towels with fruit."[103] Medical personnel considered patients too demanding.[104] At a trade union meeting of the sanatorium, the worker A. Kassina claimed that attendants were overworked.[105] Another, the meeting's chairperson, O. N. Bogaevskaia, bought newspapers and dominos for patients with her own money, an admission that showed how medical workers picked up institutional slack at personal expense.[106]

Soviet medical workers and the public were not blind to the problems in their country. Foreign contact under Khrushchev had opened their eyes. The Moscow Youth Festival in the summer of 1957, a US exhibition in Moscow two years later, and a loosening of the restrictions on travel abroad introduced Soviet citizens to life beyond Soviet borders. At the 1959 American National Exhibition in Moscow, the Soviet public was surprised to learn that US mothers were encouraged to stay at home with their children, US doctors could cure all forms of tuberculosis, and the United States had low infant and maternal mortality rates. The paper towels "delighted" Soviet visitors, and they "loved" the Band-Aids. Some of those present realized that the Soviet Union had much to do if it was to catch up with US healthcare standards.[107] The problems in healthcare were abundantly clear to Soviet medical workers. They were also evident to the public.

Nurses in the Botkin hospital were not slow in elucidating some of these problems. In August 1961, a senior Botkin nurse annoyingly found that she was without the buffet worker and the nanny when she arrived to work.[108] Even a major Moscow hospital such as the Botkin suffered from staff shortages. Other problems included a scarcity of oxygen supplies as well as trouble with the parquet flooring—staff and patients repeatedly tripped on the newly laid, but not secured, timber. One nurse complained that needles were "too thin or too thick."[109] A senior nurse added that her department's main problem was transporting patients: it was not always possible for orderlies to bring patients to the x-ray or urology department because the special trolley for transporting them "had specific hours." If medical workers missed this window, they could not transport the patient.[110] One of the problems arising from the litany of complaints was the issue of responsibility and accountability. In the 1920s and 1930s, so-called enemies of the people were scapegoats. In the late 1950s and 1960s, the onus was on assuming collective responsibility. But that had its own problems—if everyone was at fault, then nobody was at fault, and therefore problems tended to remain unresolved.

Other nurses complained that they could not buy an electrocardiogram (EKG) machine. A senior nurse in the surgical department noted that their main problem was flies, especially in the postoperative ward.[111] In the dressing station there was no cold water, so "surgeons ended up scalding their hands." The complaints at the meeting went on and on. The head doctor, B. G. Darevskii, drew proceedings to a close, noting that he did not expect senior nurses to work in these conditions. He added that cadres "had it bad because of the low pay"—an issue that he wanted resolved.[112] How he proposed to resolve the matter was not clear. It is likely that complaints made their way through the bureaucracy and remained unresolved. Individual workers had to manage the problems themselves on an everyday basis.

Many medical workers seemed worn-out and in no way ready to contribute to the last great push for communism. Social and ideological values ("collective solidarity" and "the dignity of labour" versus "personal dignity") divided Soviet society.[113] These contradictions also connect to perceptions of individual and collective understandings of happiness under socialism.[114] What was an acceptable level of self-sacrifice for nurses to make on behalf of patients? How long were they supposed to prioritize collective interests? If their hard work ruined their health and undermined their family's material circumstances, how was that in the public good? Many of these questions were part of the paradoxes of Soviet life. Medical workers had to resolve these themselves.

The Botkin nurses' complaints seemed pretty typical of hospital meetings across the Soviet Union. Vladimir A. Tsesis, a Soviet doctor working in a rural hospital in the Moldovan republic in the 1960s, found the morning *piatiminutka*—a supposedly five-minute briefing session attended by all physicians, head nurses, and representatives from housekeeping and so forth—to be "spirited and democratic."[115] The session usually lasted an hour, and everyone could contribute.[116] That was where the positive appraisals ended. "The Soviet practice of medicine," Tsesis wrote, was "built around improper and inconsistent training, shortages in equipment and medicine, and brilliantly incompetent and illusory bureaucratic policies and procedures."[117]

If the 1930s saw the emergence of oppositional narratives between the caring state, on the one hand, and callous workers, on the other, then the 1960s saw a similar oppositional binary that asked medical workers to behave in a moral and ethical fashion while stretching them to their physical, material, and emotional limits. Indeed, in the over sixty-six thousand letters of complaint that the Ministry of Health received in 1965, patients blamed individual healthcare workers for "corruption, laziness, and lack of compassion."[118] Once again it was medical workers who were personally held to account for flaws in the system. But medical workers pushed back against criticism, pleading understaffing and overwork. And they often defended each other, with doctors coming to the defense of middle and junior medical workers. Medical workers in hospitals, sanatoria, and clinics worked as a collective. This meant that they rooted out those perceived to have transgressed norms, but, inversely, it also meant that they often defended one another when criticized.

The Patient Experience: Focus on Sanatoria

Although seemingly quite simple, two factors—service and care—when carried out properly, hugely affected a patient's experience. The archives of Sochi sanatoria go some way in illustrating how patients evaluated their experiences. A patient from Sochi's Primorye considered that sanatorium the best because daytime activities were well thought out and because all personnel had a "warm attitude" to treatment and rest.[119] One pensioner staying in Metallurg, newly constructed in the 1950s with 375 beds, called it a "palace," and another patient considered it one of the best on the Black Sea coast.[120] This latter patient arrived with an "unidentified illness and almost lost hope," but departed "content and renewed." Another wrote in the Metallurg comment book that when a person feels unwell "a kind word and friendly attitude" means a great deal and that the service personnel played an important role in that.[121] But these repair shops for Soviet people were not uniformly good. The head of the trade union health section, M. Kaziev, wrote in 1960 that delivering an adequate health service to sanatorium patients was still an issue. Sometimes, he noted, patients' health actually deteriorated after a sanatorium stay.[122]

In the Soviet Union the "culture of complaint" persisted into the late socialist years, and many Soviet citizens were familiar with the practice.[123] People wrote letters to local and central officials, newspapers, journals, and anyone who they deemed likely to assist them in their quest for help, be that in healthcare, housing, education, or another area. Indeed, Moscow's Ostroumova hospital, one of the best in the Soviet Union, received complaints, most of which concerned a rude attitude toward patients.[124] In the mid-1970s, patients in the Metallurg sanatorium complained about bad organization, while doctors complained that nurses did not prepare patients' medical histories sufficiently well, did not go on rounds, and did not offer patients enough opportunity to see the nurse.[125]

One disgruntled former patient wrote to *Black Sea Resort* (Chernomorskoe zdravnitse) in November 1976 to complain about his experience in Sochi's Kavkazkaia Riviera. The piece, titled "Forgetting about the Person" (Zabyli o cheloveke), outlined the shortcomings of middle medical personnel and criticized their work.[126] The nurse council meeting that convened to discuss the matter concluded with an agreement to strengthen educational, or *vospitanie*, work among nurses accused of inattention to "answer for their serious shortcomings."[127] Patient experiences were by this stage very much personalized and defined by their encounters with individual medical personnel. Nurses in Kavkazskaia Riviera were aware of the importance of making the right impression on sanatorium patients. They wanted to give patients a "warm welcome" and "create conditions for good rest."[128] Reputation and prestige mattered. Sanatoria were the beacons of Soviet care, and Soviet citizens expected the best from their stay, particularly in Sochi. There was thus considerable pressure on medical workers and sanatoria administrators to live up to these high expectations.

For patients, it was often the little things that mattered. Providing patients with a warm welcome and kind word as soon as they entered the sanatorium was part of the larger process of care and treatment. All medical personnel had a "moral and professional responsibility" to understand the patient's "mind" and "heart."[129] The comment books in Kavkazskaia Riviera contained many notes of praise and gratitude.[130] Patients were grateful because their moods had improved and they had confidence in their health. People felt they had "become younger."[131] The language employed by patients to describe their sanatorium experience was largely formulaic (especially positive comments) and engaged with the kinds of image of medical care represented by the state.[132] The Soviet state, particularly under developed socialism, promoted high ideals of Soviet life, and people's expectations of standards of care were consequently high.

Similar to the culture of complaints, Soviet citizens followed social convention in how they responded to issues that affected their lives. Bad service, "unsocialist" care, or examples of outstanding care motivated people to write to local and central authorities as well as the press. But those who complained were unlikely to cross the line "between criticizing local power and indicting the entire system."[133] Patients did not criticize socialism or the state but rather complained about individual medical workers. For "great numbers of Soviet citizens," writes the anthropologist Alexei Yurchak, "many of the fundamental values, ideals, and realities of socialist life (such as equality, community, selflessness, altruism, friendship, ethical relations, safety, education, work, creativity, and concern for the future) were of genuine importance" even if they did not always adhere to these norms in their everyday lives.[134] Others have reached similar conclusions in assessments of public opinion in the Soviet Union: many people shared the state's goals but "ignored these in their own behavior."[135] These values existed on a "mythological" level, and people applied them as "values for others."[136] Patients who held these kinds of social values had basic "mythological" expectations about Soviet healthcare and socialism: when these expectations were not met in practice, they felt obliged to take action to criticize medical workers.

Countdown to Communist Paradise

Although scrutinized by patients and pressed to their limits, medical workers had some reason for optimism. Their material conditions were set to improve slightly after their inclusion in the general wage increases in the 1960s. Salary increases in 1964 granted nurses a 40 percent pay increase, more than the 17–26 percent increase for physicians. Consequently, their monthly salary increased from 45.00–76.50 rubles to 60–110 rubles, not dissimilar to teachers' salaries, which increased from 52–131 rubles to 80–137 rubles per month (depending on experience, qualifications, and location).[137] Based on 1962 prices, nurses could afford basic foodstuffs relatively comfortably with their higher salary, but purchasing consumer goods would have presented greater difficulty.[138] Salary increases alongside efforts to reorganize the medical bureaucracy signaled positive moves toward change in the 1960s and hopes for further consolidation in the 1970s. Brezhnev's government continued to endorse the Third Party Program and the state's commitment to improving social welfare and greater egalitarianism: indeed, every Five-Year Plan under Brezhnev provided for wage increases.[139]

But the Brezhnev years were also marked by disillusionment following Soviet military intervention in Prague in 1968, a belligerent response to Czechoslovakian leader Aleksandr Dubcek's "socialism with a human face," and a growing sense that people were losing faith in socialist ideology. Brezhnev's government rolled out "developed socialism" at the Twenty-Fourth Party Congress in March 1971 to revitalize ideology and to "reaffirm the correctness of the party's chosen historical course."[140] The salary increases for medical workers formed part of the Brezhnev government's broader efforts to improve standards of living and people's well-being, as Khrushchev had also set out to do. But developed socialism was as much about reaffirming people's spiritual connection to communism as it was about economics.[141] Instilling morality and humanism into people's everyday lives would achieve that. And, as people's experience of staying in a sanatorium indicated, Soviet citizens believed that they had a right to good quality care provided in a kind and meaningful way.

Coverage of an international healthcare conference held in Moscow in 1975 to discuss the living and working conditions of workers in public healthcare, titled "Unity and Solidarity—in the Name of Humanism," symbolized state efforts to marry economic and spiritual causes.[142] As such, healthcare acted as a kind of barometer for developed socialism. How was it faring? Although Minister of Public Health B. V. Petrovskii acknowledged that the scientific-technical revolution posed some challenges for medical workers, N. N. Grigor'eva, representative of the trade unions Central Committee, noted that progress was made in the early 1970s. She then outlined the benefits that medical workers studying in medical institutes received.[143] In the eyes of the state, medical workers received opportunities and incentives aplenty to improve their qualifications.

Conference delegates had traveled from over thirty countries and included doctors and nurses from international medical unions, nursing associations, and societies. David Stark Murray, president of the British Socialist Medicine Association, and Anne Zimmerman, president of the American Nurses Association, were among the guests. All were also invited to attend two installations at the Exhibition of Achievements of the National Economy (VDNKh): one on Soviet healthcare and the other on labor and rest.[144] They no doubt left Moscow with positive impressions of socialist healthcare.

Grigor'eva and some her colleagues seemed a little out of touch with the realities of life for medical workers. Not long after the salary increases introduced by Khrushchev, two nurses from Kuibyshev called for nurse attestation and higher salaries in 1968.[145] They wanted a tiered system for nurses and greater professional opportunities—further signs of nurses advocating for change. Doctors had wide professional networks, they claimed, but nurses did not. These nurses were eager to learn and progress further in their career. But they also wanted professional and financial recognition. These nurses had to wait some time for this, because the Ministry of Health did not issue a decree on nurse attestation until the 1970s. Even then, it was limited.[146] Praise for achievements in Soviet healthcare concealed widespread "behind the scenes" dissatisfaction and inadequacies. Rural healthcare was plagued by problems: middle medical workers often took the place of doctors, medical workers had to work more than one job, or unsatisfactory living conditions caused high turnover rates.[147] In many parts of the Soviet Union the absence of suitable premises and instructors, or the inability of medical workers to travel to course locations on a regular basis, meant that conferences and seminars became vital for nurse training and education. In Krasnodar there were four hundred annual places in specialization and further education courses for thirty-one thousand medical workers.[148] To deal with the shortfall in course places, lectures, seminars, conferences, and mentoring were "just as effective," especially if senior figures and experts participated and if they took place regularly.[149] These were hardly ideal conditions for producing highly trained medical workers who could deliver the kind of quality of care the state promoted.

Even the head of the Sklifosovskogo hospital, the surgeon Leonid Sul'povar, interviewed in a 1990 documentary film about public healthcare, spoke about how he entered the first year of medical school and worked as an orderly, then a medical brother, then a feldsher.[150] Although morale was good, he said, he remained financially dependent on his parents "practically his whole life." Even the head of a prestigious Moscow hospital could barely scrape a living in the late socialist years. The Soviet state was increasingly relying on people's sense of duty and humanity to keep public healthcare running.

Interest and achievements in science might have reached their zenith in the 1960s and 1970s, but that did not translate fully into the everyday lives of the 2.7 million middle medical workers who had to cope with both the intellectual and physical challenges of their work.[151] Their labor seemed to go largely unnoticed, so much so that the national press attempted to champion the cause of nurses, reminding readers that they provided crucial care. "Compassion is their main weapon against illness," *Pravda* proclaimed on its front page in October 1973.[152] Readers were told, "Humanism—the basic achievement of modern medicine—is a new feature [*sushchestvo*] of this old profession." But— the article informed its readers—nurses rarely featured on the radio, on television, or in film because journalists and writers were "more interested in doctors and surgeons." The newspaper (a.k.a. the government's mouthpiece) called on the party, trade unions, and heads of medical institutions to raise the prestige of nurses, improve their living and working conditions, and provide opportunities for them to advance professionally.[153] The spiritual mission of the Brezhnev period found in medical workers an ideal outlet to champion socialist values of humanism and compassion.

This newly found press attention was a welcome development for nurses, who seemed to be near breaking point in the 1970s, tested by the pressures of their work every day. Their plight suggested a lengthy pit stop on the road to communism rather than a direct route to utopia. Even a most basic form of developed socialism seemed out of their reach. Medical workers found the strain of lifting and transporting patients to be particularly arduous, a problem some claimed to owe as much to "organizational" problems as to science or economics.[154] The national newspaper *Izvestiia* had a "raid brigade" investigate the reality of technical advancements after the international exhibition

Public Healthcare–74, and the brigade members reported that nurses in the Ostroumova's traumatology department often struggled to move beds with virtually immovable wheels.[155] New machines designed to clean hospital corridors were useless because they were too "noisy." The hard physical labor of scrubbing and cleaning "forced young, capable nurses to leave after a year or two," sighed one older nurse.[156] The Soviet Union had managed to send a man into space in 1961, but it still struggled to produce functional hospital beds.

Although Soviet nurses had to master an increasingly complex and growing body of knowledge, they were often not able to do this for reasons beyond their control. The head of the Russian medical technical service (Rosmedtekhnika) wrote about the problem in 1973. He noted that EKG machines, surgical instruments, ultrasound devices, and other equipment all required specific training and expertise, but nurses had limited knowledge of how to deal with basic faults.[157] Sometimes medical colleges did not teach much in the way of electronics or technical issues, even though nurses were expected to know about these.[158] Another problem, noted by a Riazan nurse, was that outdated equipment was often dumped in medical colleges.[159] Such problems were rife. Recalling the long-anticipated arrival of an EKG machine in rural Moldova in the 1960s, the Soviet doctor Tsesis noted that it repeatedly broke down and nobody had hired an EKG technician.[160] Once again, the issue of accountability, or lack thereof, arose.

Middle medical workers continued to experience the physical, intellectual, and emotional strain that Prof. A. A. Kasparov, deputy director of scientific work at the Institute of Labor Hygiene and Work-Related Illness AMN SSSR, mentioned at the international healthcare conference in Moscow in 1975, but they did not seem to get many benefits.[161] Conditions were so difficult that turnover—a huge and ongoing problem in the Soviet Union—showed no signs of resolution. Medical workers were hunting for a bright communist future that seemed to lay elsewhere in another medical institution. Even one of Moscow's largest hospitals, the Ostroumova, saw turnover increases in the mid-1970s.[162] It was not alone in its plight. The harried head doctor of a Moscow polyclinic, featured in the film *Did You Call for a Doctor?* similarly struggled to hold onto medical workers. We see him pleading with a "star" orderly who is intent on leaving for better, "equal" conditions in another clinic, in spite of the fact that she earns the same salary as doctors working there.[163] But a glance at the statistics in the Ostroumova hospital would suggest that better childcare facilities and improved conditions for mothers with young children, as well as part-time work for retired staff, might go a long way in helping to retain its medical workers. This brings us to the issue of women at work.

Women at Work: A Closer Look

Scholarship on women has already attested to the huge workload, paid and unpaid, borne by Soviet women. Among female industrial workers in Leningrad during the years 1956–1962, dissatisfaction with living and working conditions, especially the lack of childcare facilities, led to high turnover levels.[164] It was common for women to quit their jobs to find better childcare provisions.[165] Rising alcoholism and associated poor health among men in the late Soviet period placed additional pressure on women to work and financially support dependents. The moral decline and crisis of identity that Soviet men experienced thus had a direct impact on women.[166] Yet men retained privileged positions at home and at work.[167]

Natalia Baranskaia's story of a typical week in the life of the Moscow scientist and mother Olga Voronkova in the 1969 short story "A Week Like Any Other" depicts the hardship and inequality Soviet women faced.[168] Nurses shared many of these difficulties too. Although nurses were educated women who performed physical and emotional labor, they constantly struggled to find a job that provided satisfactory living and working conditions. This problem continued in the 1970s. By the early part of that decade over three quarters of medical workers in the Soviet Union were women. Medical institutions consequently needed to adapt to the needs of their predominantly female workforce. The Ostroumova's administration looked into easing the workload for women, improving services, and showing some form of assistance for those raising children.[169] The head doctor, T. N. Amaratova, outlined the major problems confronting the hospital and the initiatives undertaken to improve conditions for workers and patients.

Some 1,173 workers were women, including department supervisors, doctors, nurses, orderlies, and domestic workers.[170] Women's massive workload incorporated prophylactic work to "restore and preserve the health of Soviet people," participation in social work, as well as work in the party bureau, local committee, and union and the Communist Youth League.[171] Some 75 percent of women employees had children, the care (*zabota*) of whom was "one of the most important aspects in the work of the administration and local committee." The hospital's administrative and social organizations wanted to address the work and everyday lives of working women and the leisure opportunities available to them.[172] This included efforts to raise women's qualifications, allow them to exert more control over their work conditions, reduce illness among women, implement better nutrition in the hospital, and improve the ideological, political, and cultural level of working women.[173]

Excursions around Moscow and other cities, cultural trips to the Museum of the Revolution, and group visits to the cinema were to help "raise their cultural level."[174] This plan fed into the objectives of developed socialism by reinvigorating people's connection to ideology and communism. Finally, more concrete ideological and political work took the form of lectures by the voluntary association Znanie (whose remit was atheist work) and lectures on the international situation.[175] The hospital established a woman's committee under the leadership of L. N. Petrova, the senior nurse of the department of functional diagnostics. The committee was to "examine the conditions of work, life and rest" for women working at the hospital.[176] Nursing activity in the late 1970s focused on improving conditions for the hospital collective and women themselves. The medical world was almost exclusively female. Women, as guardians of Soviet health, were empowered to oversee hospitals, clinics, and other medical institutions through their work as department heads, doctors, and nurses. But whether any of the hospital administration's plans were fully realized, or if they were of any actual use to women, is another question.

It is more likely that women identified with Baranskaia's character and struggled to balance the demands of work and home. And even if hospitals such as the Ostroumova attempted to improve the lot of its female workforce, such initiatives were at the discretion of individual clinics and hospitals. By the late 1980s, women seemed to be no better off. In the 1990 documentary film *Oh, Thank You Doctor* (*Oi, spasibo doctor*), one woman, L. I. Novak, a representative of the trade union central committee for medical personnel, speaks about the hardship endured by workers. In the interview, she bemoans the daily grind of taking on extra workloads and, for women, household duties: professional qualifications, she concludes, comes "in sixth or seventh place."[177] Women might have received some comfort from the fact that their plight was being acknowledged, but that did not help to reduce their workloads or domestic chores. For many, the drudgery of work limited their capacity to assume advanced training and education.

Moral Crisis: The Politics of Care

By the mid-1960s there was a growing awareness of ethics, morality, and deontology. This increased further over the next twenty years. Nurses and other medical workers frequently dropped these terms into discussions of patient care and professional relations between medical workers, but especially between doctors and middle- or junior-level personnel. Ethics became linked to culture; that is, the more cultured a nurse, the higher her or his ethical standards. A section on ethics and deontology appeared regularly in *Nurse* in the 1980s, a sure sign that the subject was there to stay. Medical ethics applied to workers' interactions with patients and each other.[178] Debates about ethics also fed into the wider ideological issues of the Brezhnev government and "developed socialism." The New Soviet Person was to be of high moral standing, after all.[179] Medical workers, and especially medical students, were to remain ideologically vigilant.

Indeed, discussions about ethics were also a sign of serious concern for a healthcare system crippled with many shortcomings, including medical workers' indifference.[180] Widespread discussion of deontology, ethics, and the moral character of nurses showed that this was a conversation that was still very much necessary in the 1970s and 1980s. Publications gave nurses the chance to read about the language of humanity in action. One article, for example, presented the nurse Vera Petrovna Bezukh as a dedicated nurse who understood that "a living person lies in the hospital bed."[181] Readers learned that nurses such as Bezukh worked from the soul and heart to create an atmosphere of "warmth and optimism." But nurses like Bezukh seemed the exception rather than the norm. William A. Knaus wrote in the 1970s that Soviet hospital nurses were a "disagreeable lot" who assumed "a degree of officiousness which is out of proportion to their responsibilities."[182] They did not take an interest in the patient, in his view, and rarely checked a patient's pulse or vital signs.[183] While harsh generalizations are not particularly helpful, the constant propaganda designed to portray the "good" Soviet nurse suggested that all was far from ideal.

Although the medical press made much of humanity, ethics, and professional commitment, serious mistakes still occurred, and these continued to be attributed to inattention and carelessness. A *Medical Gazette* (*Meditsinskaia gazeta*) correspondent in the Ukrainian SSR received a letter from a nurse who seemed to be at her wit's end. The nurse, Ekaterina Fedorovna Andrushchenko, wrote that many of the mistakes in her hospital involved medication: nurses mixed up drugs, did not know the correct dosages, used medicine that had long expired, or did not understand the labeling.[184]

Even the Botkin had problems. Consider the case of the nurse Anna Ivanova. After finishing the Botkin medical college, she went to work in the hospital's gynecological department in August 1975.[185] During Ivanova's time in this post, the head of the department found that she showed "complete professional incompetence" and repeatedly transgressed medical ethics. The hospital accused Ivanova of frequently failing to fulfill or correctly follow doctor's instructions, misinforming doctors about medications, and "forgetting" to take notes when observing the critically ill. She allegedly went home without checking the instructions of the doctor "on more than one occasion," and she "forgot" to take notes on the history of the illness: all this was construed to be a testament to her "careless attitude to duty." Ivanova reportedly did not "participate in the social life of the collective" and was deemed unfit to work in the hospital.[186] The case of Ivanova was only one in an emerging healthcare crisis. Some commentators criticized Moscow hospitals for dangerous use of x-ray and anesthesia equipment, shortages of equipment, and a lack of supervision of medical personnel.[187] The high standards of care and morality espoused in the 1970s left no room for error, but on the whole, the progress made in the 1960s seemed to be stalling.

Middle medical workers were found guilty of a range of transgressions against the morally upright society supposedly being created during late socialism. Concern with the moral and ethical behavior of medical workers and the quality of care increased significantly from the mid-1970s on. Perhaps in response, in 1976 the Ministry of Health oversaw the introduction of a course on medical ethics that would bring together different aspects of ethics and deontology taught in medical institutes.[188] The Ministry of Health was well aware of the problems with standards of care. It called on nurses in clinics to work more closely with junior nurses in caring for patients and listed a whole spate of other measures to improve public healthcare in the late 1970s and first half of the 1980s.[189] A flurry of calls for greater attention to be paid to ethical issues was indicative of the rising tide of indifference and malpractice. It might also have signaled a greater political willingness to recognize and address the problems. There were so many "scandalous cases of malpractice" that Brezhnev attacked corruption in the public healthcare service in his 1981 speech to the party congress.[190] Corruption and the black market had become a common feature of people's lives in the later years of Soviet power. Healthcare workers pilfered "medicine and equipment from factories, hospitals, polyclinics, and pharmacies" where they worked and then sold these items on the black market.[191] Brezhnev's calls for reform in the early 1980s had fallen on deaf ears: in 1988 and 1989, some thirty-three thousand medical workers were reprimanded on charges of bribery and theft.[192] Corruption, nepotism, and patronage pervaded Soviet medical education too, with incompetent students often graduating as a result.[193] Some scholars have asserted that "ideological commitment to the collective, and to socialist goals in general" could no longer avert the favoritism and corruption that were so rife in the late 1970s.[194] Economic stagnation and bureaucracy forced many nurses and medical workers, as well as Soviet citizens more broadly, to engage in extralegal activities to make ends meet.

By 1981 Soviet healthcare expenditures dropped to negative figures and "health conditions in Soviet society demonstrably worsened."[195] Although the Tenth Five-Year Plan provided nurses with an 18 percent pay increase by 1980[196] the rate of inflation and corruption likely negated it. Nurses and other junior- and middle-level workers continued to feel the pinch. Often working weekends and holidays and doing the work of others because of high turnover and staff shortages, the Soviet Union's over two million nurses were no better off than before and searched for easier work for a similar salary.[197] Low pay meant that half of all junior and middle medical worker positions remained vacant by 1984.[198]

Indeed, the exodus of nurses from the profession precipitated a great deal of concern, so much so that the national press again devoted considerable attention to the issue.[199] One elevator operator interviewed in *Izvestiia* in 1984 referred to the nurse's salary as "ridiculous" and claimed that he would never let his daughter enter the profession.[200] But when asked if they regretted their career choice or wished they could change it, nurses generally replied in the negative and regretted only that their multitude of various responsibilities "left little time for them to care for patients."[201] Despite these mounting problems and worsening conditions in the early 1980s, nurses and nurse councils continued to organize "best nurse" competitions to reward nurses for good "cultural behavior" and a "communist attitude to work."[202] Political, ideological, and economic mobilization was so deeply embedded in the culture of medical institutions and the lives of their workers that they betrayed no signs of a political system about to unravel. Problems had always existed, after all.

At the Twenty-Sixth Party Congress in 1982, Brezhnev stated that the Soviet person should "always and everywhere receive timely, qualified, and sensitive medical assistance."[203] One of the issues identified in Brezhnev's speech was letters of complaint from patients citing medical worker infringements and lack of attention toward people. To this end, the party wanted to improve the quality of medical service and "moral relations in the sphere of public healthcare."[204] Students in medical institutes were to learn that "knowledge and morality" went hand in hand.[205] Medical ethics essentially concerned norms of "behavior and morals, professional duty, honor, conscience, and dignity."[206] These norms or ethics were to inform how medical workers interacted with patients, their relatives, their colleagues, and society more generally. They were most often discussed in detail with regard to professionalism and humanity and as a response to party calls to improve the standard of public healthcare. Nurse publications had discussed the "moral character" of medical workers since the 1950s. By the 1980s a "deontological code" that spoke more specifically to nurse-patient relations guided contributors.[207] A. L. Ostapenko, a professor who worked in the Ministry of Health administration in Moscow and a regular contributor to medical journals, argued that nurses did not show enough compassion to patients. He wanted readers to understand that "mercy" was an important element in ethical and moral discussions.[208] He also differentiated between legal and deontological norms between the nurse and the patient: medical institutes taught legal standards and included doctor-patient confidentiality, while deontology was more connected to care and "humanism."[209] The difference between capitalist and socialist medical workers, Ostapenko wrote elsewhere, was that, in the former, a person's duty was an individual rather than a collective issue, whereas the opposite was true in socialist ethics. Quoting Friedrich Engels, he stated: "Every class and even every profession has their own morals."[210]

But these efforts seemed to be in vain. One of Yuri Andropov's first tasks in power in 1982 was to prevent Soviet people sliding into "an abyss of complete demoralization."[211] In 1985 a group of patients from an unidentified but "well-known clinic" wrote a letter to a nurse that was published in *Komsomol Truth* (*Komsomol'skaia pravda*). The patients informed the nurse that they dreaded her shifts and could not wait for them to end: her presence nullified the efforts of doctors and other nurses, so that the patients had "no peace of mind."[212] They told her to either change her behavior or get a different job.[213] Patients had complained throughout the Soviet period (and the above incident is reminiscent of the Lesnikov and Prokof'eva case from chapter 2), but the situation was so bad under Gorbachev that some argued it undermined his leadership.[214] The Soviet Union was by now a vast, creaking entity. The war in Afghanistan following Soviet military intervention in 1979 was costing lives, and Brezhnev himself had become an embarrassment for Russians, who mocked his bemedaled chest and incoherence when delivering public speeches. Andropov (until February 1984) and Konstantin Chernenko (until March 1985) did not live or remain in power long enough to make a difference.

Gorbachev's rise to power in 1985 wrought radical political change and a worsening crisis in the healthcare service. By this time, the moral and ethical bar had lowered considerably. In major hospitals such as the Botkin, home to that seemingly propitious meeting with *Nurse* editors in 1952, "problems with labor discipline," including punctuality, leaving work early, and unfulfilled doctors' orders, seemed rife.[215] Senior nurses agreed that they needed to be "more strict and principled about these violations" and should promptly review all cases of misconduct.[216] Senior nurses also reported a lowering of nurse discipline during night shifts.[217] To tackle the problems, the Botkin's council of nurses proposed "strengthening discipline during night work by establishing a brigade of senior nurses for night-time attendance to check sanitary

conditions and raise work discipline."[218] Those who violated ethics and deontology faced disciplinary measures.[219] Some of the violations included being
drunk at work. Two nurses, who had worked in the neurological department
for a year and a half, were drunk while on duty in February 1987.[220] The Soviet government and the Ministry of Health were under no illusions about
the problems plaguing healthcare. Decrees issued in 1986 and 1987 made direct
connections between improvements in public healthcare and medical workers, specifically their standard of living and qualifications. The decrees finally
acknowledged that attestation was necessary for a wider range of middle medical workers, including nurses in various specializations.[221]

Patient care seemed to be at an all-time low, and good care now came at
considerable cost for patients. Payment for medical service had become a common and problematic feature of public healthcare. One patient's hospital expenses in 1987 came to 100 rubles: 60 rubles for treatment and the rest for
nursing care. Relatives covered the costs of food, and his mother paid a nanny
to wash him. The patient was a head engineer and feared that others might
not be in a position to pay for care.[222] A woman complained that her husband's
hospital stay for medical tests cost the family 300 rubles (50 rubles for a place
in the ward, 1 ruble for clean sheets, and so on). Worst of all was the maternity hospital, which could cost 500 rubles.[223] Medical personnel traditionally
received a small token after a child was born, but typically this was a ruble.[224]
By the late 1980s, nurses expected 25 rubles for a newborn boy and 10 for a
girl.[225] Blaming bribery and corruption in socialist society on "old tsarist ways"
would no longer fly. Communism was getting further out of reach.

Still, there were those who fervently continued to believe in communism
and Lenin. The nurse Anna Andreevna Avseeva was one such person. She
wrote a letter to a Leningrad newspaper setting out plans for a communist
utopia "in the spirit of Chernyshevsky" and told her story in the 1988 documentary film *The Fourth Sleep of Anna Andreevna (Chetvertyi son Anny Andreevny)*.[226] Born on the day the Soviet state was established, she was a true
believer in communism and the Communist Party, which she also explained
in a letter to Brezhnev. Talking about her life, including time spent in the labor
camps and her firm commitment to setting up and running a medical station
in the town of Bratsk, Irkutsk Province, nurse Avseeva demonstrates resilience
and firmness and is dedicated to her dream of building a communist utopia.
Far away in a remote part of Russia, we see glimpses of her daily life and work.
Even though she sterilizes syringes by boiling them, and clearly has a difficult
life, she does not seem to grow despondent but argues that building communism is complicated. "Confused" by Gorbachev's perestroika and not impressed by Khrushchev, Avseeva has her own ideals.

Back in Moscow, Minister of Health Yevgeny Chazov was scathing in his comments about Soviet healthcare in 1987 and 1988. In several publications and speeches, he criticized its poorly trained doctors, dilapidated facilities, the lack of equipment and medicines, low wages, corruption, and an inattentive attitude to patients.[227] Polls also indicated high levels of public dissatisfaction since the beginning of the 1980s.[228] The main reasons for the problems in the healthcare sector—namely, wage leveling, hierarchies, and corruption—had long been self-evident to many medical workers. Interviewed in the 1990 film, *Oh, Thank You Doctor,* an impassioned Chazov called "shame on the state and on himself as minister" for failing medical workers.[229] In the same film, Sul'povar (the impoverished surgeon) rails against those in leadership positions who talked about the need for improvement—he was "not able to listen to this" and "didn't believe any slogans about free medicine" because it did not exist; in fact, he said, medicine was "getting more expensive" and perestroika was "just conversations"—"something needed to be done." Seventy years of socialism had not managed to produce an effective, functional healthcare system that provided good quality care to Soviet citizens. The closing scene of *Oh, Thank You Doctor* captured the desperation and hope. Commenting on the birth of quadruplets, the narrator wonders which baby will be the future president—a president who can solve all the problems in Soviet public healthcare.

The hope and optimism of the mid-1950s and the 1960s quickly fizzled out. Ongoing spending on defense and military needs overshadowed consumer interests. Increased spending on healthcare did not translate into better living and working conditions for medical workers or higher standards of care for Soviet citizens. Initiatives to rally people around collective activism in the public interest could go only so far in masking deeper problems. People might have believed in Khrushchev's and Brezhnev's ideological crusades to make the Soviet Union a more humanist place, asserting the superiority of communism, but widespread corruption, bureaucracy, and negligence undermined the credibility of these campaigns. The literary critic Vera Dunham famously described the "Big Deal" in late Stalinist society, that is, a kind of social contract between the state and members of society, namely, the nomenclature and the intelligentsia.[230] Medical workers were not part of any deal. The state did not depend on the loyalty of medical workers—they were hardly a powerful entity, and hence nurses and other middle and junior medical workers continued to cope with low incomes and negotiated the system on their own terms.

But there were telltale signs that something was amiss with socialism, or at least the Soviet brand of socialism. Harking back to the good old days of the Sisters of Mercy and Pirogov—anathema to the original Soviet project—indicated that socialism might have been morally barren at its core. Victoria Smolkin has shown that atheism never really took root in Soviet society because people remained drawn to religious rituals and traditions, a void that atheism never quite filled.[231] When the dust settled after the Great Patriotic War, the harsh realities of life under socialism returned. What could the Soviet state really offer its people? After the initial euphoria of success in space and scientific progress, the unrelenting everyday problems in securing housing, access to good healthcare, and consumer shortages, as well as rising alcoholism and divorce rates, left a bitter taste.

The world's worst nuclear disaster in Chernobyl in 1986 was illustrative of ongoing disregard for people's health and well-being. But the scale of Chernobyl, and especially the slow official response in dealing with its aftermath, was a deeper manifestation of the widespread lack of responsibility in Soviet politics and society. Problems were shunted aside or ignored. For nurses and other medical workers, the consequences of socialist policy since the revolution took their toll. The physical and mental scars of terror, industrialization, famine, and war; the aging population; high levels of drug abuse, alcoholism, and HIV, all placed medical workers and the healthcare system under enormous strain. Within a few years, the Soviet state would be no more.

Epilogue

In the 1980s, Soviet public healthcare suffered from the wider sociopolitical crisis that engulfed the country. At a special international nursing conference in Vienna in 1988, nurses from thirty-two European countries—including the Soviet Union—gathered to discuss issues affecting the profession.[1] The conference led to a recommendation to the World Health Organization (WHO) whereby the governments of all participant countries would introduce reforms in nursing. Some assert that the Vienna conference instigated changes in Russian nursing in the form of All-Union conferences and meetings called to discuss the profession.[2] In November 1987 the Ministry of Health issued a resolution on the development and reconstruction of Soviet healthcare in a twelve-year plan. The following year it introduced a new study plan recognizing the "fundamentals of nursing" as a discipline for the first time.[3] While the nursing profession underwent reforms, the daily lives of nurses continued to meet with hardship during and after perestroika. As the Soviet state foundered economically (not to mention politically), medical professionals and patients struggled to cope with rapidly deteriorating conditions.

Nonetheless, reforming nursing was necessary and important. Welfare benefits and public healthcare were, after all, usually thought of highly by Soviet citizens, who valued free access to medical care. Those interviewed as part of the Soviet interview project[4] considered public healthcare to be one of the features of the Soviet system worth keeping if the Bolshevik regime ended.[5] Although satisfaction levels depended on generation, gender, education, location, and economics, Soviet people on the whole appreciated socialized medicine.[6] Nursing reforms could represent an important step to more wide-ranging healthcare reforms and better standards of care.

But the proposed reforms of the late 1980s were not the first major efforts to overhaul nursing in line with international norms. The Soviet Union attempted to address nursing problems a decade earlier when it signed up to implement international nursing standards alongside a host of other countries. In 1979 it ratified the International Labor Organization (ILO) and WHO's Nursing Personnel Convention C 149 (1977), a response to the global shortage of nurses.[7] It is worth citing the convention's rationale:

> Recognizing the vital role played by nursing personnel, together with other workers in the field of health, in the protection and improvement of the health and welfare of the population, and . . . noting that the present situation of nursing personnel in many countries in which there is a shortage of qualified persons and existing staff are not always utilized to best effect, is an obstacle to the development of effective health services.[8]

To be sure, some of the problems the Soviet Union was experiencing, at least in terms of nursing, were endemic to the Soviet system and had been for a long time. And while Soviet efforts to reform nursing require scrutiny in light of a rapidly deteriorating economic and political situation at home, it is worth noting that reforms also took place within the context of an unfavorable global climate for nursing. The nursing crisis was Soviet and international. The crisis also outlived the Soviet Union and major geopolitical shifts. As the ILO stated in its 2002 version of the Nursing Personnel Convention, large numbers of trained personnel do not practice and shortages only lead to increased patient morbidity and mortality, violence in the workplace, and job dissatisfaction.[9] We need to view the serious problems that plagued the Soviet healthcare system, and nursing in particular, through a broader lens.

Once released from the ideological constraints of the Soviet Union and the debilitating military-industrial complex, nurses set about instigating change and engaging with colleagues in Europe and North America. Education and training were addressed first. In 1991, faculties of nursing were established in the Sechenov Medical Academy in Moscow and the Samara State Medical Institute.[10] Over a period of four years, nurses, midwives, and feldshers would train as nursing lecturers and organizers.[11] Russian nurses formed their own professional association in 1992 (legally registered in 1994), with Valentina

Sarkisova at its helm, and they joined the International Council of Nurses (ICN) in 2005.[12] When I asked Sarkisova about Russian nurses' knowledge of the profession in the West, she explained that Soviet nurses were aware of nurse movements abroad and that this knowledge helped shape Russian nursing in the 1990s:

> We always heard about the professional nursing movement in the world. We were familiar with the work of Florence Nightingale and knew the domestic history as well, the efforts of the Pirogov movement to advance nursing during the Crimean War. When we established our professional association, we knew about nursing associations in the world, in America, Canada, England, in many other countries—associations that could strongly influence nursing professionalism. So when we met American colleagues, we had a desire to develop a project titled "New Nurse for the New Russia," aimed at [an] increased influence of nurses on their profession. Establishing the association was a natural step in implementing the project and toward strengthening the nurses' voice.[13]

Russian nurses were and continue to be in dialogue with nurses elsewhere. Like nurses around the world, Russian nurses celebrate International Nurses Day on May 12, the anniversary of Florence Nightingale's birth. They welcome international links and exchanges. Indeed, after interviewing Sarkisova, her colleagues offered me Danish cookies, a gift from nurses in Denmark who had recently met with Russian Nurses Association members.

The Russian Nurses Association liaises with the Russian Ministry of Health, trade unions, and other organizations. It also has regional branches across the Russian Federation. Nurses in Russia finally have their own professional representation. A nursing code of ethics followed in 1997, and discussions of ethics and deontology continue to this day.[14] The Russian Nurses Association's section on ethics deals with patient complaints at the regional level; complaints deemed serious are dealt with at the national level by the Ministry of Health.[15] Nowadays, nurses also have a much wider literature to read; when I asked a group of three nurses from a cardiology unit in a St. Petersburg clinic if they read *Nurse* or *Medical Worker*, and if they found these beneficial, they were quick to let me know about the variety of nursing literature available to them, including regional publications.[16] And they said the literature is very helpful to them.

Reforms have undoubtedly improved the nursing profession in Russia. Steps toward offering higher education to nurses have helped to stem the tide of nurses moving into medicine after they qualify as nurses. This was a positive development. In Sarkisova's words: "If you love the nursing profession, you have the opportunity to improve your qualification in that profession, and not become a doctor but a good nurse. It's better to be a good nurse [*laughs*] than a bad doctor. It means that if you love your profession, you can remain in it."[17] Baccalaureate degrees in nursing were approved only in 2013, although physicians continue to teach in nursing programs. After four years of study, student doctors can work as nurses, as they did in the Soviet period; thus a tendency to see nursing as a stepping-stone to medicine remains. Although, this has benefits—nurses I interviewed said that doctors who worked as orderlies and nurses before qualifying as doctors had a good understanding of the subtleties of each profession.[18] Still, this is a hangover of the Soviet system, whether for good or bad.

Nursing in Russia, and globally, is confronted with many problems. Loving one's profession is important, but medical workers also need to be sufficiently remunerated for their commitment to what is an intellectually, physically, and emotionally difficult job. While some doctors and nurses receive good salaries, disparities nonetheless exist across the sector. Some Russian nurses in online forums complain about "miserly" wages, and others claim to earn their salaries elsewhere, treating their nursing work as a hobby that gives them spiritual rather than material reward.[19] While physicians maintain or increase their average salaries internationally, nurses continue to see their salaries and purchasing power drop.[20] According to the ICN, "There is an urgent need to give the world's nurses a pay rise and better working conditions in order to address the attractiveness of the profession." It further warns that "all governments have a responsibility to ensure the safety and security of their citizens and this includes having a sufficient number of healthcare professionals, because the consequences of not are detrimental to human health and mortality."[21] When we are the patient lying in a hospital bed, do we really want to be cared for by an overworked and exhausted nurse? And if countries continue to undervalue nurses, paying them meager salaries, few will be drawn to the profession.

Coda

Almost fifty years after war and revolution, public healthcare standards remained low. An *American Journal of Nursing* article, published in 1966, described a composite profile of a Soviet nurse, written by an US nurse who had been living in Moscow for ten months. The nurse, "Nadia," was "intensely proud of both her profession and her country."[1] The author attributes this sense of pride to the "system" or "tradition" of free medical care that dated back to the nineteenth century and that was still considered to be the root of the high degree of humanitarianism present in the medical professions in the 1960s. But pride could go only so far; the spirit of humanitarianism was being suffocated by worsening economic and political conditions by the late 1970s.

Like socialism itself, the nursing profession in the Soviet Union underwent a crisis of morality in the 1980s. The sense of public hopelessness in Soviet healthcare was palpable by the end of that decade. The public healthcare system had managed to survive the early 1920s, another time of immense desperation, and recovered from the devastation of the Great Patriotic War. But the world was a very different place in the 1980s, and the Soviet brand of socialism seemed to be of a different time. People traveled abroad and listened to foreign radio; they knew the Soviet Union lagged behind European and North American standards of living. The state could conceal the contradictions no longer. It was trapped in the false dichotomies it had created.

Nurses such as "Nadia" show us that people were committed to their jobs and to helping others. But there is no doubt that nurses and other medical workers were disillusioned with socialism and the revolution. They were disappointed with the Soviet state and felt that they had been let down. Low salaries and miserable working and living conditions undermined their satisfaction with politics and ideology. Their daily lives seemed to be a constant battle to make ends meet, and while the public health authorities recognized their difficulties in principle, they continued to fail their medical workers in practice. Workers in industry were lauded for their achievements, but medical workers did not quite fit that proletarian mold. Medical workers were overwhelmingly women, and female emancipation largely resulted in nurses and other medical workers carrying a double burden. Class and gender obstacles marginalized many medical workers, and even the opportunities that the Soviet state granted, such as upward mobility, had its limitations as the medical profession as a whole was not well remunerated. Upward mobility also tended to devalue nursing and create cadre deficits.

Questions around care under communism tell us much about social values and responsibilities. In many ways, the Bolshevik revolution did not cause many of the problems afflicting public healthcare. Turnover, issues about junior medical workers as primary caregivers, difficult living and working conditions, and low pay already made life very hard for nurses and other medical workers. But successive governments never managed to sufficiently deal with these matters. The struggle to balance medicine and care remained ongoing. Providing pay increases meant little when wages already started from a low base and inflation was rising. That said, the principles and values underlying socialist healthcare were admirable, and the mission to provide high standards of care was always present. Envisioning care under communism was not completely utopian but often pragmatic and sometimes innovative. And while some Soviet citizens—not just the elites, but ordinary people—did experience genuine care at the hands of nurses, that was not a guarantee for all. The various stakeholders in Soviet public healthcare spent a great deal of time discussing patient care, but these discussions often remained just that. The military-industrial complex reigned supreme. Consequently, resources for areas such as healthcare suffered. Care is a basic human right, not a utopian fantasy. Irrespective of ideology, states need to properly provide for their nurses and patients.

NOTES

Introduction

1. B. M. Potulov, *V. I. Lenin i okhrana zdorov'ia sovetskogo naroda* [V. I. Lenin and the health protection of the Soviet people] (Moscow: Meditsina, 1980), 266–267.

2. Potulov, *V. I. Lenin*, 266–267.

3. N. L. Rutkevich, "Otlichnaia meditsinskaia sestra" [An excellent nurse], *Meditsinskaia sestra*, no. 4 (1948): 29–30.

4. Rutkevich, "Otlichnaia meditsinskaia sestra," 29–30. See also V. F. Egorov, "Zhizn', dostoinaia prekloneniia" [A life worthy of worship], *Meditsinskaia sestra*, no. 10 (1969): 57–58.

5. Rutkevich, "Otlichnaia meditsinskaia sestra," 30.

6. Karl Schlögel, *Moscow, 1937*, trans. Rodney Livingstone (Cambridge, UK: Polity Press, 2012).

7. Much of the literature on nursing focuses on the late nineteenth and early twentieth centuries. See, for example, Natalia L. Lopatkina, *Kul'turologicheskie aspekty v razvitii sestrinskogo dela* [Cultural studies aspects in the development of nursing], (Kemerovo: Aksioma, 2009); A. V. Posternak, *Ocherki po istorii obshchin sester miloserdiia* [Essays on the history of the sister of mercy communities], (Moscow: Sviato-Dmitrievskoe uchilishche sester miloserdiia, 2001); Elena Kozlovtseva, *Moskovskie obshchiny sester miloserdiia v XIX–nachale XX veka* [Moscow sister of mercy communities in the nineteenth century to the beginning of the twentieth century] (Moscow: Pravoslavnyi Sviato-Tikhonovskii gumanitarnyi universitet, 2010); V. P. Romaniuk, V. A. Lapotnikov, and Ia. A. Nakatis, *Istoriia sestrinskogo dela v Rossii* [The history of nursing in Russia], (St. Petersburg: Sankt-Peterburgskaia gosudarstvennaia meditsinskaia akademiia, 1998); and Laurie Stoff, *Russia's Sisters of Mercy and the Great War: More than Binding Men's Wounds* (Lawrence: University Press of Kansas, 2015).

8. They especially targeted the field feldshers, who had little training other than that gained during war. Schooled feldshers received more substantive training and continued to do so into the Soviet period.

9. Sheila Fitzpatrick, *Everyday Stalinism: Ordinary Life in Extraordinary Times; Soviet Russia in the 1930s* (New York: Oxford University Press, 1999).

10. Royal College of Nursing, "Setting Appropriate Ward Nurse Staffing Levels in NHS Acute Trusts," accessed April 13, 2018, https://www.rcn.org.uk/about-us/policy-briefings/br-0518.

11. Royal College of Nursing, "Ward Nurse Staffing Levels."

12. Royal College of Nursing, "Briefing: Patient Safety Adjournment Debate—Wednesday 28 March 2018," accessed April 13, 2018, https://www.rcn.org.uk/about-us/policy-briefings/br-0518.

13. American Nurses Association, "Safe Staffing," discussion of the Safe Staffing for Nurse and Patient Safety Act (S. 2446, H.R. 5052), accessed November 30, 2018, https://ana.aristotle.com/SitePages/safestaffing.aspx. Similar arguments about care and nursing are made in Sioban Nelson and Suzanne Gordon, introduction to *The Complexities of Care: Nursing Reconsidered*, ed. Sioban Nelson and Suzanne Gordon (Ithaca, NY: ILR Press, an imprint of Cornell University Press, 2006), 1–12.

14. See Suzanne Gordon, *Nursing against the Odds: How Health Care Cost Cutting, Media Stereotypes, and Medical Hubris Undermine Nurses and Patient Care* (Ithaca, NY: ILR Press, an imprint of Cornell University Press, 2005), especially discussion on 4–16.

15. A "deficit of 25,000 doctors in the ambulatory-polyclinic section." Statistics from Rosstat, Schetnaia palata [Accounts chamber], 17, cited in Nataliia Nekhlebova, "Na grani izzhivaniia" [On the verge of extinction], *Ogonek*, no. 37 (October 23, 2019): 14–17. My thanks to Botakoz Kassymbekova for this article.

16. Nekhlebova, "Na grani izzhivaniia," 15–16. The Ministry of Health attributed the decision to qualifications and standards.

17. Susan M. Reverby, "The Duty or Right to Care? Nursing and Womanhood in Historical Perspective," in *Circles of Care: Work and Identity in Women's Lives*, ed. Emily K. Abel and Margaret K. Nelson (Albany: State University of New York Press, 1990), 133.

18. Altruism is "assumed to be the basis of caring," while autonomy is "assumed to be the basis of rights." Reverby, "Duty or Right to Care?," 133.

19. See Hafeeza Anchrum, Taryn Pochon, and Julie Fairman, "Gender: A Useful Category of Analysis for the History of Nursing," in *Russian and Soviet Health Care from an International Perspective: Comparing Professions, Practice and Gender, 1880–1960*, ed. Susan Grant (London: Palgrave Macmillan, 2017), 127–128.

20. See Rosemary Pringle, *Sex and Medicine: Gender, Power and Authority in the Medical Profession* (Cambridge: Cambridge University Press, 1998), 4.

21. See Susan Grant, introduction to *Russian and Soviet Health Care from an International Perspective: Comparing Professions, Practice and Gender, 1880–1960*, ed. Susan Grant (London: Palgrave Macmillan, 2017), 10–14. On gender and prestige, see Chris Burton, "Medical Welfare During Late Stalinism. A Study of Doctors and the Soviet Health System, 1945–53" (PhD diss.: University of Chicago, 2000), 176–184.

22. This problem is still evident in contemporary international nursing, where tensions in professional healthcare relationships can have harmful outcomes on a patient's health. See Gordon, *Nursing against the Odds*, especially 4–16.

23. Here I am drawing on the psychologist Nancy Eisenberg's definition, as discussed in Robert C. Solomon, *True to Our Feelings: What Our Emotions Are Really Telling Us* (New York: Oxford University Press, 2007), 66.

24. Susan E. Reid discusses the meanings of care in "'Palaces in Our Hearts': Caring for Khrushchevki," in *Architecture, Democracy, and Emotions: The Politics of Feeling since 1945*, ed. Till Grossmann and Philipp Nielson (London: Routledge, 2019), 141–174.

25. Nelson and Gordon, introduction to *Complexities of Care*, 5.

26. Nelson and Gordon, introduction to *Complexities of Care*, 7. Such narratives of care relate to the "virtue script." For more discussion, see Susan Grant, "Creating Cadres of Soviet Nurses, 1936–1941," in *Russian and Soviet Health Care from an International*

Perspective: Comparing Professions, Practice and Gender, 1880–1960, ed. Susan Grant (London: Palgrave Macmillan, 2017), 60.

27. For discussion of identities, see Charles Taylor, *Sources of the Self: The Making of the Modern Identity* (Cambridge, MA: Harvard University Press, 1989), 35–37. Thanks to Anatoly Pinsky for bringing Charles Taylor's book to my attention.

28. For discussion of the origin of nursing and the role of virtue and ethics, see Suzanne Gordon and Sioban Nelson, "Moving beyond the Virtue Script in Nursing: Creating a Knowledge-Based Identity for Nurses," in *The Complexities of Care: Nursing Reconsidered*, ed. Sioban Nelson and Suzanne Gordon (Ithaca, NY: ILR Press, an imprint of Cornell University Press, 2006), 18–19.

29. On Eliot Freidson, Andrew Abbott, and others, see Robert Dingwall, Anne Marie Rafferty, and Charles Webster, *An Introduction to the Social History of Nursing* (London: Routledge, 1988), 5.

30. Janice Ryder Ellis and Celia Love Hartley, *Nursing in Today's World: Challenges, Issues, and Trends*, 7th ed. (1980; Philadelphia: Lippincott Williams & Wilkins, 2001), 170–171. Here the authors discuss the criteria for a profession as outlined by Abraham Flexner in 1915, see A. Flexner, in Bernard LA, Walsh M: *Leadership: The Key to Professionalism of Nursing* (New York: John Wiley & Sons, 1981); Bixler and Bixler (1959), in Bixler GK, Bixler RW, "The professional status of nursing," *The American Journal of Nursing* 45 (9): 730, 1945; and Ronald M. Pavalko (1971), in Pavalko RM, *Sociology of Occupations and Professions* (Itasca, IL: Peacock Publishers, 1971). For excellent discussion of the Flexner Report and its impact on medical education, including in the Soviet Union, see Chris Burton, "Medical Welfare During Late Stalinism. A Study of Doctors and the Soviet Health System, 1945–53," (PhD dissertation: University of Chicago, 2000), 163–164.

31. Ellis and Hartley, *Nursing in Today's World*, 170–174.

32. Ellis and Hartley, *Nursing in Today's World*, 175.

33. Nelson and Gordon, introduction to *Complexities of Care*, 3.

34. Nelson and Gordon, introduction to *Complexities of Care*, 4. Nelson and Gordon's discussion of problems in narratives of nursing care can apply just as easily to the Soviet context.

35. Ellis and Hartley, *Nursing in Today's World*, 164.

36. Ellis and Hartley, *Nursing in Today's World*, 166.

37. Virginia Henderson, *The Nature of a Science of Nursing* (New York: Macmillan, 1966), 15, cited in Ellis and Hartley, *Nursing in Today's World*, 167.

38. Ellis and Hartley, *Nursing in Today's World*, 168.

39. Ellis and Hartley, *Nursing in Today's World*, 168–169.

40. V. V. Murashko and L. S. Tapinskii (eds.), preface to *Uchebnik dlia podgotovki mladshikh meditsinskikh sester po ukhody za bol'nymi* [Textbook for training junior medical nurses in patient care], ed. V. V. Murashko and L. S. Tapinskii, 2nd ed. (Moscow: Meditsina, 1979), 3.

41. Murashko and Tapinskii, preface to *Uchebnik dlia podgotovki*, 18. The preface is only pp. 3–4, and the writers of it are also the editors.

42. See *Meditsinskaia sestra* and legislation from December 19, 1969, "Ob utverzhdenii Osnov zakonodatel'stva Soiuza SSR i soiuznykh respublik o zdravookhranenii." A full list is available on the *Large Medical Encyclopedia* website, accessed November 26, 2020, https://бмэ.орг/index.php/ЗАКОНОДАТЕЛЬСТВО_О_ЗДРАВООХРАНЕНИИ.

43. Murashko and Tapinskii, *Uchebnik dlia podgotovki*, 19.

44. Murashko and Tapinskii, *Uchebnik dlia podgotovki*, 19–20.

45. M. K. Sh., "Pochemu ia ne prazdnovala 1–3 maia?" [Why did I not celebrate 1–3 May?] *Meditsinskii rabotnik*, no. 8 (1923): 18.

46. Sh., "Pochemu ia ne prazdnovala."

47. Sioban Nelson, "Ethical Expertise and the Problem of the Good Nurse," in *The Complexities of Care: Nursing Reconsidered*, ed. Sioban Nelson and Suzanne Gordon (Ithaca, NY: ILR Press, an imprint of Cornell University Press, 2006), 76. Here Nelson discusses the work of the nursing theorist Patricia Benner and the neo-Aristotelians.

48. Nelson, "Ethical Expertise," 78.

49. In the classic tradition morality is the question of right or wrong, whereas ethics is concerned with the good life. See Solomon, *True to Our Feelings*, x. Solomon categorizes emotions as personal and in the realm of ethics.

50. See Taylor, *Sources of the Self*, 3–4. Taylor argues against a reductionist understanding of morality and is critical of moral philosophy that focuses too narrowly on right and wrong rather than on "what it is good to be" or the good life. Taylor, *Sources of the Self*, 3; see also 4–9.

51. Taylor, *Sources of the Self*, 13–14. As Taylor notes, this argument goes back to Aristotelian ethics. See also Solomon, *True to Our Feelings*, x.

52. These could be described as the twelve commandments for communism, introduced under Nikita Khrushchev. Moral Code of the Builders of Communism, Seventeen Moments in Soviet History, Macalester College and Michigan State University, accessed December 18, 2020, http://soviethistory.msu.edu/1961-2/moral-code-of-the-builder-of-communism/moral-code-of-the-builder-of-communism-texts/moral-code-of-the-builder-of-communism/.

53. Suzanne Gordon, "The New Cartesianism: Dividing Mind and Body and Thus Disembodying Care," in *The Complexities of Care: Nursing Reconsidered*, ed. Sioban Nelson and Suzanne Gordon (Ithaca, NY: ILR Press, an imprint of Cornell University Press, 2006), 106–107.

54. See, for example, Suzanne Gordon and Sioban Nelson, "Moving Beyond the Virtue Script in Nursing," in *The Complexities of Care: Nursing Reconsidered*, ed. Sioban Nelson and Suzanne Gordon (Ithaca, NY: ILR Press, an imprint of Cornell University Press, 2006), 26.

55. Harvard Project on the Soviet Social System Online (hereafter HPSSS), accessed November 18, 2020, https://library.harvard.edu/sites/default/files/static/collections/hpsss/about.html#about; I Remember / Ia pomniu, accessed November 18, 2020, https://iremember.ru/about/.

56. For example, see Alessandro Portelli, *The Death of Luigi Trastulli, and Other Stories: Form and Meaning in Oral History*, Suny Series in Oral and Public History (Albany: State University of New York Press, 1991).

1. War and Revolution

1. Adele Lindenmeyr, *Poverty Is Not a Vice: Charity, Society, and the State in Imperial Russia* (Princeton, NJ: Princeton University Press, 1996), 125. Eighteenth- and nineteenth-century institutions of care included "educational houses" (*vospitatel'nye domov*), established in 1715, and the House of Compassionate Widows, established in 1818.

2. Dasha Sevastopolskaia (Daria Lavrentievna Mikhailovna) was a fifteen-year-old orphan who assisted doctors during the war and received a silver medal and gold cross, inscribed "Sevastopol." See Natalia L. Lopatkina, *Kul'turologicheskie aspekty v razvitii sestrinskogo dela* [Cultural studies aspects in the development of nursing] (Kemerovo: Aksioma, 2009), 94–95. Grand Duchess Elena Pavlovna was born in Stuttgart as Princess Charlotte Marie of Württemberg. The Russian Orthodox Church gave her the name Elena Pavlovna in 1823, and the following year she married Grand Duke Mikhail Pavlovich of Russia. Bakunina was from St. Petersburg, where her father was governor. Pirogov was a prominent physician. For fuller biographies and analysis of the three figures, see Inge Hendriks, Dmitry Zhuravlyov, James Bovill, Fredrik Boer, and Pancras Hogendoorn, "Women in Healthcare in Imperial Russia: The Contribution of the Surgeon Nikolay I. Pirogov," *Journal of Medical Biography* 29, no. 1 (2019): 9–18.

3. Nikolai Pirogov from a letter to E. F. Raden, February 27, 1876, in *Vishnia. Pirogov, Sevastopol'skie pis'ma i vospominaniia* [Cherry. Pirogov, Sevastopol' letters and memoirs], (Moscow, 1950), 209, cited in A. V. Posternak, *Ocherki po istorii obshchin sester miloserdiia* [Essays on the history of the sister of mercy communities] (Moscow: Sviato-Dmitrievskoe uchilishche sester miloserdiia, 2001), 89–90.

4. Pirogov to Raden, 209, cited in Posternak, *Ocherki po istorii obshchin*, 89–90.

5. Pirogov to Raden, 209, cited in Posternak, *Ocherki po istorii obshchin*, 90.

6. See Posternak, *Ocherki po istorii obshchin*, 54, 55. Biller arrived in St. Petersburg in 1820, responding to the tsar's general call to set up a school for poor girls. For more on Quakers in Russia, see Barbara Addison, comp., "Recent Scholarship in Quaker History, 2010," Friends Historical Association, accessed January 25, 2021, https://static1 .squarespace.com/static/565478bfe4b0d39ff6af7738/t/566f25f705f8e23e24cd1975 /1450124791156/FHA_booklist_2010.pdf.

7. Posternak, *Ocherki po istorii obshchin*, 55.

8. *Istoricheskii ocherk Sviato-Troitskoi obshchiny sester miloserdiia v Peterburge za 50-letie (1844–1894)* [Historical essay on the Saint Trotsky sister of mercy community in St. Petersburg over 50 years (1844–1894)] (St. Petersburg: 1898), cited in V. P. Romaniuk, V. A. Lapotnikov, and Ia. A. Nakatis, *Istoriia sestrinskogo dela v Rossii* [The history of nursing in Russia], (St. Petersburg: Sankt-Peterburgskaia gosudarstvennaia meditsinskaia akademiia, 1998), 35.

9. A. A. Shibkov, *Pervye zhenshchiny-mediki Rossii* [The First women-medics in Russia] (Leningrad, 1961), 51. These included the Sturdzovskaia (1850), Pokrovkaia (1858), Saint Georgiia (1870), Kharkovskaia (1872), Blagoveshchenskaia (1875), and Tiflisskaia (1876) communities.

10. P. V. Vlasov, *Istoriia obrazovaniia meditsinskikh sester v Rossii* [The history of nursing education in Russia], (Medsestra, 1987), cited in Romaniuk, Lapotnikov, and Nakatis, *Istoriia sestrinskogo dela v Rossii*, 39.

11. See John Shelton Curtiss, "Russian Sisters of Mercy in the Crimea," *Slavic Review* 25, no. 1 (1966): 84–100; Posternak, *Ocherki po istorii obshchin*, 67; and Central State Archive of the Supreme Organs of Government and Administration of Ukraine (hereafter TsDAVO), f. R-4616, op. 1, d. 109, l. 59, 1957.

12. Shibkov, *Pervye zhenshchiny-mediki Rossii*, 19. Most of the Exaltation of the Cross community's 202 members in 1854–1856 were lower nobility (primarily from families in the bureaucracy)—a figure that stood at 77. A further 48 members were from military families (officers) and 38 were from bourgeois, middle-class families (*meshchanskii*).

13. Evelyn R. Benson, "On the Other Side of the Battle: Russian Nurses in the Crimean War," *Journal of Nursing Scholarship* 24, no. 1 (1992): 66. The charters of each Sisters of Mercy community varied slightly.

14. Benson, "Other Side of the Battle," 66.

15. A. G. Katsnel'bogen, *Geroinia trekh voin* [The heroine of three wars] (Klin. med: 1990, no. 2), 139–142, cited in Romaniuk, Lapotnikov, and Nakatis, *Istoriia sestrinskogo dela v Rossii*, 40.

16. Katsnel'bogen, *Geroinia trekh voin*, cited in Romaniuk, Lapotnikov, and Nakatis, *Istoriia sestrinskogo dela v Rossii*, 40 (italics in secondary source).

17. Benson, "Other Side of the Battle," 67.

18. For a different perspective, see Elizabeth Murray, "Russian Nurses: From the Tsarist Sister of Mercy to the Soviet Comrade Nurse; A Case Study of Absence of Migration of Nursing Knowledge and Skills," *Nursing Inquiry* 11, no. 3 (2004): 121.

19. See Michelle D. DenBeste-Barnett, "Earnestly Working to Improve Russia's Future: Russian Women Physicians, 1867–1905" (PhD diss., Southern Illinois University at Carbondale, 1997), 25–26.

20. A. A. Shibkov, *Zhenshchiny Rossii v meditsinskoi shkole i na voine* [Russian women in medical school and in war] (Leningrad: 1957), 14, cited in Romaniuk, Lapotnikov, and Nakatis, *Istoriia sestrinskogo dela v Rossii* [The history of nursing in Russia], 68, 72. Six received silver medals for their bravery.

21. Posternak, *Ocherki po istorii obshchin*, 97.

22. P. P. Shcherbinin, *Voennyi faktor v povsednevnoi zhizni russkoi zhenshchiny v XVIII–nachale XX v* [The war factor in the everyday lives of Russian women in the eighteenth to the beginning of the twentieth century] (Tambov: Izdatel'stvo Iulis, 2004), 364.

23. For statistics, see Shibkov, *Pervye zhenshchiny-mediki Rossii*, 50.

24. Shibkov, *Pervye zhenshchiny-mediki Rossii*, 50. Some thirty-six women's committees with twelve hundred members existed across Russia by 1876.

25. DenBeste-Barnett, "Working to Improve Russia's Future," 89–90.

26. See Michelle DenBeste, "Gender and Russian Health Care, 1880–1905: Professionalism and Practice," in *Russian and Soviet Health Care from an International Perspective: Comparing Professions, Practice and Gender, 1880–1960*, ed. Susan Grant (London: Palgrave Macmillan, 2017), 165–190.

27. DenBeste-Barnett, "Working to Improve Russia's Future," 160, 163.

28. Thomas Neville Bonner, *To the Ends of the Earth: Women's Search for Education in Medicine* (Cambridge, MA: Harvard University Press, 1995), 99.

29. Citation from *Vestnik ROKK* (1882), cited in Shibkov, *Pervye zhenshchiny-mediki Rossii*, 106.

30. *Vestnik ROKK*, cited in Shibkov, *Pervye zhenshchiny-mediki Rossii*, 106–108. Qualified midwives were rare in spite of medical college midwifery courses of two years' duration. Shibkov, *Pervye zhenshchiny-mediki Rossii*, 108.

31. Shibkov, *Pervye zhenshchiny-mediki Rossii*, 108.

32. Benson, "Other Side of the Battle," 67.

33. The feldsher-midwife schools accepted women between the ages of eighteen and twenty-eight years for courses of four years' duration. Shibkov, *Pervye zhenshchiny-mediki Rossii*, 108.

34. Shibkov, *Pervye zhenshchiny-mediki Rossii*, 108.

35. Romaniuk, Lapotnikov, and Nakatis, *Istoriia sestrinskogo dela v Rossii*, 63. The Russian Society for the Care of Injured and Sick Troops during War became the Russian Society of the Red Cross (ROKK) in 1873.

36. Elena Kozlovtseva's work on the Moscow communities provides an excellent example of the differences and commonalities between the communities. Elena Kozlovtseva, *Moskovskie obshchiny sester miloserdiia v XIX–nachale XX veka* [Moscow sister of mercy communities in the nineteenth century to the beginning of the twentieth century] (Moscow: Pravoslavnyi Sviato-Tikhonovskii gumanitarnyi universitet, 2010).

37. Romaniuk, Lapotnikov, and Nakatis, *Istoriia sestrinskogo dela v Rossii*, 43.

38. Romaniuk, Lapotnikov, and Nakatis, *Istoriia sestrinskogo dela v Rossii*, 66. These efforts were in St. Petersburg.

39. Romaniuk, Lapotnikov, and Nakatis, *Istoriia sestrinskogo dela v Rossii*, 66. Feldshers and midwives studied for three years.

40. Posternak, *Ocherki po istorii obshchin*, 122–123. Posternak cites S. A. Arendt and F. I. Feigan. S. A. Arendt, *Vospominaniia sestry miloserdiia (1877–1878)* [Memoirs of a sister of mercy (1877–1878)] (Russkaia starina, 1887, vol. 7), 99, and F. I. Feigan, *Nedostatki vrachebnoi pomoshchi v nashei deistvuiushchei armii v kampanii 1877–1878 gg.* [Shortcomings of medical care in our active army in the campaign of 1877–1878] (St. Petersburg, 1885), 35–36.

41. The new structure included a patron representing a committee of workers, nonpaying members, patrons, and ROKK members. Posternak, *Ocherki po istorii obshchin*, 129.

42. *Normal'nyi ustav obshchin sester miloserdiia Rossiiskogo obshchestvo Krasnogo Kresta* [The normal charter of the sisters of mercy communities of the Russian Society of the Red Cross] (Moscow, 1903), 66–67 [no. 39–40].

43. *Normal'nyi ustav*, 66–67. The theoretical course included lectures on anatomy, physiology, pathology, pharmacology, epidemiology, women's and children's diseases, and skin, nervous, and psychological illnesses. The practical course was to cover subjects such as internal and surgical illnesses, bandaging, minor surgical operations, and smallpox vaccination.

44. Kozlovtseva, *Moskovskie obshchiny*, 96.

45. See Greta Bucher, *Daily Life in Imperial Russia* (Westport, CT: Greenwood Press, 2008), 170–171. The shift is broadly in line with the rise of the professional classes in Europe at the turn of the twentieth century.

46. Ellen Albin, "Nursing in the USSR," *American Journal of Nursing* 46, no. 8 (1946): 525.

47. Albin, "Nursing in the USSR," 525.

48. Lopatkina, *Kul'turologicheskie aspekty*, 83.

49. Russian Sisters of Mercy received only meager subsistence allowances, and women often joined the Sisters of Mercy communities for various reasons, seeing the work as a release from societal duties, an adventure, a means to survive, or an altruistic endeavor. See Christina Danilovna Alchevskaia, cited in Kozlovtseva, *Moskovskie obshchiny*, 112–114.

50. Indeed, the dropout rate for the communities was extremely high, sometimes up to 60 percent. See Kozlovtseva, *Moskovskie obshchiny*, 101.

51. Shcherbinin, *Voennyi faktor*, 359.

52. Posternak, *Ocherki po istorii obshchin*, 209.

53. O. A. Baumgarten, *V osazhdennom Port-Arture: Dnevnik sestry miloserdiia Olgi Apollonovnyi fon Baumgarten* [In besieged Port-Arthur: Diary of sister of mercy Olga Apollonova von Baumbarten] (St. Petersburg, 1906), cited in *Angely khraniteli. Stranitsy istorii Otechestva* [Guardian Angels: Pages of the History of the Fatherland], ed. Yuri Khechinov (Moscow: Reklam-izdatel'stvo agenstvo "Dium," 1996), 16.

54. V. V. Veresaev, "Na yaponskoi voine. Zapiski" / / Veresaev V. *Ukaz. soch.*, 231 (In the Japanese war. Notes), cited in Shcherbinin, *Voennyi faktor*, 364–365.

55. For more on Sisters of Mercy in the Russo-Turkish War, 1877–1878, and particularly relations between them, see Posternak, *Ocherki po istorii obshchin*, 128–129. Boris Kolonitskii also makes this point about the "amoral behavior" of Sisters of Mercy before the Russo-Japanese War. Boris Kolonitskii, *Tragicheskaia erotika: Obrazy imperatoskoi sem'i v gody Pervyi mirovoi voiny* [Tragic erotica: images of the Imperial family during the First World War] (Moscow: New Literary Review, 2010), 336.

56. V. Mandel'berg, *Iz perezhitogo* [From experience] (Davos, 1910), 57, cited in Shcherbinin, *Voennyi factor*, 383.

57. N. V. Kozlova, "Pod voennoi grozoi (vospominaniia sestry-volonterki)" [Under a military storm (memoirs of a volunteer nurse)], *Istoricheskii vestnik*, no. 12 (1913): 944, cited in Shcherbinin, *Voennyi factor*, 381.

58. Shcherbinin, *Voennyi factor*, 387, originally cited in Varnek T. *Vospominaniia sestry miloserdiia / / Dobrovolitsy. Sbornik vospominanii* (Moscow, 2001) (Memoirs of a Sisters of Mercy, in Volunteers. A collection of memoirs), 7.

59. Jane Delano, "Red Cross Work," *American Journal of Nursing* 9, no. 8 (1909): 582–583.

60. Lavinia Dock, "Foreign Department," *American Journal of Nursing* 12, no. 12 (1912): 1023–1024; 17, no. 8 (1917): 721–722.

61. Lopatkina, *Kul'turologicheskie aspekty*, 80, 83.

62. Romaniuk, Lapotnikov, and Nakatis, *Istoriia sestrinskogo dela v Rossii*, 28–29. Other historians put this figure at 65 feldsher-midwifery schools in 1915, with a total of 8,750 students. A. S. Artiukhov, G. Ya. Klimenko, and A. V. Nikitin, *Istoriia sestrinskogo dela v Rossii i za rubezhom* [The history of nursing in Russia and abroad] (Voronezh, 1998), 7.

63. Lopatkina, *Kul'turologicheskie aspekty*, 80.

64. Kozlova, "Pod voennoi grozoi," 533, cited in Shcherbinin, *Voennyi faktor*, 362–363.

65. Posternak, *Ocherki po istorii obshchin*, 205.

66. See Ruth Harris, *Lourdes: Body and Spirit in the Secular Age* (London: Penguin Books, 1999), 320–366.

67. On women workers, see Bucher, *Daily Life in Imperial Russia*, 175.

68. Victoria Smolkin, *A Sacred Space Is Never Empty: A History of Soviet Atheism* (Princeton, NJ: Princeton University Press, 2018), 26. On religion, see Posternak, *Ocherki po istorii obshchin*, 205.

69. The Red Cross–trained nurses fell into four categories: Sisters of Mercy of the Russian Red Cross; Red Cross reserve Sisters of Mercy, formerly Red Cross community nurses; Red Cross reserve Sisters of Mercy who had completed a nine-month training course; and wartime Sisters of Mercy who had completed a short-term course of two month's duration.

70. Posternak, *Ocherki po istorii obshchin*, 177; *Kratkii obzor deiatel'nosti ROKK po oka-zaniiu pomoshchi ranenym i bol'nym voinam na teatrakh voiny s Avstro-Vengriei, Germaniei i Turtsiei v 1914–1915 gg* [A short review of ROKK activities in helping injured and sick soldiers in theaters of war from Austria-Hungary, Germany, and Turkey in 1914–1915], (Petrograd, 1916), 11–12.

71. On the "romantic ideal," see Christine E. Hallett, "Russian Romances: Emotionalism and Spirituality in the Writings of 'Eastern Front' Nurses, 1914–1918," *Nursing History Review* 17 (2009): 121.

72. Margaret H. Darrow, "French Volunteer Nursing and the Myth of War Experience in World War I," *American Historical Review* 101, no. 1 (1996): 100.

73. For an excellent example, see Laurie Stoff, *Russia's Sisters of Mercy and the Great War: More than Binding Men's Wounds* (Lawrence: University Press of Kansas, 2015). Stoff mines the archives and a wide range of sources.

74. T. A. Varnek, published in *Dobrovolitsy: Sbornik vospominanii* (Moscow: Russkii put', 2001), 7–39. For an in-depth analysis of diaries and the Russian nurse experience during World War I, see Stoff, *Russia's Sisters of Mercy*.

75. St. Petersburg was renamed Petrograd in 1914, and from 1924–1991 it was named as Leningrad.

76. Sophie Botcharsky and Florida Pier, *The Kinsmen Know How to Die* (New York: William Morrow, 1931), 7.

77. Tatiana Alexinsky, *With the Russian Wounded*, trans. Gilbert Canaan (London: T. Fisher Unwin, 1916), 97.

78. Botcharsky and Pier, *Kinsmen*, 222.

79. Darrow, "French Volunteer Nursing," 92.

80. Alexinsky, *With the Russian Wounded*, 11. See also Laurie Stoff, "The 'Myth of the War Experience' and Russian Wartime Nursing during World War I," *Aspasia: The International Yearbook of Central, Eastern, and Southeastern European Women's and Gender History* 6 (2012): 102.

81. Sophie Botcharsky and Florida Pier, *They Knew How to Die: Being a Narrative of the Personal Experiences of a Red Cross Sister on the Russian Front* (London: P. Davies, 1931), 66–68.

82. "Raznye postanovleniia Glavnogo Upravleniia" [Various resolutions of the General Directorate], *Vestnik Krasnogo Kresta*, no. 2–3 (1917): 628.

83. Alexinsky, *With the Russian Wounded*, 71–72.

84. Elsa Brandstrom, *Among Prisoners of War in Russia and Siberia*, trans. C. Mabel Rickmers (London: Hutchinson, 1929), 40. Brandstrom, the daughter of the Swedish ambassador, lived in Petrograd prior to the war. My thanks to Alistair Dickins for drawing my attention to this source.

85. See Santanu Das, *Touch and Intimacy in First World War Literature* (Cambridge: Cambridge University Press, 2005), 185–186.

86. Brandstrom, *Among Prisoners of War*, 40.

87. Darrow, "French Volunteer Nursing," 103.

88. Darrow, "French Volunteer Nursing," 103.

89. M. I. Deviz (Okhotina), "Iz dnevnika sestry miloserdiia" [From the diary of a nurse], *Istoricheskii vestnik* 115, no. 3 (1909): 1029. The soldiers also told Deviz that there were many "genuine" nurses who were good and kind.

90. Anne Summers, *Angels and Citizens: British Women as Military Nurses, 1854–1914* (London: Routledge & Kegan Paul, 1988), 261.

91. Florence Farmborough, Oral History, 000312/17/06, reel 8, Imperial War Museum, London.

92. "Otchislenie sester miloserdiia ot Zemskogo i Gorodskogo soiuzov" [Expulsions of sisters of mercy from the Zemstvo and City unions], *Vestnik Krasnogo Kresta*, no. 2–3 (1917): 532–533.

93. "Otchislenie sester miloserdiia," 532–533.

94. "Otchislenie sester miloserdiia," 533.

95. "Sestry miloserdiia i ikh kostiumy" [Sisters of mercy and their uniforms], *Damskii mir*, no. 1 (1915): 40.

96. "Sestry miloserdiia i ikh kostiumy," 40.

97. "Sestry miloserdiia i ikh kostiumy," 40.

98. "Zhenshchiny i voina" [Women and war], *Zhenskii vestnik*, no. 5–6 (1915): 113.

99. See *Zhenskoe delo*, no. 3 and no. 4 (1915).

100. Ia. I. Akodus and A. A. Skoriukova, *Meditsinskaia sestra Sovetskogo Krasnogo Kresta* [The Soviet Red Cross Nurse] (Moscow: Medgiz, 1955), 32.

101. See Kolonitskii, *Tragicheskaia erotica*, 342. Kolonitskii cites officers at the front in 1916 to illustrate. See State Archive of the Russian Federation (hereafter GARF), f. 102, op. 265, d. 1057, l. 730, cited in Kolonitskii, *Tragicheskaia erotica*, 343.

102. Anna Haines, *Health Work in Soviet Russia* (New York: Vanguard Press, 1928), 155–156.

103. Haines, *Health Work in Soviet Russia*, 156.

104. Stoff, *Russia's Sisters of Mercy*.

105. See Kolonitskii, *Tragicheskaia erotica*, chap. 5.

106. See Akodus and Skoriukova, *Meditsinskaia sestra Sovetskogo Krasnogo Kresta*, 32.

107. The union was officially "approved" on September 1, 1917, and its Central Administration had fifteen members and five candidate members. GARF, f. 5532, op. 1, d. 5, September 3, 1917–August 15, 1918. For more discussion of the All-Russian Society of the Union of Sisters of Mercy, see Susan Grant, "From War to Peace: Russian Nurses, 1917–22," in *Russia's Home Front in War and Revolution, 1914–22*, bk. 2, *The Experience of War and Revolution*, ed. Adele Lindenmeyr, Christopher Read, and Peter Waldron (Bloomington, IN: Slavica Publishers, 2016), 251–272.

108. A. Aluf, *Spravochnik srednego medpersonala* [Handbook for middle medical personnel], (Moscow: TsK Medsantrud, 1928), 11. Aluf lists the various unions.

109. A. Aluf, *Kratkaia istoriia professional'nogo medrabotnikov* [A short history of professional medical workers] (Moscow: TsK Medsantrud, 1927), 49. Aluf noted that "mobilization, professional needs, and cultural enlightenment," as well as the circumstances of the communities, dominated discussions, but that was "not unusual."

110. GARF, f. 5532, op. 1, d. 1, l. 3, August 26–September 3, 1917. For more in-depth analysis of the All-Russian Union of Sisters of Mercy, see Grant, "From War to Peace."

111. "Ofitsial'nyi otdel'" [Official department], *Pervyi vestnik*, no. 7 (1918): 2–3.

112. Central State Archive of St. Petersburg (hereafter TsGASPb), f. 2916, op. 1, d. 13, l. 6. See also TsGASPb, f. 2916, op. 1, d. 13, l. 28, Protocol of February 17, 1928; TsGASPb, f. 2738, op. 1, d. 2, l. 8.

113. GARF, f. 5532, op. 1, d. 19, l. 12 ob, January 16, 1918.

114. GARF, f. 5532, op. 1, d. 19, l. 12 ob.

115. They included nurses Filippova, Sobolewski, and Bazilevskaia. GARF, f. 5532, op. 1, d. 19, l. 12 ob.

116. GARF, f. 5532, op. 1, d. 19, l. 12 ob.

117. *Pervyi vestnik sestry miloserdiia*, no. 7 (1918): 2, February 14–15, 1918.

118. GARF, f. 5532, op. 1, d. 19, l. 5, 1918.

119. GARF, f. 5532, op. 1, d. 19, l. 5 ob, Sister Servirova, January 4, 1918.

120. GARF, f. 5532, op. 1, d. 19, l. 5 ob.

121. For detailed discussion of the Commissariat of Health, see Neil B. Weissman, "Origins of Soviet Health Administration, Narkomzdrav, 1918–1929," in *Health and Society in Revolutionary Russia*, ed. Susan Gross Solomon and John F. Hutchinson (Bloomington: Indiana University Press, 1990), 95–120.

122. Red Cross reorganization in summer 1918 raised the question of a merger between the Union of Sisters and the Red Cross communities to enter into on "professional union." GARF, f. 5532, op. 1, d. 19, l. 12, no. 31.

123. TsGASPb, f. 2916, op. 1, d. 13, l. 20 ob, January 17, 1918.

124. GARF, f. 1565, op. 7, d. 31, l. 33, August 25–December 20, 1918.

125. GARF, f. 1565, op. 7, d. 31, l. 33.

126. GARF, f. 1565, op. 7, d. 31, l. 36, October 21, 1918.

127. GARF, f. 1565, op. 7, d. 31, l. 36. See also GARF, f. 1565, op. 7, d. 31, l. 58; GARF, f. 1565, op. 7, d. 31, l. 36.

128. GARF, f. 1565, op. 7, d. 31, l. 36.

129. GARF, f. R-5532, op. 1, d. 32, l. 223, November and December 1918.

130. See Grant, "From War to Peace," 263–264. See also Weissman, "Origins of Soviet Health Administration," 103.

131. GARF, f. 3341, op. 1, d. 103, l. 45, August 7, 1918–October 30, 1919.

132. GARF, f. 3341, op. 1, d. 103, l. 47.

133. GARF, f. 3341, op. 1, d. 103, l. 47.

134. GARF, f. 3341, op. 1, d. 103, l. 48.

135. See Grant, "From War to Peace," 264–265.

2. Creating Order out of Chaos

1. Lynne Viola, *The Best Sons of the Fatherland: Workers in the Vanguard of Soviet Collectivization* (New York: Oxford University Press, 1987), 11. On war communism and the red terror, see also James Ryan, *Lenin's Terror: The Ideological Origins of Early Soviet State Violence* (London: Routledge, 2012), 100–119.

2. Evan Mawdsley, *The Russian Civil War* (1987; Edinburgh: Birlinn, 2008), 4.

3. Tricia Starks, *The Body Soviet: Propaganda, Hygiene, and the Revolutionary State* (Madison: University of Wisconsin Press, 2008), 3.

4. The Russian civil war or "wars" pitted the Bolshevik Red Army against a host of national and international forces known collectively as the White Army. The confederation included former imperial officers and anti-Bolsheviks within Russia as well as British, US, and Czech forces.

5. See Christopher Read, *The Making and Breaking of the Soviet System* (Basingstoke: Palgrave Macmillan, 2001), 36.

6. On competing interests, see Susan Gross Solomon, "The Limits of Government Patronage of Sciences: Social Hygiene and the Soviet State, 1920–1930," *Social History of Medicine* 3, no. 3 (1990): 407. See also Michael David, "The White Plague in the Red Capital: The Control of Tuberculosis in Russia, 1900–1941" (PhD diss., University of Chicago, 2007), 145.

7. See Mark G. Field, *Soviet Socialized Medicine: An Introduction* (New York: Free Press, 1967), 50–58. The Proletarian Red Cross, established before the revolution, had short courses to train sanitary brigades. See Irzhi Toman, *Rossiia i Krasnyi Krest (1917–1945)* [Russia and the Red Cross (1917–1945)] (Moscow: MKKK [Mezhdunarodnyi komitet Krasnogo Kresta / International Committee of the Red Cross], 2002), 20; and L. A. Khodorkov, "Osnovnye etapy razvitiia sovetskogo obshchestva Krasnogo Kresta i Krasnogo Polumesiatsa" [The main stages of the development of the Soviet Society of the Red Cross and Red Crescent], in *Materialy nauchnoi konferentsii, posviashchennoi 100-letiiu Krasnogo Kresta v SSSR* [Scientific conference material in honor of 100 years of the Red Cross in the USSR] (Moscow: Izdatel'stvo "Meditsina," 1968), 39.

8. V. A. Rybasov, "Krasnye sestry v grazhdanskoi voine" [Red nurses in the civil war], *Meditsinskaia sestra* 3 (1949): 22; see also Susan Grant, "From War to Peace: Russian Nurses, 1917–22," in *Russia's Home Front in War and Revolution, 1914–22*, bk. 2, *The Experience of War and Revolution*, ed. Adele Lindenmeyr, Christopher Read, and Peter Waldron (Bloomington, IN: Slavica Publishers, 2016), 260. For similar developments in pharmacy, see Mary Schaeffer Conroy, *In Health and in Sickness: Pharmacy, Pharmacists, and the Pharmaceutical Industry in Late Imperial, Early Soviet Russia* (Boulder, CO: East European Monographs; distributed by Columbia University Press, 1994), 414–415.

9. "Kursy dlia sanitarov" [Courses for orderlies], *Meditsinskii rabotnik*, no. 7–10 (1919): 41. Three-week courses in Moscow would be organized according to district.

10. For the full program, see Russian State Archive of Socio-Political History (hereafter RGASPI), f. 17, op. 10, d. 33, l. 57, 1919–1921. The Soviet state did not officially exist until December 30, 1922, but references to "Soviet" power and so forth abound in the source material.

11. RGASPI, f. 17, op. 10, d. 33, l. 41.

12. Richard Stites, *The Women's Liberation Movement in Russia: Feminism, Nihilism, and Bolshevism* (Princeton, NJ: Princeton University Press, 1978), 318. See also Susan Grant, "Nurses in the Soviet Union: Explorations of Gender in State and Society," in *The Palgrave Handbook of Women and Gender in Twentieth-Century Russia and the Soviet Union*, ed. Melanie Ilic (London: Palgrave Macmillan, 2018), 249–265.

13. K. S. Baturina, S. A. Davydovskaia, and A. S. Shutskever, *Pravda, stavshaia legendoi* [The truth that has become legend], (Moscow: Voennoe izdatel'stvo Ministerstva oborony SSSR, 1964), 116–117.

14. O. L. Mokievskaia-Zubok, introduction to the chapter on Zinaida Mokievskaia-Zubok, in *Dobrovol'tsy: Sbornik vospominanii* [Volunteers: Collection of memoirs], (Moscow: Russkii put', 2001), 240.

15. Joshua A. Sanborn, *Drafting the Russian Nation: Military Conscription, Total War, and Mass Politics, 1905–1925* (DeKalb: Northern Illinois University Press, 2003), 154.

16. A. G. Katsnel'bogen, *Podvig miloserdiia* [Feat of mercy], (Moscow: Meditsina, 1991), 24–25. Katsnel'bogen has the number of women awarded the Red Cross medal at ninety; other scholars put the figure at thirty-eight. E. N. Zhelikhovskii and F. V.

Pasiukov, "Meditsinskie sestry na frontakh grazhdanskoi i Velikoi Otechestvennoi voin" [Nurses at the front of the civil war and First World War], *Meditsinskaia sestra* 6 (1969): 51.

17. Katsnel'bogen, *Podvig miloserdiia*, 24–25.

18. Anna Haines, *Health Work in Soviet Russia* (New York: Vanguard Press, 1928), 101.

19. Report on the Medical Conditions of Russia, October 1922, reel 106, box 92, folder 13, Lillian Wald Papers, Rare Book & Manuscript Library, Columbia University in the City of New York.

20. *Dobrovolitsy*, 254. Mokievskaia-Zubok worked as a volunteer for three months, until it was possible to receive short-term training at a Sisters of Mercy community. *Dobrovolitsy*, 255.

21. *Dobrovolitsy*, 254.

22. GARF, f. 3341, op. 1, d. 2, l. 71 ob, April 28, 1919.

23. State Archive of Tambov Oblast (hereafter GATO), f. 1512, op. 1, d. 49, December 15, 1919.

24. Daniel R. Brower, "'The City in Danger': The Civil War and the Russian Urban Population," in *Party, State, and Society in the Russian Civil War: Explorations in Social History*, ed. Diane P. Koenker, William G. Rosenberg, and Ronald Grigor Suny (Bloomington: Indiana University Press, 1989), 62; Conroy, *In Health and in Sickness*, 421–443; Nikolai Krementsov, *Revolutionary Experiments: The Quest for Immortality in Bolshevik Science and Fiction* (New York: Oxford University Press, 2014), 27–29. Krementsov refers to the years 1914–1923 as the "decade of death."

25. GARF, f. 5465, op. 1, d. 69, l. 33, May 1919.

26. GARF, f. 5465, op. 1, d. 69, l. 33, April 30, 1919.

27. GARF, f. A-482, op. 2, d. 43, l. 8, June 29, 1921.

28. GARF, f. A-482, op. 2, d. 43, l. 8.

29. Katsnel'bogen, *Podvig miloserdiia*, 24.

30. On science and education, see Starks, *Body Soviet*, 21.

31. GARF, f. 5465, op. 1, d. 60, l. 16, correspondence from July 24, 1919.

32. The Commissariat of Public Health requested information (usually in the form of questionnaires) about the schools (e.g., number of students, resources, curricula) from the provincial health departments (*gubzdravotdely*). GARF, f. A-482, op. 14, d. 24–34 (see especially op. 14, d. 34, l. 42, June 5, 1920). For details on the nursing schools position, see RGASPI, f. 17, op. 10, d. 33, ll. 58–60, Semashko and Raukhvarger's "Polozhenie o shkolakh sester miloserdiia" [Position on nursing schools].

33. GARF, f. 5465, op. 1, d. 60, l. 16, July 24, 1919.

34. The International Red Cross and Crescent officially recognized the Soviet Red Cross in 1921. See Khodorkov, "Osnovnye etapy," 39–44; and Toman, *Rossiia i Krasnyi Krest*, 37–38.

35. When Glavprofobr assumed control of medical education in 1922, there were 29 feldsher-midwifery schools, 22 midwifery schools, 33 nursing schools, and a host of courses. These encompassed 13,000 people, largely from the working class and peasantry. N. A. Vinogradov, *Printsipy raboty s meditsinskimi kadrami* [Principles of working with medical personnel], (Moscow: Medgiz, 1955), 38–40.

36. *Plan obucheniia i programmy shkol sester miloserdiia* [Study plan and program for nurse schools], (Moscow, 1919), 1. A joint work by the Red Cross (which compiled it) and the Commissariat of Public Health, the textbook was published in February 18, 1919.

37. Decree, published in *Izvestiia Narodnogo komissariata zdravookhraneniia*, no. 3–4 (1920), cited in A. V. Flint, "Po povodu dvukh iubelinykh dat" [On the occasion of two anniversary dates], *Sestrinskoe delo*, no. 4 (2010): 12. See also Grant, "From War to Peace," 269–270.

38. Anastasiia Sergievna Konokhova, "Sestry miloserdiia v gody revolutsii i grazh-danskoi voiny" [Nurses in the years of revolution and civil war], *Noveishaia istoriia Rossii*, no. 1 (2012): 93. See also Grant, "From War to Peace," 269.

39. Iu. E. Sorkin, "Iz istorii meditsinskaia obrazovaniia" [From the history of medical education], *Meditsinskaia sestra*, no. 4 (1987): 47–53, cited in Elizabeth Murray, "Russian Nurses: From the Tsarist Sister of Mercy to the Soviet Comrade Nurse; A Case Study of Absence of Migration of Nursing Knowledge and Skills," *Nursing Inquiry* 11, no. 3 (2004): 136. Ia. I. Akodus and A. A. Skoriukova put the number of nursing schools and nursing courses in 1922 at 38 (increasing to 123 in 1927 and 260 in 1932). Ia. I. Akodus and A. A. Skoriukova, *Meditsinskaia sestra Sovetskogo Krasnogo Kresta* [Soviet Red Cross nurse], (Moscow: Medgiz, 1955), 38.

40. Murray, "Russian Nurses," 136; Field, *Soviet Socialized Medicine*, 135.

41. N. I. Propper, "Podgotovka meditsinskoi sestry prezhde i teper'" [Nurse training past and present], *Meditsina*, no. 9 (1927): 14. Propper argued that the new study program produced below-par nurses.

42. *Plan obucheniia*, 145–154.

43. *Plan obucheniia*, 8. For another example of handbooks for nurses, see GARF, f. A-482, op. 14, d. 105.

44. *Plan obucheniia*, 4–5.

45. Susan McGann, "Collaboration and Conflict in International Nursing, 1920–39," *Nursing History Review* 16 (2008): 52. The Russians discussed nursing in England, the United States, and Australia. GARF, f. 5465, op. 1, d. 60, l. 28 ob, 1919, Mezernitskii.

46. Diane P. Koenker, *Republic of Labor: Russian Printers and Soviet Socialism, 1918–1930* (Ithaca, NY: Cornell University Press, 2005), 29. See also Conroy, *In Health and in Sickness*, 433.

47. The *kassa*-based insurance medicine also began to appropriate facilities including factories' medical facilities and "even contemplated requisitioning Red Cross facilities." See Sally Ewing, "The Science and Politics of Soviet Insurance Medicine," in *Health and Society in Revolutionary Russia*, ed. Susan Gross Solomon and John F. Hutchinson (Bloomington: Indiana University Press, 1990), 74.

48. Ryan, *Lenin's Terror*, 140.

49. For more discussion about transferring former ROKK property to the new healthcare authority, see GARF, f. 4094, op. 1, d. 255, ll. 13 ob–14 ob.

50. GARF, f. 3341, op. 1, d. 57, l. 36, June 3, 1918.

51. GARF, f. 3341, op. 1, d. 57, l. 36.

52. GARF, f. 3341, op. 1, d. 57, l. 36. On January 6, 1918, the Council of People's Commissars (Sovnarkom) issued a decree to nationalize the property and assets of the Russian Red Cross and establish a committee to oversee this process. In June of that year another decree stated that the "Soviet government recognized all conventions on the wounded and prisoners of war and that the Soviet Red Cross consider[ed] itself a member of the International organization of the Red Cross." Ia. I. Akodus, *Kratkii ocherk istorii Sovetskogo Krasnogo Kresta* [Brief essay on the history of the Soviet Red Cross], (Moscow: Moskovskii gorodskii komitet obshchestva Krasnogo Kresta, 1958),

cited in V. P. Spasokukotskii, *O vneshnei deiatel'nosti Sovetskogo Krasnogo Kresta* [On the external activities of the Soviet Red Cross], (Moscow, 1958), 7.

53. Daniel T. Orlovsky, "State Building in the Civil War Era: The Role of the Lower-Middle Strata," in *Party, State, and Society in the Russian Civil War: Explorations in Social History*, ed. Diane P. Koenker, William G. Rosenberg, and Ronald Grigor Suny (Bloomington: Indiana University Press, 1989), 197.

54. GARF, f. 3341, op. 1, d. 31, l. 33, November 21, 1919. In certain circumstances some public organizations such as the public health insurance fund could use Red Cross communities and their institutes. GARF, f. 3341, op. 1, d. 31, l. 17, March 2, 1918–September 13, 1919. A commission would develop "temporary rules for the administration of the Sisters of Mercy communities of the Red Cross." Two of the commission's members (M. A. Kossovich and N. S. Obolenskaia) were formerly of the All-Russian Union of Sisters of Mercy.

55. GARF, f. 3341, op. 1, d. 31, l. 33.

56. Orlovsky, "State Building," 197.

57. GARF, f. 3341, op. 6, d. 73, l. 67, December 20, 1925–December 12, 1928.

58. GARF, f. 3341, op. 6, d. 73, l. 67.

59. This transfer likely involved Moscow's Aleksandrovskaia Soothe My Sorrows community. GARF, f. 3341, op. 5, d. 91, ll. 1- 2, 1922. V. M. Mikhailov took part in the discussions, along with the former head doctor of the community. In these discussions the representative of the Central Committee of the Russian Society of the Red Cross (Tsentrokrest), Z. P. Soloviev, was responding to an address about the transfer of the Aleksandrovskaia community to the Red Cross by the head of the Medical Department, A. S. Puchkov). See Elena Kozlovtseva, *Moskovskie obshchiny sester miloserdiia v XIX–nachale XX veka* [Moscow sister of mercy communities in the nineteenth century to the beginning of the twentieth century], (Moscow: Pravoslavnyi Sviato-Tikhonovskii gumanitarnyi universitet, 2010), 150–151. For difficulties with the transfer of the Pokrovskaia community in Petrograd in 1918–1919, see Maria Kunkite, "Petrogradskie obshchiny sester miloserdiia v pervye gody sovetskoi vlasti: K voprosu o pravopreemstvennosti sovremennykh LPU i srednikh medshkol Peterburga Obshchinam sester miloserdiia" [Petrograd sisters of mercy communities in the first years of Soviet power: On the question of the succession of contemporary LPU and middle medical schools in the Petersburg sisters of mercy community] in *Iubileinyi sbornik*, chast' 2, *Nauchno-issledovatel'skaia rabota Muzeia istorii sestrinskogo dela v Peterburge: 2007–2010* [Anniversary collection, part 2, Scientific-research work on the museums of the history of nursing in Petersburg: 2007–2010], (St. Petersburg: Sankt Peterburgskoe gosudarstvennoe obrazovatel'noe uchrezhdenie srednego professional'nogo obrazovaniia Meditsinskii Tekhnikum No. 2, 2010), 29–30. Thanks to Maria Kunkite for sharing her work. The Sisters of Mercy communities were also renamed around this time. See Konokhova, "Sestry miloserdiia," 93.

60. GARF, f. 3341, op. 5, d. 91, l. 2.

61. GARF, f. 3341, op. 5, d. 91, l. 2.

62. GARF, f. A-482, op. 14, d. 34, l. 41, June 30, 1920.

63. GARF, f. 3341, op. 5, d. 91, l. 2 ob.

64. GARF, f. 3341, op. 5, d. 91, l. 2 ob.

65. GARF, f. 3341, op. 5, d. 91, l. 2 ob, 1922.

66. GARF, f. 3341, op. 5, d. 91, l. 8 ob.

67. GARF, f. 3341, op. 5, d. 91, l. 9.

68. GARF, f. 3341, op. 5, d. 91, l. 9, April 1922. For similar discussion on financial challenges in healthcare in 1918 and 1919, see Conroy, *In Health and in Sickness*, 417.

69. GARF, f. 3341, op. 5, d. 91, l. 9.

70. In adopting the economic policy of war communism during the civil war, the Bolsheviks nationalized industry and facilitated forceful grain appropriation to help address the massive food supply problems.

71. Samuel C. Ramer, "Feldshers and Rural Health Care in the Early Soviet Period," in *Health and Society in Revolutionary Russia*, ed. Susan Gross Solomon and John F. Hutchinson (Bloomington: Indiana University Press, 1990), 132–133.

72. Peter Holquist, *Making War, Forging Revolution: Russia's Continuum of Crisis, 1914–1921* (Cambridge, MA: Harvard University Press, 2002), 282.

73. GARF, f. A-1565, op. 7, d. 41, l. 29, February 20, 1922.

74. GARF, f. A-1565, op. 7, d. 41, l. 29.

75. GARF, f. A-1565, op. 7, d. 41, l. 29.

76. GARF, f. A-1565, op. 7, d. 41, l. 29.

77. GARF, f. A-1565, op. 7, d. 41, l. 51.

78. GARF, f. A-1565, op. 7, d. 41, l. 29; Holquist, *Making War, Forging Revolution*, 283. In early 1919, orders to conduct mass terror in the Cossack regions accompanied devastating economic policies. Holquist, *Making War, Forging Revolution*, 180–182.

79. GARF, f. A-1565, op. 7, d. 41, l. 29.

80. GARF, f. A-1565, op. 7, d. 41, l. 29.

81. GARF, f. A-1565, op. 7, d. 41, ll. 49–51 ob.

82. GARF, f. A-1565, op. 7, d. 41, l. 51.

83. L. Raukhvarger, "Voprosy meditsinskogo obrazovaniia" [Questions of medical education], *Meditsinskii rabotnik*, no. 5–8 (1920): 10.

84. For discussion of courses, see M. Gol'dberg, "K voprosu o kursakh kvalifikatsii mladshego medpersonala" [On the question of courses for qualified junior medical personnel], *Meditsinskii rabotnik*, no. 9 (1923): 11.

85. GARF, f. 5465, op. 1, d. 60, l. 85, November 1919. See also GARF, f. 5465, op. 1, d. 69, l. 32 (April 30, 1919).

86. Raukhvarger, "Voprosy meditsinskogo obrazovaniia," 10.

87. Raukhvarger, "Voprosy meditsinskogo obrazovaniia," 10.

88. Over the course of 1918–1919 the medical union was contained through the efforts of Semashko and the Bolshevik party, both keen to limit union power and autonomy. Neil B. Weissman, "Origins of Soviet Health Administration, Narkomzdrav, 1918–1929," in *Health and Society in Revolutionary Russia*, ed. Susan Gross Solomon and John F. Hutchinson (Bloomington: Indiana University Press, 1990), 104.

89. GARF, f. 5465, op. 3, d. 202, l. 2, 1921.

90. Raukhvarger, "Voprosy meditsinskogo obrazovaniia," 12.

91. Raukhvarger, "Voprosy meditsinskogo obrazovaniia," 12. Pharmacognosy is the study of medicinal drugs derived from plants and other natural resources.

92. Haines, *Health Work in Soviet Russia*, 156.

93. Boris Kolonitskii, *Tragicheskaia erotika: Obrazy imperatoskoi sem'i v gody Pervyi mirovoi voiny* [Tragic erotica: Images of the Imperial family in the years of the First world war], (Moscow: New Literary Review, 2010), 262; Anne E. Gorsuch, *Youth in*

Revolutionary Russia: Enthusiasts, Bohemians, Delinquents (Bloomington: Indiana University Press, 2000).

94. Haines, *Health Work in Soviet Russia*, 154.

95. Haines, *Health Work in Soviet Russia*, 157.

96. Haines, *Health Work in Soviet Russia*, 157.

97. GARF, f. A-482, op. 14, d. 135, l. 36, September 1922.

98. GARF, f. A-482, op. 14, d. 135, l. 36.

99. GARF, f. A-482, op. 14, d. 135, l. 36. For more discussion about feldsher-midwife schools, see Susan Grant, "Nurses across Borders: Displaced Russian and Soviet Nurses after World War I and World War II," *Nursing History Review* 22 (2014): 13–36.

100. GARF, f. A-482, op. 14, d. 55, l. 1, July 3, 1920.

101. N. I. Propper, "K voprosu o reforme srednego medobrazovaniia" [Towards the question of reforming middle medical education], *Meditsina*, no. 3 (1927): 16.

102. GARF, f. A-482, op. 14, d. 31, l. 14, July 1920.

103. GARF, f. A-482, op. 14, d. 35, l. 17, June 21, 1920.

104. L. M. Kurakina put the number of company/field feldshers at 56 percent. L. M. Kurakina, "Reforma srednego-meditsinskogo obrazovaniia" [Reforms in middle medical education], *Biulleten' Narkomzdrava*, no. 11 (1924): 28.

105. Samuel C. Ramer, "Professionalism and Politics: The Russian Feldsher Movement, 1891–1918," in *Russia's Missing Middle Classes: The Professions in Russian History*, ed. Harley D. Balzer (Armonk, NY: M. E. Sharpe, 1996), 117–142; Samuel C. Ramer, "Who Was the Russian Feldsher?," *Bulletin of the History of Medicine* 50, no. 2 (1976): 213–225.

106. GARF, f. A-482, op. 14, d. 135, l. 28.

107. GARF, f. A-482, op. 14, d. 135, l. 28.

108. GARF, f. A-482, op. 14, d. 135, l. 35, 1921–1922.

109. GARF, f. A-482, op. 14, d. 45, l. 2. October 20, 1920.

110. P. Logina, *Rabotnitsa sovetskoi meditsiny* [A Woman worker of Soviet medicine], (Leningrad: Gosizdat, 1920), 18.

111. S. V. Leonov, *Rozhdenie sovetskoi imperii: gosudarstvo i ideologiia 1917–1920gg* [Birth of the Russian Empire: state and ideology 1917–1920], (Moscow: Dialog MGU, 1997), cited in Ryan, *Lenin's Terror*, 110–111.

112. Natalia Smillie, 1959, 4, International Council of Nurses (ICN) Refugee Nurses Series, MC112, box 16, Barbara Bates Center for the Study of the History of Nursing, University of Pennsylvania School of Nursing.

113. Andrea-Aleksandra Stegman Memoirs, 1954–1968, Bakhmeteff Archive, Rare Book & Manuscript Library, Columbia University in the City of New York.

114. Grant, "Nurses across Borders."

115. *Dobrovolitsy*, 327.

116. TsGASPb, f. 2738, op. 1, d. 2, l. 29, October 29, 1918.

117. TsGASPb, f. 2738, op. 1, d. 2, l. 29.

118. TsGASPb, f. 2738, op. 1, d. 2, l. 29 ob.

119. GARF, f. 3341, op. 1, d. 19, l. 43, March 10, 1918.

120. GARF, f. 3341, op. 1, d. 19, l. 43.

121. GARF, f. 5465, op. 1, d. 63, l. 7, 1919.

122. GARF, f. 5465, op. 1, d. 65, l. 97, October 10, 1919.

123. S. A. Smith, *Red Petrograd: Revolution in the Factories, 1917–1918* (Cambridge: Cambridge University Press, 1983), 3.

124. GATO, f. 1512, op. 1, d. 52, ll. 13–14, March 13, 1919.

125. GATO, f. 1512, op. 1, d. 52, l. 14.

126. GARF, f. 3341, op. 1, d. 55, l. 72, March 1919.

127. GARF, f. 1565, op. 7, d. 31, l. 38 ob, October 1918.

128. GARF, f. 1565, op. 7, d. 31, l. 38 ob.

129. GARF, f. 4094, op. 1, d. 152, l. 52, May 7, 1918.

130. TsGASPb, f. 2916, op. 1, d. 2, l. 307, October 1917.

131. TsGASPb, f. 2916, op. 1, d. 2, l. 307 ob.

132. TsGASPb, f. 2916, op. 1, d. 2, l. 316–316 ob.

133. Koenker, *Republic of Labor*, 28.

134. Report on the Medical Conditions of Russia, Lillian Wald Files. See also Haines, *Health Work in Soviet Russia*, 81–82.

135. GARF, f. A-482, op. 35, d. 38, l. 134, March 10, 1922; GARF, f. A-482, op. 35, d. 38, ll. 35 ob–136. For further discussion of the medical conditions, see Grant, "From War to Peace"; and Susan Grant "The American Hospital in Moscow: A Lesson in International Cooperation, 1917–1923," *Medical History* 59, no. 4 (2015): 554–574.

136. GARF, f. A-482, op. 35, d. 38, l. 137 ob.

137. GARF, f. A-482, op. 35, d. 38, l. 14, American Medical Aid to Russia, Frances Witherspoon.

138. Central State Archive of Historico-Political Records of St. Petersburg (hereafter TsGAIPD Spb), f. 1, op. 1, d. 962, l. 68.

139. TsGAIPD Spb, f. 1, op. 1, d. 962, ll. 68, 69.

140. TsGAIPD Spb, f. 1, op. 1, d. 962, ll. 68, 69.

141. Smith, *Red Petrograd*, 265.

142. GATO, f. 1512, op. 1, d. 52, l. 126 ob, August 28, 1919.

143. GATO, f. 1512, op. 1, d. 52, l. 126 ob.

144. GARF, f. 3341, op. 1, d. 103, l. 64, 1918/1919; GARF, f. 3341, op. 1, d. 103, l. 64; GARF, f. 3341, op. 1, d. 103, l. 64; GARF, f. 3341, op. 1, d. 103, l. 64 ob.

145. GARF, f. A-1565, op. 7, d. 14, l. 113, February 28–March 1, 1921.

146. GARF, f. A-1565, op. 7, d. 14, l. 113.

147. GARF, f. A-1565, op. 7, d. 14, l. 113.

148. GARF, f. 4094, op. 1, d. 152, l. 51.

149. GARF, f. 4094, op. 1, d. 152, l. 53.

150. Smith, *Red Petrograd*, 228.

151. GARF, f. 4094, op. 1, d. 152, l. 51 ob, May 10, 1918.

152. GARF, f. 4094, op. 1, d. 152, l. 54; l. 51 ob.

153. GARF, f. 4094, op. 1, d. 152, l. 54.

154. GARF, f. 4094, op. 1, d. 152, l. 54.

155. GARF, f. 4094, op. 1, d. 152, l. 54 ob; l. 58 ob.

156. GARF, f. 4094, op. 1, d. 152, l. 55; l. 60.

157. GARF, f. 4094, op. 1, d. 152, l. 55 ob; l. 58 ob.

158. GARF, f. 4094, op. 1, d. 152, l. 64 ob.

159. GARF, f. 4094, op. 1, d. 152, l. 58.

160. GARF, f. 4094, op. 1, d. 152, l. 58.

161. GARF, f. 4094, op. 1, d. 152, l. 58 ob.

162. GARF, f. 4094, op. 1, d. 152, l. 62.

163. GARF, f. 4094, op. 1, d. 152, l. 63, June 19, 1918, Vologda.

164. GARF, f. 4094, op. 1, d. 152, l. 66 ob.

165. GARF, f. 4094, op. 1, d. 152, l. 66 ob.

166. David L. Hoffmann, *Stalinist Values: The Cultural Norms of Soviet Modernity, 1917–1941* (Ithaca, NY: Cornell University Press, 2003), 58–62.

167. Maria Cristina Galmarini-Kabala, *The Right to Be Helped: Deviance, Entitlement, and the Soviet Moral Order* (DeKalb: Northern Illinois University Press, 2016), 12.

168. TsGASPb, f. 2745, op.1, d. 3, l. 9, January 1919.

169. GARF, f. A-482, op. 58, d. 18, l. 2 ob.

170. GARF, f. A-482, op. 58, d. 18, l. 2 ob. The inspectors found that nannies and orderlies were often "from nearby villages and not able to cope with their work." GARF, f. A-482, op. 58, d. 18, l. 4 ob.

171. On the "roughening" of speech patterns as a result of the possible brutalization of social life, see S. A. Smith, "The Social Meanings of Swearing: Workers and Bad Language in Late Imperial and Early Soviet Russia," *Past and Present* 160 (1998): 191.

3. Black Star, Red Star

1. Christopher Read, *The Making and Breaking of the Soviet System* (Basingstoke: Palgrave Macmillan, 2001), 54–55.

2. For more on foreign contacts, see, for example, Susan Gross Solomon, "Knowing the 'Local': Rockefeller Foundation Officers' Site Visits to Russia in the 1920s," *Slavic Review* 62, no. 4 (2003): 710–732.

3. Solomon, "Knowing the 'Local.'"

4. Social hygiene became an established discipline in Russia in 1922. See Susan Gross Solomon, "Social Hygiene and Soviet Public Health, 1921–1930," in *Health and Society in Revolutionary Russia*, ed. Susan Gross Solomon and John F. Hutchinson (Bloomington: Indiana University Press, 1990), 175–199; Susan Gross Solomon, "The Limits of Government Patronage of Sciences: Social Hygiene and the Soviet State, 1920–1930," *Social History of Medicine* 3, no. 3 (1990): 405–435.

5. For more on the insider/outsider relationships, but especially the Russian-German relationship, see Susan Gross Solomon, ed., *Doing Medicine Together: Germany and Russia between the Wars* (Toronto: University of Toronto Press, 2006).

6. Anne Marie Rafferty, "Internationalising Nursing Education during the Interwar Period," in *International Health Organisations and Movements, 1918–1939*, ed. Paul Weindling (Cambridge: Cambridge University Press, 1995), 268.

7. The Rockefeller Foundation commissioned the investigation that became known as the Goldmark Report. In 1918 the Foundation tasked the "social investigator Josephine Goldmark" with preparing a study of public health nursing in the United States. Susan Reverby has neatly summed up its findings: "It pointed to the need for nurses with postgraduate course work to the public-health field; similar additional training for educators, supervisors, and superintendents; the maintenance of high educational standards, including more basic science courses; a properly funded training school with a graded curriculum of twenty-eight months; and the endowment of a university based school of nursing to train the profession's future leadership." It also "called for the replacement of student nurses by graduates in hospitals and the training of 'hospital

helpers' in the execution of routine duties of a 'non-educational character.'" Susan Reverby, *Ordered to Care: The Dilemma of American Nursing, 1850–1945* (Cambridge: Cambridge University Press, 1987), 164–165.

8. Nor was there any doubt about US interest in Soviet science and medicine. For more on the Rockefeller Foundation and Alan Gregg's visit to the Soviet Union, see Susan Gross Solomon, "Building Bridges: Alan Gregg and Soviet Russia, 1925–1928," *Minerva* 41 (2003): 167–176. In a report to the Rockefeller Foundation, Gregg noted that Soviet science and medicine compared favorably to western Europe. Solomon, "Building Bridges," 174. Gregg worked in the Foundation's International Health Division from 1919 and in 1922 he became Associate Director of its Division for Medical Education. For more on Gregg, see Alan Gregg—Biographical—The Rockefeller Foundation: A Digital History, https://rockfound.rockarch.org/biographical/-/asset_publisher/6ygcKECNI1nb/content/alan-gregg, accessed July 8, 2021.

9. Anna Haines, *Health Work in Soviet Russia* (New York: Vanguard Press, 1928), 16.

10. On the threat of the NEP to female emancipation, see Elizabeth A. Wood, *The Baba and the Comrade: Gender and Politics in Revolutionary Russia* (Bloomington: Indiana University Press, 1997), 175.

11. Christie Watson, *The Language of Kindness: A Nurse's Story* (London: Chatto & Windus, 2018), 113.

12. For an examination of these exchanges, see Susan Gross Solomon, "'The Power of Dichotomies': The Rockefeller Foundation's Division of Medical Education, Medical Literature, and Russia, 1921–1925," in *American Foundations in Europe: Grant-Giving Policies, Cultural Diplomacy and Trans-Atlantic Relations, 1920–1980*, ed. Giuliana Gemelli and Roy MacLeod (Brussels: Peter Lang, 2003), 31–51.

13. GARF, f. A-482, op. 35, d. 55, l. 37, October 25, 1923.

14. GARF, f. 5465, op. 5, d. 179, l. 38, February 13, 1923, Aluf.

15. GARF, f. 5465, op. 5, d. 179, l. 7.

16. GARF, f. 5465, op. 5, d. 179, l. 19, August 20, 1923.

17. GARF, f. A-482, op. 35, d. 69, l. 114, August 7, 1924.

18. GARF, f. A-482, op. 35, d. 69, l. 153; program, GARF, f. A-482, op. 35, d. 69, l. 154, 1924. This course "placed particular emphasis on training nurses for social health work." Rafferty, "Internationalising Nursing Education," 275.

19. Susan McGann, "Collaboration and Conflict in International Nursing, 1920–39," *Nursing History Review* 16 (2008): 35.

20. See V. M. Banshchikov and N. I. Propper, *Srednee meditsinskoe obrazovanie* (Moscow, 1928), 129–130. The physician Sapir drew up the curriculum.

21. David L. Hoffmann, *Stalinist Values: The Cultural Norms of Soviet Modernity, 1917–1941* (Ithaca, NY: Cornell University Press, 2003), 15.

22. Jaime Lapeyre, "Public Health Nursing Education in the Interwar Period," in *Russian and Soviet Health Care from an International Perspective: Comparing Professions, Practice and Gender, 1880–1960*, ed. Susan Grant (London: Palgrave Macmillan, 2017), 217–242.

23. Aeleah Soine, "'The Relation of the Nurse to the Working World': Professionalization, Citizenship, and Class in Germany, Great Britain, and the United States before World War I," *Nursing History Review* 18 (2010): 61.

24. Violetta Thurston, *Field Hospital and Flying Column: Being the Journal of an English Nursing Sister in Belgium and Russia* (London; New York: G. P. Putnam's Son [Pranava Books], 1916), 120.

25. From 1915 to 1955, the Rockefeller Foundation helped nursing in Europe in the form of equipment, salaries, scholarships, and so forth. For a "list of nursing grants" for 1915–1955, see Rockefeller Archive Center (hereafter RAC), Rockefeller Foundation Records (RF), record group (RG) 1.1, series 100C, box 38, folder 341.

26. The Rockefeller Foundation was also keen to obtain reliable information about medical education and healthcare in Russia. Solomon, "Knowing the 'Local,'" 712–715.

27. International School of Nursing and Child Welfare for Russia, reel 106, box 92, folder 13, Lillian Wald Papers, Rare Book & Manuscript Library, Columbia University in the City of New York.

28. Copies of the agreement, signed in September 1922, are in GARF; the Library of the Society of Friends / Quakers in Britain (hereafter LSF); the RAC; and the AFSC Archive. For the RAC copy, see Translation of the Agreement between the Commisarate [*sic*] of Medical Education and the English Mission, October 1922, RAC, RF, RG 1.1, series 785A, box 2, folder 17.

29. See Muriel Payne to E. Crowell, October 17, 1922, RAC, RF, RG 1.1, series 785A, box 2, folder 17.

30. Notes on Infant Mortality in Russia (1922) and Translation of the Agreement between the Comisarate [sic] of Medical Education and the English Mission, represented by Lady Muriel Paget (no date but copied for E. Crowell October 1922); RAC, RF, RG 1.1, series 785A, box 2, folder 17. This document was signed by Anatoly Lunacharsky, head of the People's Commissariat for Education.

31. Report on Visit to Moscow and Need for Child Welfare—Programme in Russia. RAC, RF, RG 1.1, series 785A, box 2, folder 17 Paget had gone to Moscow to discuss Russian support for the nursing school scheme. Copies of the agreement are in the RAC and GARF. They signed the agreement on October 4, 1922.

32. Bertrand M. Patenaude, *The Big Show in Bololand: The American Relief Expedition to Soviet Russia in the Famine of 1921* (Stanford, CA: Stanford University Press, 2002), 234.

33. Report on Visit to Moscow.

34. Report on Visit to Moscow.

35. Report on Visit to Moscow.

36. GATO, f. 1512, op. 3, d. 117, l. 14, May 3, 1920.

37. Notes on Infant Mortality in Russia (1922), RAC, RF, RG 1.1, series 785A, box 2, folder 17; Translation of the Agreement between the Commisarate [*sic*] of Medical Education and the English Mission, represented by Lady Muriel Paget. Lunacharsky signed the agreement, and the scheme was accepted on September 6, 1922. A copy was sent to Crowell. For details about the scheme, see Muriel Payne to Frances Elisabeth Crowell, October 16, 1922, RAC, RF, RG 1.1, series 785A, box 2, folder 17. Crowell was a social worker and nurse who was based in Europe as part of her work for the Rockefeller Foundation. She joined the International Health Board in 1917 and from 1923 she was involved in the Division of Studies Program. For her professional biography, see Frances Elisabeth Crowell—Biographical—The Rockefeller Foundation—A Digital History, https://rockfound.rockarch.org/biographical/-/asset_publisher/6ygcKECNI1nb /content/frances-elisabeth-crowell, accessed 8 July 2021. Crowell and Paget also discussed nurse training in Russia in November and December 1922, RF 1.1, series 785 USSR. Box 3, Folder 28. My thanks to Susan Gross Solomon for this source.

38. A copy of the syllabus is available in the Lillian Wald Papers, reel 106, box 92, folder 13, Lillian Wald Papers, Rare Book & Manuscript Library, Columbia University

in the City of New York.. See also Scheme for the Establishment of a Public Health and Child Welfare Training in Connection with Medical Relief for Russian Children, RAC, RF, RG 1.1, series 785A, box 2, folder 17. The scheme was signed by Paget, representing the Lady Muriel Paget Mission, on September 1, 1922.

39. See Michael David-Fox, *Showcasing the Great Experiment: Cultural Diplomacy and Western Visitors to the Soviet Union, 1921–1941* (Oxford: Oxford University Press, 2012), 47.

40. Tricia Starks, *The Body Soviet: Propaganda, Hygiene, and the Revolutionary State* (Madison: University of Wisconsin Press, 2008), 136.

41. Starks, *Body Soviet*, 137.

42. Between November 1920 and 1922, Model Dispensary nurses made 1,845 home visits. Michael David, "The White Plague in the Red Capital: The Control of Tuberculosis in Russia, 1900–1941" (PhD diss., University of Chicago, 2007), 248.

43. A. Sholomovich, *Meditsinskii rabotnik*, no. 7 (1923): 23. For more on disease and the Bolshevik efforts to tackle it, see Starks, *Body Soviet*, 37–69.

44. The Rockefeller Foundation remained firm in its decision not to become involved in supporting the nursing scheme in Russia. George E. Vincent to John D. Rockefeller Jr., August 9, 1921, RAC, RF, RG 1.1, series 785A, box 2, folder 17. For more on the Rockefeller Foundation's engagement in Russia, see Solomon, "'Power of Dichotomies'"; F. E. Crowell to Embree (Rockefeller Foundation secretary), November 3, 1922, RAC, RF, RG 1.1, series 785C, box 3, folder 28. My thanks to Susan Gross Solomon for sharing this source. Mary Beard traveled to Moscow and Leningrad June 14–18, 1937, but during her visit did not see any hospitals or public health institutes. Mary Beard Diary, April 15, 1937, 58, RAC, RF, RG 1.1, disc 2. My thanks also to Jaime Lapeyre for sharing the Beard and Crowell sources.

45. Payne established an organization called the International School of Nursing and Child Welfare in Russia. GARF, f. A-482, op. 35, d. 53, l. 64, June 5, 1923 (English translation of name as in the original); GARF, f. A-482, op. 35, d. 53, l. 65. Lady Paget's mission was not in a position to offer financial assistance and seemingly withdrew its support. See GARF, f. A-482, op. 35, d. 53, l. 63, June 26, 1923. See also GARF, f. A-482, op. 35, d. 53, l. 65; GARF, f. A-482, op. 35, d. 53, l. 65. For a list of patrons, see GARF, f. A-482, op. 35, d. 54, l. 160 (November 2, 1923).

46. GARF, f. A-482, op. 35, d. 62, l. 138, 1924.

47. GARF, f. A-482, op. 35, d. 53, l. 65; GARF, f. A-482, op. 35, d. 53, l. 67; C. Heath, January 8, 1915 (1922 version), LSF, FEWVRC.

48. David L. Ransel, *Village Mothers: Three Generations of Change in Russia and Tataria* (Bloomington: Indiana University Press, 2000), 47.

49. Payne to Carl Heath, March 5, 1924, LSF. The Quakers favored providing equipment and advice. Nicholson to AFSC, June 17, 1924, AFSC, Foreign Service (FS), Russia General.

50. On discussions about Russia between the Rockefeller Foundation secretary Edwin Embree and Lillian Wald, see Europe in general (report), January 6, 1924, RAC, RF, RG 1.1, series 100C, box 37, folder 314. Wald established the Henry Street Settlement in New York.

51. GARF, f. A-482, op. 35, d. 56, l. 24, February 28, 1924; December 31, 1924. The Russian Commissariat of Public Health representative in New York, Mikhailovskii, and Anna Louise Strong arranged the visit.

52. GARF, f. A-482, op. 35, d. 56, l. 31, January 16, 1923. Mikhailovskii would send these materials to Moscow. The exhibition opened in a library in Moscow, before moving on to other parts of the country.

53. Lillian Wald, *Windows on Henry Street* (Boston: Little, Brown, 1934), 265.

54. The entourage included Elizabeth Farrell, who worked with "subnormal children in public schools," and Lillian Hudson, professor of nursing at Teachers College, Columbia University. Wald, *Windows on Henry Street*, 262.

55. David-Fox, *Showcasing the Great Experiment*, 47.

56. Wald, *Windows on Henry Street*, 262–263.

57. Wald, *Windows on Henry Street*, 264–265.

58. Wald, *Windows on Henry Street*, 266.

59. David-Fox, *Showcasing the Great Experiment*, 87–88.

60. Maria Cristina Galmarini-Kabala, *The Right to Be Helped: Deviance, Entitlement, and the Soviet Moral Order* (DeKalb: Northern Illinois University Press, 2016), 134.

61. On peasants, see Ransel, *Village Mothers*, 57; on abortion, see Galmarini-Kabala, *Right to Be Helped*, 134.

62. From October 1, 1925, the American Women's Hospital Association, headed by Esther Lovejoy, had an interest in Russia and funded a total of six nurses. WKT to D. White, Philadelphia–Moscow, September 28, 1925, letter no. 594, AFSC, FS, Russia General, Correspondence.

63. Education Department, Annual Report 1924, Society of Friends and American Women's Hospital Association, Buzuluk Uezd, Russia, May 1923–May 1, 1924, 15, AFSC, FS, Russia General.

64. See Hoffmann, *Stalinist Values*, 15–23; Galmarini-Kabala, *Right to Be Helped*, 133–145.

65. L. M. Nisnevich and N. I. Propper, "O sostoianii uchebnykh zavedenii po podgotovke srednego meditsinskogo personala v RSFSR" [On the state of educational institutes in the training of medical personnel in the RSFSR], *Meditsina*, no. 8 (1926): 8. There were a total of 10,000 nurses and 15,500 feldshers in the RSFSR. During the period 1926–1928, all middle medical institutes, schools, and courses were reorganized into medical colleges, with branches for two-year nursing courses, three-year courses in midwifery, and special two-and-a-half-year courses for mother and child welfare nurses. Course length was still below the international standard of at least three years set by the ICN, of which the Soviet Union was not a member. McGann, "Collaboration and Conflict," 37. N. A. Vinogradov, *Printsipy raboty s meditsinskimi kadrami* [Principles of work with medical personnel] (Moscow: Medgiz, 1955), 38.

66. N. N. Semenkov, "Etapy razvitiia sestrinskogo obrazovaniia" [Stages of development in nursing education], *Sovetskoe zdravookhraneniia*, no. 7 (1983): 53.

67. Semenkov, "Etapy razvitiia sestrinskogo obrazovaniia," 53–54.

68. For more on nurse types, see N. I. Propper, "Kakie nuzhny sestry—obshchie ili spetsial'nye" [Types of nurses needed—general or specialist], *Meditsina*, no. 3 (1928): 14. For an extensive list, see *Trud i byt' medrabotnikov g. Moskvy i Moskovskoi guberniya* [The work and life of medical workers in Moscow city and Moscow province] (Moscow: Izdatel'stvo Moskovskogo gubotdela soiuza Vsemedsantrud, 1923), 1:42–50.

69. Propper, "Kakie nuzhnyi sestry," 14–15.

70. G. A. Miterev, ed., *Dvadtsat' piat' let sovetskogo zdravookhraneniia* [Twenty-five years of Soviet healthcare] (Moscow: Gos. Izd-vo Meditsinskoi literatury, 1944), 235–236.

71. Miterev, *Dvadtsat' piat' let sovetskogo zdravookhraneniia.*

72. On universalism in medical education, see Susan Gross Solomon, "Social Hygiene in Soviet Medical Education, 1922–30," *Journal of the History of Medicine and Allied Sciences* 45 (1990): 615–616, 639; Propper, "Kakie nuzhny sestry," 14. Local rather than central authorities would finance the new departments for medical specializations. Propper, "Kakie nuzhny sestry," 15. On new specializations and the structure of medical institutes, including schools for workers (*rabfaki*), see V. M. Banshchikov, *Meditsinskie kadry i ikh podgotovka* [Medical personnel and their training] (Moscow-Leningrad: Gosmedizdat, 1931), 17, 27–46.

73. A. P. Zhuk, "Meditsinskaia sestra k 25-i godovshchie Velikoi Oktiabr'skoi sotsialisticheskoi revoliutsii" [The nurse on the 25th anniversary of the Great October socialist revolution], *Meditsinskaia sestra*, no. 11–12 (1942): 7.

74. N. I. Propper, "Podgotovka meditsinskoi sestry prezhde i teper'" [Nurse training past and present], *Meditsina*, no. 9 (1927): 14. In the first year nurses and midwives studied the same course together. On the important role of nurses, see M. Lukomskii, "Rol' srednego personala v dele medpomoshchi" [The role of middle medical personnel in the matter of medical assistance], *Meditsina*, no. 2 (1926): 10–11.

75. On science and medical workers, see Starks, *Body Soviet*, 137.

76. David, "White Plague," 161. The total number of female physicians in 1926 was 20,049. David, "White Plague," 162.

77. David, "White Plague," 163. For the statistics on women and men in healthcare in the mid-1920s, see *Statisticheskie materialy po sostianiiu narodnogo zdravookhraneniia i organizatsii meditsinskoi pomoshchi v SSSR za 1924–1925 gg.* [Statistical material on the state of national healthcare and the organization of medical assistance in the USSR for 1924–1925], (Moscow: Izdatel'stvo Narkomzdrava RSFSR, 1927), 55.

78. GARF, f. A-482, op. 35, d. 144, ll. 128–130, March 12, 1925.

79. GARF, f. A-482, op. 35, d. 144, l. 130. On ideas for "nurse-investigators" and tuberculosis dispensaries, see David, "White Plague," 211–213.

80. GARF, f. A-482, op. 35, d. 144, l. 130.

81. GARF, f. A-482, op. 35, d. 144, l. 130.

82. Haines, *Health Work in Soviet Russia*, 153.

83. Haines, *Health Work in Soviet Russia*, 154.

84. For discussion of the negative imagery associated with the midwife, see Starks, *Body Soviet*, 151. On the patronage nurse, see David, "White Plague," 211. Young women seemed drawn to this kind of work: 48 percent of the 842 nurses for maternal and infant care working in the city and province of Moscow were between twenty and thirty years old, whereas only 16 percent were over age forty. V. M. Banshchikov, "Litso srednego medrabotnika" [The face of the medical worker], *Meditsina*, no. 2 (1930): 11–12.

85. See the discussion on patronage nurses and "schools of motherhood" in Galmarini-Kabala, *The Right to Be Helped*, 133–144.

86. Starks, *Body Soviet*, 126.

87. A. Haines to WKT, August 26, 1925, AFSC, FS, Russia General. See Susan Grant, "Nurses in the Soviet Union: Explorations of Gender in State and Society," in *The Pal-*

grave Handbook of Women and Gender in Twentieth-Century Russia and the Soviet Union, ed. Melanie Ilic (London: Palgrave Macmillan, 2018), 254.

88. AH to WKT, May 27, 1925, AFSC, FS, Russia General, Anna Haines Letters.

89. AH to WKT, August 26, 1925, AFSC, FS, Russia General, Anna Haines Letters.

90. AFSC, Committee Minutes, November 17, 1926.

91. Starks, *Body Soviet*, 154, 155. David also discusses dispensarization, introduced in Moscow in 1924, as a form of surveillance. David, "White Plague," 228–229.

92. Starks, *Body Soviet*, 156.

93. Katrin Schultheiss, *Bodies and Souls: Politics and the Professionalization of Nursing in France, 1880–1922* (Cambridge, MA: Harvard University Press, 2001), 90.

94. Because it was illegal for Russians to send money abroad, Lebedeva needed the AFSC to buy the material on behalf of the clinic and she would then transfer funds to the AFSC training school account in Moscow. DW to WKT, October 26, 1926, letter no. 290, AFSC, FS, Russia General, Correspondence.

95. DW to WKT, November 19, 1926, letter no. 292, AFSC, FS, Russia General.

96. AFSC Committee Minutes, June 16, 1926.

97. Helen R. Bryan, AFSC Committee Minutes, November 1926. On expenditure, see AFSC Minutes, Foreign Service Section (FSS), November 16, 1927, Committee Meetings.

98. AFSC Committee Minutes, March 16, 1927. So as not to jeopardize its continued existence in Russia, the committee agreed to undertake interim work in the nurses' training school, attended by Alice Davis and a Russian nurse, Danielevskaia. This would help maintain links with the Commissariat of Health and assist student nurses in Moscow. See also AFSC Minutes, November 16, 1927.

99. AFSC Minutes, November 1926.

100. GARF, f. A-482, op. 35, d. 62, l. 114.

101. GARF, f. A-482, op. 35, d. 62, l. 114.

102. Haines to Thomas, June 26, 1926, AFSC, FSS, Russia.

103. Susan M. Reverby, *Ordered to Care: The Dilemma of American Nursing, 1850–1945* (Cambridge: Cambridge University Press, 1987), 109.

104. Reverby, *Ordered to Care*, 109.

105. Haines to Thomas, June 26, 1926.

106. Michael David-Fox, *Crossing Borders: Modernity, Ideology, and Culture in Russia and the Soviet Union* (Pittsburgh: University of Pittsburgh Press, 2015), 8.

107. AFSC Minutes, March 16, 1927. L. Hollingsworth Wood, reporting on an interview with "Dr. Pearce of the Rockefeller Foundation," claimed there were still interested parties. See also AFSC Minutes, January 19, 1927. Other potential funders referred Haines back to the Rockefeller Foundation. Mary Beard Diary, October 28, 1927, 151, disc 1. In any event, the Rockefeller Foundation had a preference for sending Russian medical personnel to train in the United States. D. White to WKT, December 29, 1927, AFSC, FS, Russia General, Correspondence. AFSC members also made appeals in England. See Nancy Babb's interview, in "Appeal for Funds to Build School for Training Nurses," *Manchester Guardian*, November 24, 1927, LSF, News 066.39.

108. RF; RG 1.1 Projects; Officer Diaries RG 12RF, Mary Beard Diary, October 28, 1927, 151.

109. Progress Report (Nursing Education Program 1926–1928), vol. 3, 8–29, Europe, RAC, RF, RG 1.1, series 100C, box 38, folder 332. Alan Gregg reported this conversation with Alice Davis during his trip to Moscow in December 1926.

110. Progress Report (Nursing Education Program 1926–1928), vol. 3, 8–29. See also Alan Gregg Diary, Tuesday, December 13, 1927 (Moscow), RAC, RF, RG 1.1, disc 1.

111. Anna Haines to Lillian Wald, January 14, 1928, Lillian Wald Files, reel 106, box 92, folder 13, Columbia University Rare Book and Manuscript Library.

112. The Model Dispensary for tuberculosis patients was one such scheme, facing delays of up to seven months before opening in 1921. David, "White Plague," 216.

113. A. Davis to WKT, May 17, 1928, AFSC, FS, Russia General.

114. Haines, preoccupied with fundraising in the United States, was not interested in going to Russia to work in Yasnaya Polyana, despite the best efforts of Alice Davis and British Qauker Dorice White to persuade her. Dorice White to Alice Nike, March 21, 1928, letter no. 266, LSF, FSC/RU/PO/2, 6362. Davis and Russian nurse Danielevskaia wanted to work in the hospital.

115. WKT to Alice Nike (London), October 19, 1928, AFSC, FS, Russia General.

116. WKT to Nike, October 19, 1928.

117. The war scare was a complex intermingling of foreign and domestic issues. In April–May tensions between the Soviet Union and Britain were tense with Britain cutting off contact with the Soviets in late May. In July 1927 Stalin wrote about a war scare. For a full treatment of the 1927 war scare, see David R. Stone, *Hammer and Rifle: The Militarization of the Soviet Union, 1926–1933* (Lawrence: University Press of Kansas, 2000), 43–64.

118. David, "White Plague," 266.

119. AFSC Committee Minutes, March 20, 1929.

120. WKT to Alice Davis, November 9, 1928, AFSC, FS, Russia General.

121. AFSC, General Administration, April 22, 1929. For more on Quaker work with the OMM, see cable from White to the AFSC, AFSC Minutes, June 19, 1929, Committee Meetings. On Quaker plans, see AFSC Minutes, April 25, 1929.

122. Conditions of Work of the Foreign Nurses in the Proposed Clinic for Baby Diseases (translation). AFSC, FS Russia General, May 28, 1929.

123. To Philadelphia from Russia, letter translated and dated May 28, 1929, AFSC, FS, Russia General.

124. AFSC Minutes, April 25, 1929. See also AFSC Minutes, June 19, 1929, Committee Meetings, 1929.

125. White to William Eves, Russia–Philadelphia, July 12, 1929, letter no. 348, AFSC, FS, Russia General. It was proving quite difficult for the Quakers to find nurses meeting the very specific criteria (Friends, trained nurses, with special training in children's diseases, and, if possible, a knowledge of the Russian language). [William] Eves 3rd, chairman FSS, to DW, August 31, 1929, letter no. 881, AFSC, FS, Russia General.

126. Clarence E. Pickett, AFSC executive secretary, AFSC Minutes, September 1929, Committee Meetings. The AFSC would contribute $2,000 toward expenses once the nurses were dispatched.

127. Dorice White to Friends' Service Committee, Russia–Philadelphia, June 19, 1929, letter no. 347, AFSC, FS, Russia General.

128. AFSC Minutes, August 1931.

129. Marta Aleksandra Balinska, "Assistance and Not Mere Relief: The Epidemic Commission of the League of Nations, 1920–1923," in *International Health Organisations and Movements, 1918–1939*, ed. Paul Weindling (Cambridge: Cambridge University Press, 1995), 99.

4. Proletarian Paradise

1. V. M. Banshchikov, "O zvanii srednikh medrabotnikov" [About the rank of middle medical workers], *Meditsina*, no. 11 (1928): 14.

2. At the Eighth Party Congress in March 1919, Lenin proclaimed that the party must "learn humility and respect for the work of specialists in science and technology." Neil B. Weissman, "Origins of Soviet Health Administration, Narkomzdrav, 1918–1929," in *Health and Society in Revolutionary Russia*, ed. Susan Gross Solomon and John F. Hutchinson (Bloomington: Indiana University Press, 1990), 104.

3. Banshchikov, "O zvanii srednikh medrabotnikov," 14.

4. Diane P. Koenker, *Republic of Labor: Russian Printers and Soviet Socialism, 1918–1930* (Ithaca, NY: Cornell University Press, 2005), 197.

5. *Direktivy KPSS i sovetskogo pravitel'stva po khoziastvennym voprosam: 1917–1928 gody*, 1, (Moscow: Gos. Izd-vo polit. Lit-ry, 1956), 588–590; 1, 573 [CPSU and Soviet government directives on economic issues: 1917–1923, 1], cited in William J. Chase, *Workers, Society, and the Soviet State: Labor and Life in Moscow, 1918–1929* (Urbana: University of Illinois Press, 1989), 189 (67n210).

6. A.L., "Kak zhivut moskovskie medrabotniki. Bol'nitsa imeni D-ra Botkina (byvshaia Soldatenkovskaia)" [How do medical workers live. The hospital named after Botkin (the former Soldatenkovskaia], *Meditsinskii rabotnik*, no. 11 (1924): 12.

7. A.L., "Kak zhivut moskovskie medrabotniki," 12–13.

8. A.L., "Kak zhivut moskovskie medrabotniki? Sokol'nicheskaia bol'nitsa," *Meditsinskii rabotnik*, no. 14 (1924): 11.

9. For membership figures, see A. Aluf, *Spravochnik srednego medpersonala* [Handbook for middle medical workers], (Moscow: TsK MST, 1928), 13. Doctors made up 11.4 percent of members and Sisters and Brothers of Mercy 8.1 percent. Junior medical workers claimed the highest membership, at 25.2 percent. Aluf, *Spravochnik srednego medpersonala*, 13–14.

10. Chase, *Workers, Society, and the Soviet State*, 188. Chase notes that complaints about workers' living conditions appeared in the press after 1925.

11. Living space in Moscow went from 9.3 square meters in 1920 to 5.5 square meters in 1927. Chase, *Workers, Society, and the Soviet State*, 185.

12. GARF, f. 5465, op. 10, d. 129, l. 176.

13. GARF, f. 5465, op. 10, d. 129, l. 176. From Gerasimov in the Chuvash SSR's Commissariat of Health, March 3, 1927, to Sovnarkom RSFSR.

14. I. Dobreitser, "Izuchenie professional'nykh zabolevanii sredi meditsinskikh rabotnikov" [A study of occupational illnesses among medical workers], *Biulleten' Narodnogo Kommissariata zdravookhraneniia*, no. 3 (1926): 11.

15. Dobreitser, "Izuchenie professional'nykh zabolevanii," 11.

16. Chase, *Workers, Society, and the Soviet State*, 192.

17. P. I. Nemkovskaia, "Kartinki byta" [Pictures of everyday life], *Meditsinskii rabotnik*, no. 15 (1925): 10.

18. For discussion of religion and science, see Nikolai Krementsov, *Revolutionary Experiments: The Quest for Immortality in Bolshevik Science and Fiction* (New York: Oxford University Press, 2014), 28–34; on science as the "new religion," see 189–191.

19. Nemkovskaia, "Kartinki byta," 10.

20. The majority of medical workers were from the peasantry. At the medical union / Medsantrud (Vsemedikosantrud became Medsantrud in the mid-1920s) congress in July 1926, just 4.4 percent of the 317 delegates were nurses. A. Aluf, *Itogi shestogo Vsesoiuznogo S''ezda Soiuza Medsantrud* (Konspekt doklada dlia populiarizatsii reshenii VI Vsesoiuznogo S''ezda Medsantrud) [Results of the sixth All-Union Congress of Medsantrud (Summary of a report for popularizing decisions of the VI All-Union Congress of Medsantrud)], (Moscow: Izd. TsK Medsantrud, 1926), 3. The largest group was feldshers, at 25.5 percent. Of the delegates (237 men and 80 women), 239 were party members, 4 were Communist Youth League members, and 74 were nonparty.

21. *Statisticheskii sbornik (Vsesoiuznii professional'nyi soiuz medsantrud)* [Statistic collection. The All-Union professional union of medsantrud], (Moscow: IsK Soiuza Medsantrud, 1928, 1930), Edition 1–3. 156. These numbers represent only those who provided information about their training to the union, or in all, 9,423 middle medical workers.

22. "Chto dolzhen znat' rabotnik" [What a worker should know], 10; F. Kogan, "Srednee meditsinskoe obrazovanie i potrebnosti zdravookhraneniia" (K itogam IV Vserossiiskoi konferentsii po srednemu meditsinskomu obrazovaniiu—iiun' 1929 g.) [Middle medical education and healthcare needs (On the results of the IV All-Russian conference on middle medical education—June 1929)], *Na fronte zdravookhraneniia / Voprosy zdravookhraneniia*, no. 15 (1929): 32.

23. Kogan, "Srednee meditsinskoe obrazovanie," 32.

24. N. A. Vinogradov, *Printsipy raboty s meditsinskimi kadrami* [Principles of working with medical personnel], (Moscow: Medgiz, 1955), 43. Vinogradov noted a drop to 39.9 percent in 1939. Statistics on education showed that 55 percent of the nurses had prerevolutionary education, 31 percent had attended wartime courses, and 13 percent had taken retraining courses. Some 56 percent of Moscow nurses were over 30 years of age (37% were 30–40 years and 21% were over 40), while 44 percent of the nurses had work experience longer than 10 years. V. M. Banshchikov, "Litso srednego medrabotnika" [Face of the middle medical worker], *Meditsina*, no. 2 (1930): 11.

25. TsGAIPD Spb, f. 235, op. 1, d. 34, l. 6, September 18, 1926.

26. TsGAIPD Spb, f. 235, op. 1, d. 34, ll. 2–4, 1925/1926.

27. Hiroaki Kuromiya, *Stalin's Industrial Revolution: Politics and Workers, 1928–1932* (Cambridge: Cambridge University Press, 1988), 235.

28. GARF, f. 5465, op. 20, d. 344, l. 8, 1932, Avdeeva to Sovnarkom representative Molotov, Medsantrud Central Committee.

29. E. Thomas Ewing, *The Teachers of Stalinism: Policy, Practice, and Power in Soviet Schools of the 1930s* (New York: Peter Lang, 2002), 7.

30. Liumkis, "Bezrabotitsa medpersonala i bor'ba s nei" [Unemployed medical personnel and the struggle with it], *Meditsinskii rabotnik*, no. 5 (1924): 4. In particular Liumkis feared a loss of qualified medical personnel. His concerns were based on information from thirty-six gubernia labor exchanges for November 1923.

31. Chase, *Workers, Society, and the Soviet State*, 163.

32. Diane P. Koenker, "Fathers against Sons / Sons against Fathers: The Problem of Generations in the Early Soviet Workplace," *Journal of Modern History* 73, no. 4 (2001): 793.

33. Liumkis, "Bezrabotitsa medpersonala," 4. Unemployment for medical workers in twenty gubernia (including Moscow and Petrograd) amounted to 10,542 in 1923, but the medical sections of fifty gubernias had not submitted their unemployment statistics. M. Chernikov, "Bezrabotitsa i bor'ba s nei" [Unemployment and the struggle with it], *Meditsinskii rabotnik*, no. 19 (1923): 4.

34. We know that among doctors, some 4,000 were unemployed out of a total number of 33,869 in the RSFSR on January 1, 1924—in other words, 8.47 percent of doctors were unemployed. Liumkis, "Bezrabotitsa medpersonala," 4.

35. Those unemployed were mainly wartime nurses and field feldshers. L. M. Nisnevich and N. I. Propper, "O sostoianii uchebnykh zavedenii po podgotovke srednego meditsinskogo personala v RSFSR" [On the state of educational institutions in training middle medical personnel in the RSFSR], *Meditsina*, no. 8 (1926): 8–9. The Commissariat of Health required a minimum of 35,000 doctors and a maximum of 95,000 for the RSFSR. For more statistics, see B. D. Vladimirov, "Polozhenie medpersonala i organy zdravookhraneniia" [The position of medical personnel and the healthcare authorities], [*Na fronte zdravookhraneniia*] *Biulleten' NKZ*, no. 11 (1924): 3.

36. Kuromiya, *Stalin's Industrial Revolution*, 201. When the situation in industry worsened by 1930, an irritated Stalin duly apportioned blame for the labor shortages to the Commissariat of Labor and the All-Union Central Council of Trade Unions (VTsSPS). See also Chase, *Workers, Society, and the Soviet State*, 163.

37. Nisnevich and Propper, "O sostoianii uchebnykh zavedenii," 9.

38. Nisnevich and Propper, "O sostoianii uchebnykh zavedenii," 9.

39. "Ne khvataet sester" [Not enough sisters (nurses)], *Meditsinskii rabotnik*, no. 8 (1927) 11.

40. Vladimir Gsovski, *Soviet Civil Law* (2 vols.; Ann Arbor: University of Michigan Law School, 1948), I, 800 in Mark G. Field, *Doctor and Patient in Soviet Russia* (Cambridge, MA: Harvard University Press, 1957), 3n247. This move did not necessarily resolve the issue. Ewing shows that one-half of newly trained graduates from a teacher training program in Moscow did not show up for their rural assignment in Azerbaijan. Ewing, *Teachers of Stalinism*, 70–71. For more information, see Field's chapter "Allocation of Medical Personnel: The Administrative Solution," 78–101.

41. Chernikov, "Bezrabotitsa i bor'ba s neiu," 4. See also Henry E. Sigerist, *Socialized Medicine in the Soviet Union* (New York: W. W. Norton, 1937), 122; Koenker, "Fathers against Sons," 793.

42. Chernikov, "Bezrabotitsa i bor'ba s neiu," 4.

43. Chase, *Workers, Society, and the Soviet State*, 144.

44. Chase, *Workers, Society, and the Soviet State*, 144.

45. Chernikov, "Bezrabotitsa i bor'ba s neiu," 5. Chernikov was referring to an article published in a *Meditsinskii rabotnik* issue the previous year (presumably by Liumkis).

46. GARF, f. 5515, op. 15, d. 15, l. 32, 1926, F. M. Seniushkin (Medsantrud Central Committee secretary) and N. B. Bakhmutskii (deputy head of the Department of Technical Use or OTE (Otdel tekhnicheskoi ekspluatatsii) to NKT USSR. In 1925–1926 a doctor's monthly salary was 65 rubles and a nurse's was 32 rubles.

47. GARF, f. 5515, op. 15, d. 15, l. 31.

48. Wendy Z. Goldman shows that the NEP reasserted traditional gender divisions in industry and women remained in the lowest-paid jobs. Wendy Z. Goldman, *Women at the Gates: Gender and Industry in Stalin's Russia* (Cambridge: Cambridge University Press, 2002), 15; for unemployment figures, see 17 and 26.

49. GARF, f. 5515, op. 15, d. 15, l. 32 ob, 1926.

50. GARF, f. 5515, op. 15, d. 15, l. 31.

51. For a good synopsis of changing material conditions during the period of NEP and the First Five-Year Plan, see David L. Hoffmann, *Stalinist Values: The Cultural Norms of Soviet Modernity, 1917–1941* (Ithaca, NY: Cornell University Press, 2003), 120–127.

52. "Vrachi na fel'dsherskie mesta" [Doctors to feldsher places], *Meditsinskii rabotnik*, no. 4 (1924): 11; GARF, f. 8009, op. 14, d. 55, l. 11, May 14, 1939.

53. On feldsherism, see Kogan, "Srednee meditsinskoe obrazovanie," 32; GARF, f. 5465, op. 10, d. 150, l. 41, October 2, 1926, NKT-RSFSR, from Aluf and Margolin.

54. HPSSS, Schedule B, vol. 22, Case 1158 (interviewer M.F.), 47, Widener Library, Harvard University, accessed February 13, 2018, https://iiif.lib.harvard.edu/manifests/view/drs:5596364$47i.

55. GARF, f. 5465, op. 9, d. 98, l. 9. Similar steps were being undertaken to tackle unemployment in other industries at the same time. See Koenker, *Republic of Labor*, 220–225.

56. GARF, f. 5465, op. 10, d. 150, l. 41 ob.

57. GARF, f. 5465, op. 10, d. 150, l. 41 ob, October 2, 1926. The special medical facilities established in 1921 for schooled feldshers to retrain as physicians were abolished in 1925. Samuel C. Ramer, "Feldshers and Rural Health Care in the Early Soviet Period," in *Health and Society in Revolutionary Russia*, ed. Susan Gross Solomon and John F. Hutchinson (Bloomington: Indiana University Press, 1990), 128–129.

58. GARF, f. 5465, op. 10, d. 150, l. 41 ob.

59. GARF, f. 5465, op. 10, d. 150, ll. 41–41 ob.

60. GARF, f. 5465, op. 9, d. 98, l. 9, Seniushkin, Bakhmutskii, and Chernysheva. Lecturers and supervisors of practical classes received about 10 rubles a month in unemployment benefits. This rate was less than that of printers (typically high earners), who received just under 17 rubles in October 1927. Koenker, *Republic of Labor*, 224.

61. GARF, f. 5465, op. 9, d. 98, l. 9. The Commissariats of Labor and Education would cover all expenses for the training schools.

62. GARF, f. 5465, op. 9, d. 98, l. 9.

63. GARF, f. 5465, op. 10, d. 150, l. 20, October 20, 1927, NKT, RSFSR, from Central Committee secretary Aluf; GARF, f. 5465, op. 10, d. 150, l. 32. Subjects included general biology and clinical medicine, as well as classes on general care that would take place in the medical institute. Nurses were also to learn about vaccinations and how to administer them. The lecturer was to provide a report about the subjects, the students, and the medical college courses to Glavprofobr.

64. GARF, f. 5465, op. 10, d. 150, l. 21 ob; GARF, f. 5465, op. 9, d. 98, l. 9, 1927. For discussion of divisions between the Commissariats of Health and Labor, see Sally Ewing, "The Science and Politics of Soviet Insurance Medicine," in *Health and Society in Revolutionary Russia*, ed. Susan Gross Solomon and John F. Hutchinson (Bloomington: Indiana University Press, 1990), 69–96.

65. GARF, f. 5465, op. 10, d. 150, l. 22, in the Medsantrud Central Committee, October 20, 1927. From OTE head Bakhmutskii and the head of the cultural section, Chernysheva. The reports' details included information on which courses were opened and when, their duration, the number accepted into the courses, those graduating, and, if possible, the destination of course graduates. The Commissariat of Labor also wanted to know if the funds were used fully. If Medsantrud did not provide reports with these details, then the commissariat would not guarantee the release of funds in the future.

66. Lev Kuperman, "K voprosu o perekvalifikatsii sester voennogo vremeni" [On the question of retraining wartime nurses], *Meditsina*, no. 7 (1929): 11.

67. L.F., "O povyshenii kvalifikatsii i perekvalifikatsii srednego personala" [On raising the qualifications and retraining of middle medical personnel], *Meditsina*, no. 19 (1929): 9–10. This lack of interest was in spite of a shortage of twenty thousand middle medical workers.

68. GARF, f. 5465, op. 6, d. 161, l. 53. Zhukovitskii provided his party card number and dated the letter October 18, 1924. The signature "Gor'kii" was a play on the Russian word meaning "sad" or "bitter" and the writer Maxim Gorky.

69. GARF, f. 5465, op. 6, d. 161, l. 104. From the *uezd* (administrative subdivision) secretary of the Medsantrud union in Bolog Gubernia, March 1924. For further discussion of worker complaints and "medical horror stories," see Ewing, "Soviet Insurance Medicine," 81.

70. See Christopher M. Davis, "Economics of Soviet Public Health," in *Health and Society in Revolutionary Russia*, ed. Susan Gross Solomon and John F. Hutchinson (Bloomington: Indiana University Press, 1990), 166.

71. Davis, "Economics of Soviet Public Health," 166.

72. *Izvestiia N. K. Truda SSSR*, no. 28 (1930), cited in Kuromiya, *Stalin's Industrial Revolution*, 202. As in other commissariats, new cadres replaced 100 percent of top staff and department heads of the Commissariat of Labor. Kuromiya, *Stalin's Industrial Revolution*, 223.

73. Kuromiya, *Stalin's Industrial Revolution*, 223.

74. A. Aluf, "Vzaimootnosheniia srednego medpersonala s naseleniem" [The relationship between medical personnel and the population], *Meditsina*, no. 3 (1927): 10.

75. Dav. Khait, "Kak zhivut moskovskie medrabotniki (1-ia Gorodskaia bol'nitsa imeni Pirogova)" [How do Moscow medical workers live (the first City Hospital named for Pirogov)], *Meditsinskii rabotnik*, no. 22 (1924): 10–11.

76. Nancy Mandelker Frieden, *Russian Physicians in an Era of Reform and Revolution, 1856–1905* (Princeton, NJ: Princeton University Press, 1981), 143–153. The Soviet period saw some cases of medical workers assaulting patients, but those were less common. Kenneth Pinnow has discussed violence against doctors and medical ethics in the Soviet Union. Kenneth Pinnow, "Medical Ethics and the Crisis of the Doctor-Patient Relationship in the Early Soviet Union" (paper presented at the Jordan Center for the Advanced Study of Russia, New York University, New York, November 2, 2020).

77. Aluf, "Vzaimootnosheniia srednego medpersonala s naseleniem," 10.

78. Some in the trade union held "malicious bullies and hooligans" responsible for violent attacks. GARF, f. 5465, op. 7, d. 110, l. 1.

79. GARF, f. 5465, op. 7, d. 110, l. 1.

80. For examples, see GARF, f. 5465, op. 7, d. 110, l. 2.

81. See GARF, f. 5465, op. 10, d. 276, l. 15, l. 31, 1928.

82. GARF, f. 5465, op. 7, d. 113. See also Central State Archive of Moscow Oblast (hereafter TsGAMO), f. 975, op. 5, d. 15, l. 58.

83. Aluf, "Vzaimootnosheniia srednego medpersonala s naseleniem," 10.

84. Ramer, "Feldshers and Rural Health Care," 137.

85. Russian State Military Archive (hereafter RGVA), f. 19032, op. 1, d. 2, l. 30, April 20, 1928.

86. RGVA, f. 19032, op. 1, d. 2, l. 30, l. 30 ob.

87. RGVA, f. 19032, op. 1, d. 2, l. 30, l. 30 ob.

88. Tracy McDonald, *Face to the Village: The Riazan Countryside under Soviet Rule, 1921–1930* (Toronto: University of Toronto Press, 2011), 209.

89. GARF, f. 5465, op. 10, d. 164, l. 25, Shtess. See also for weapons found on patients, attempted escapes, and patient self-harm.

90. A. Aluf, "Izd TsK Medsantrud" [Izd TsK Medsantrud], *Meditsina*, no. 3 (1929): 14. The provincial health department put the matter of expanding medical staff in psychiatric hospitals before the provincial executive committee.

91. GARF, f. 5465, op. 10, d. 17, l. 2, 1928. Seniushkin listed five main problems in total, including illness simulation, feelings of incompetence, and dissatisfaction with treatment.

92. GARF, f. 5465, op. 10, d. 17, l. 2.

93. GARF, f. 5465, op. 10, d. 17, l. 7, 1928.

94. Peasant migration to major cities increased significantly in 1930–1931 as a consequence of collectivization. See David L. Hoffmann, *Peasant Metropolis: Social Identities in Moscow, 1929–1941* (Ithaca, NY: Cornell University Press, 1994), 35.

95. Lynne Viola, V. P. Danilov, N. A. Ivnitskii, and Denis Kozlov, eds., *The War against the Peasantry, 1927–1930: The Tragedy of the Soviet Countryside*, trans. Steven Shabad (New Haven, CT: Yale University Press, 2005), 15.

96. GARF, f. 5465, op. 17, d. 37, ll. 14–14 ob, 1931.

97. H. Davies, "Falling Public Trust in Health Services: Implications for Accountability," *Journal of Health Services Research and Policy* 4 (1999): 193–194, cited in M. W. Calnan and E. Sanford, "Public Trust in Health Care: The System or the Doctor?," *Quality and Safety in Healthcare* 13 (2004): 92.

98. McDonald, *Face to the Village*, 213.

99. GARF, f. 5465, op. 6, d. 1, l. 20, Kalinin.

100. GARF, f. 5465, op. 6, d. 1, ll. 20–21.

101. Hoffmann, *Stalinist Values*, 59–60.

102. Hoffmann, *Stalinist Values*, 59–60.

103. Iu.D., "Delo 1-go Moskovskogo rodil'nogo doma" [The case of the First Moscow maternity hospital], *Meditsinskii rabotnik*, no. 38 (1926): 14. For sensational and inaccurate accounts, see GARF, f. 5465, op. 9, d. 129, l. 134, l. 137.

104. Iu.D., "Delo 1-go Moskovskogo rodil'nogo doma," 14.

105. In the end Baron received a three-year sentence. The maternity hospital was also shut down on September 25, 1926. Iu.D., "Delo 1-go Moskovskogo rodil'nogo doma," 14.

106. For a discussion of suffering and compassion, see Elizabeth V. Spelman, *Fruits of Sorrow: Framing Our Attention to Suffering* (Boston: Beacon Press, 1997).

107. "V," "Sud i byt: Akusherka Skliarskaia," *Rabotnitsa*, no. 34 (1928): 19.

108. "V," "Sud i byt: Akusherka Skliarskaia," 19.

109. The midwife received a six-month prison term. The doctor received a one-year prison sentence.

110. Martha C. Nussbaum, *Upheavals of Thought: The Intelligence of the Emotions* (Cambridge: Cambridge University Press, 2003), 420. There were some examples of good care and compassion; see, for example, "Sem' let vo sne: Redkii sluchai entsefalita" [Seven years asleep: A rare case of encephalitis] *Meditsinskii rabotnik*, no. 27 (1929): 17.

111. Drawing on feminist debate, Elizabeth V. Spelman discusses stereotypes of women, women's treatment of each other, and the ethics of care. Spelman, *Fruits of Sorrow*, 92–94.

112. TsGAMO, f. 975, op. 2, d. 56, l. 5. In more general terms, work discipline on the part of middle medical workers was a concern. See Ia. Gal'perin, "O trudodistsipline" [On work disciple], *Meditsina*, no. 9 (1929): 1.

113. Weissman, "Origins of Soviet Health Administration," 112.

114. GARF, f. 5465, op. 13, d. 118, l. 17.

115. Kuromiya, *Stalin's Industrial Revolution*, 81.

116. Elena Osokina, *Our Daily Bread: Socialist Distribution and the Art of Survival in Stalin's Russia, 1927–1941*, ed. Kate Transchel, trans. Kate Transchel and Greta Bucher, The New Russian History (Armonk, NY: M. E. Sharpe, 2001), 16. See also Goldman, *Women at the Gates*, 76–82.

117. Kuromiya, *Stalin's Industrial Revolution*, 228–235.

118. Sheila Fitzpatrick, *Everyday Stalinism: Ordinary Life in Extraordinary Times; Soviet Russia in the 1930s* (New York: Oxford University Press, 1999), 57–58, 97. An archive report on price rises from a *"svodka"* or secret police report is discussed in Fitzpatrick, *Everyday Stalinism*, 165–172.

119. GARF, f. 5465, op. 13, d. 118, l. 17.

120. GARF, f. 5465, op. 13, d. 118, l. 17.

121. Jeffrey J. Rossman, "The Teikovo Cotton Workers' Strike of April 1932: Class, Gender and Identity Politics in Stalin's Russia," *Russian Review* 56 (1997): 44–69.

122. GARF, f. 5465, op. 13, d. 118, l. 11, September 19, 1931, S. Il'in.

123. I take this line of argument on the socioeconomic system and social identity in 1917 from William G. Rosenberg, "Identities, Power, and Social Interactions in Revolutionary Russia," *Slavic Review* 47, no. 1 (1988): 23.

124. Osokina, *Our Daily Bread*, 219n20. The highest salary was 180 rubles a month, and the lowest was 30–50 rubles a month.

125. GARF, f. 5465, op. 13, d. 118, l. 18.

126. GARF, f. 5465, op. 13, d. 118, l. 18. Private practice was common among all medical workers during the NEP period and was legal.

127. GARF, f. 5465, op. 13, d. 118, l. 18.

128. On resistance, see Donald Filtzer, *Soviet Workers and Stalinist Industrialization: The Formation of Modern Soviet Production Relations, 1928–1941* (London: Pluto Press, 1986); James C. Scott, *Weapons of the Weak: Everyday Forms of Peasant Resistance* (New Haven, CT: Yale University Press, 1987).

129. GARF, f. 5465, op. 13, d. 118, l. 18.

130. GARF, f. 5465, op. 13, d. 118, l. 18.

131. Chase, *Workers, Society, and the Soviet State*; Kuromiya, *Stalin's Industrial Revolution*; Koenker, "Fathers against Sons," 781–810.

132. GARF, f. 5465, op. 13, d. 118, l. 18.

133. GARF, f. 5465, op. 13, d. 118, l. 19.

134. GARF, f. 5465, op. 13, d. 43, l. 23. Two workers who led a group against Lotz were removed from their positions.

135. Koenker, *Republic of Labor*, 44.

136. Mikh. Sokolov, "Grimasy bol'nichnoi zhizni" [Grimaces of hospital life], *Meditsinskii rabotnik*, no. 9 (1929): 4.

137. Sokolov, "Grimasy bol'nichnoi zhizni," 4.

138. Sokolov, "Grimasy bol'nichnoi zhizni," 4.

139. Sokolov, "Grimasy bol'nichnoi zhizni," 5.

140. James Heinzen, *The Art of the Bribe: Corruption under Stalin* (New Haven, CT: Yale University Press, 2016), 113; for the complexities of differentiating between bribes, fees, and tokens of gratitude during the Stalin period, see 112–114.

141. Sokolov, "Grimasy bol'nichnoi zhizni," 5.

142. Doctors would receive 144–225 rubles per month; dentists, 110–130; middle medical personnel, 80–120; and junior personnel, 55–90. The public health authorities and the medical trade unions would work out a pay differential table for each category of medical specialty to reflect a medical worker's length of service, education, and quality of work. GARF, f. 5465, op. 13, d. 118, l.1, from *Vecherniaia Moskva*, December 16, 1931.

143. "O postanovlenii zarabotnoi platy meditsinskikh rabotnikov" [About the resolution on the salary for medical workers], *Za kadry srednego meditsinskogo personala*, no. 1–2 (1932): 45.

144. GARF, f. 5446, op. 13, d. 1957, l. 21, December 20, 1931, Sovnarkom representative.

145. GARF, f. 5465, op. 14, d. 136, l. 70, June 20, 1932. These changes took place at a time of expansion in the healthcare system: in 1932 there were 372,000 hospital beds in the Soviet Union compared to 147,700 in 1928. I. B. Rostotskii, "Istoricheskoe reshenie" [Historical decision], *Meditsinskaia sestra*, no. 8 (1955): 4. The figures excluded psychiatric hospitals; the original source is G. A. Miterev, ed., *Dvadtsat' piat' let sovetskogo zdravookhraneniia* [Twenty-five years of Soviet healthcare], (Moscow: Gos. Izd-vo Meditsinskoi literatury, 1944).

146. GARF, f. 5465, op. 14, d. 111, l. 15, May 27, 1932.

147. GARF, f. 5465, op. 14, d. 136, l. 39, October 15, 1932. This file includes a chart with differences between provisions for teachers and medical workers. The teacher would receive 800 kilos of semi-white flour, but the medical worker would receive 800 grams of rye flour. GARF, f. 5465, op. 14, d. 136, l. 37, l. 39. For comparisons with industrial workers, see Kuromiya, *Stalin's Industrial Revolution*, 249; Osokina, *Our Daily Bread*, 49–50.

148. Koenker, *Republic of Labor*, 242.

5. Stalinist Care

1. Nikolas Rose, *The Politics of Life Itself: Biomedicine, Power, and Subjectivity in the Twenty-First Century* (Princeton, NJ: Princeton University Press, 2007), 10. The clinical gaze entailed a continued focus on the body as well as the broadening of medical ju-

risdiction. Rose in his book draws on Michel Foucault's *The Birth of the Clinic*. The increase in the clinical or medical gaze tallies with Foucault's discussion of observing and seeing the visible and invisible. Michel Foucault, *The Birth of the Clinic: An Archaeology of Medical Perception*, trans. A. M. Sheridan Smith (London: Routledge, 1989), 131–151.

2. See, for example, Karen Petrone, *Life Has Become More Joyous, Comrades: Celebrations in the Time of Stalin* (Bloomington: Indiana University Press, 2000).

3. Dan Healey, "Lives in the Balance: Weak and Disabled Prisoners and the Biopolitics of the Gulag," *Kritika: Explorations in Russian and Eurasian History* 16, no. 3 (2015): 527. See also Golfo Alexopoulos, *Illness and Inhumanity in Stalin's Gulag* (New Haven, CT: Yale University Press, 2017).

4. David L. Hoffmann, *Cultivating the Masses: Modern State Practices and Soviet Socialism, 1914–1939* (Ithaca, NY: Cornell University Press, 2011), 1.

5. I. P. Pokrovskii, "Osnovnye voprosy kachestva lechebnoi pomoshchi v bol'nitse" [The main questions about the quality of medical help in the hospital], *Na fronte zdravookhraneniia*, no. 7–8 (1934): 52.

6. M. E. Zhitnitsky, "Voprosy reorganizatsii truda ukhazhivaiushchego personala bol'nichnykh uchrezhdenii" [Questions on the reorganization of labor for nursing personnel in hospital institutions], *Na fronte zdravookhraneniia*, no. 9 (1934): 28.

7. Zhitnitsky, "Voprosy reorganizatsii truda," 28–29. Zhitnitsky cites the following article: K. Kissling, "Sluzhba ukhazhivaiushchego personala, Rukovodstvo Grobera po sooruzheniiu i upravleniiu bol'nichnymi zavedeniiami" [Nursing personnel service, Grober's guide to the construction and management of hospital facilities], 745. Zhitnitsky was affiliated to the Institute of Social Hygiene and Healthcare (Commissariat of Public Health) and the Central Committee of Medsantrud.

8. Zhitnitsky, "Voprosy reorganizatsii truda," 28.

9. Zhitnitsky, "Voprosy reorganizatsii truda," 28.

10. The "woman question" of the 1920s and 1930s was a complex affair, and, in many cases, women were not especially revolutionary in the 1920s. Indeed, Elizabeth A. Wood refers to women as the "reserve army of the revolution," a group "to be dismissed when no longer needed." Elizabeth A. Wood, *The Baba and the Comrade: Gender and Politics in Revolutionary Russia* (Bloomington: Indiana University Press, 1997), 221.

11. Meryn Stuart, with Geertje Boschma, "Seeking Stability in the Midst of Change," in *Nurses of All Nations: A History of the International Council of Nurses, 1899–1999*, ed. Barbara L. Brush and Joan. E. Lynaugh (Philadelphia: Lippincott, 1999), 104.

12. Katrin Schultheiss, *Bodies and Souls: Politics and the Professionalization of Nursing in France, 1880–1922* (Cambridge, MA: Harvard University Press, 2001), 9.

13. GARF, f. 8009, op. 1, d. 97, l. 5, 1937.

14. GARF, f. 8009, op. 1, d. 97, l. 5.

15. "Meditsinskaia sestra" [Nurse], *Meditsinskaia sestra*, no. 70 (1938): 1. For more on gender and tropes of nursing, see Susan Grant, "Nurses in the Soviet Union: Explorations of Gender in State and Society," in *The Palgrave Handbook of Women and Gender in Twentieth-Century Russia and the Soviet Union*, ed. Melanie Ilic (London: Palgrave Macmillan, 2018), 249–265; and Susan Grant, "Devotion and Revolution: Nursing Values," in *Rethinking the Russian Revolution as Historical Divide*, ed. Matthias Neumann and Andy Willimott (London: Routledge, 2018), 171–185.

16. Ia. I. Akodus and A. A. Skoriukova, *Meditsinskaia sestra Sovetskogo Krasnogo Kresta* [Soviet Red Cross nurse], (Moscow: Medgiz, 1955), 52.

17. Martha C. Nussbaum, *Upheavals of Thought: The Intelligence of Emotions* (Cambridge: Cambridge University Press, 2003), 376. The other reason for assumptions about women and emotions, according to Nussbaum, is that women have less control over their social and material worlds and are consequently more vulnerable than men. Nussbaum, *Upheavals of Thought*, 377.

18. On new gender identities and deconstructing gender, see Anna Krylova, *Soviet Women in Combat: A History of Violence on the Eastern Front* (Cambridge: Cambridge University Press, 2010), 50–51.

19. Alissa Klots, "The Kitchen Maid as Revolutionary Symbol: Paid Domestic Labour and the Emancipation of Soviet Women, 1917–1941," in *The Palgrave Handbook of Women and Gender in Twentieth-Century Russia and the Soviet Union*, ed. Melanie Ilic (London: Palgrave Macmillan, 2018), 86.

20. For examples, see Frances Lee Bernstein, *The Dictatorship of Sex: Lifestyle Advice for the Soviet Masses* (DeKalb: Northern Illinois University Press, 2007); David L. Hoffmann, *Stalinist Values: The Cultural Norms of Soviet Modernity, 1917–1941* (Ithaca, NY: Cornell University Press, 2003), 89.

21. E. M. Parkhomenko, "Luchshe gotovit' srednie meditsinskie kadry" [It is better to train middle medical personnel], *Meditsinskii rabotnik*, no. 56 (1938): 3.

22. A. I. Abrikosov, "O vrachebnykh oshibkakh" [About medical mistakes], *Meditsinskii rabotnik*, no. 20 (1938): 2. It seems likely that this Abrikosov was the eminent pathologist who embalmed Lenin's body and whose son won the Nobel Prize in Physics in 2003. See "Aleksei Ivanovich Abrikosov - vidnyi rossiiskii patologoanatom" on *Professiia—vrach*, accessed January 18, 2021, https://professiya-vrach.ru/article/aleksey-ivanovich-abrikosov-vidnyy-rossiyskiy-patologoanatom/.

23. Hoffmann, *Cultivating the Masses*, 63.

24. N. I. Propper, "K voprosu o reforme srednego medobrazovaniia" [On the question of reforms in middle medical education], *Meditsina*, no. 3 (1927): 15; V. Ivanov, "Bol'nitsa—medtekhnik" [Hosptial—medical equipment], *Meditsina*, no. 17–18 (1930): 14.

25. Hiroaki Kuromiya, *Stalin's Industrial Revolution: Politics and Workers, 1928–1932* (Cambridge: Cambridge University Press, 1988), 217, 204; F. Kogan, "Srednee meditsinskoe obrazovanie i potrebnosti zdravookhraneniia" (K itogam IV Vserossiiskoi konferentsii po srednemu meditsinskomu obrazovaniiu—iiun' 1929 g.) [Middle medical education and healthcare needs (On the results of the IV All-Russian conference on middle medical education—June 1929)], *Na fronte zdravookhraneniia / Voprosy zdravookhraneniia*, no. 15 (1929): 32.

26. Michael Ryan, *Doctors and the State in the Soviet Union* (New York: St. Martin's Press, 1990), 9.

27. Ryan, *Doctors and the State in the Soviet Union*, 9.

28. G. Moskalev, "Povyshenie kvalifikatsii rabotnikov mediko-sanitarnykh uchrezhdenii, kak metod bor'by s ikh tekuchest'iu" [Raising the qualification of workers in medical-sanitary institutions, as a method of fighting against transiency], *Meditsina*, no. 13–14 (1931): 11.

29. Central State Archive of the City of Moscow—Division for Preservation of Records since 1917 (hereafter TsGAM), f. 552, op. 1, d. 13, l. 21. Instructions on the rights

and duties of nurses; based on Sovnarkom Decree No. 1649 of September 3, 1936, Banshchikov.

30. TsGAM, f. 552, op. 1, d. 13, ll. 21–22.

31. Maria Cristina Galmarini-Kabala, *The Right to Be Helped: Deviance, Entitlement, and the Soviet Moral Order* (DeKalb: Northern Illinois University Press, 2016), 167.

32. TsGAM, f. 552, op. 1, d. 13, l. 47, March 13, 1937, Commissariat of Health position on schools for nurses.

33. Hoffmann, *Stalinist Values*, 105.

34. Michael David, "The White Plague in the Red Capital: The Control of Tuberculosis in Russia, 1900–1941" (PhD diss., University of Chicago, 2007), 323–324.

35. TsGAM, f. 552, op. 1, d. 15, ll. 1–3, study plan for nurses, March 18, 1937. The plan was for two years, over a forty-eight-week period. The plan remained the same for 1938.

36. TsGAM, f. 552, op. 1, d. 31, l. 1, January 25, 1938.

37. See GARF, f. 9501, op. 3, d. 54, l.11–26; complete information with a subject breakdown on l. 26; NKZ, Kaminskii and Banshchikov, March 13, 1937, "The Rights and Duties of Nurses," and nursing curricula. G. Kaminskii, *Instruktsiia dlia starshei operatsionnoi sestry* [Instructions for a senior surgical nurse], (Moscow: Biomedgiz, 1935).

38. TsGAM, f. 552, op. 1, d. 59, l. 7 (January 18, 1939). Paula A. Michaels notes a similar trend in Kazakh medical institutes, albeit in the late 1940s. Paula A. Michaels, *Curative Powers: Medicine and Empire in Stalin's Central Asia* (Pittsburgh: University of Pittsburgh Press, 2003), 98.

39. For more on the situation for industrial workers, see Kuromiya, *Stalin's Industrial Revolution*, 227–228.

40. TsGAM, f. 552, op. 1, d. 34, l. 2, June 23, 1937.

41. TsGAM, f. 552, op. 1, d. 36, l. 4.

42. TsGAM, f. 552, op. 1, d. 36, l. 4.

43. TsGAM, f. 552, op. 1, d. 36, l. 4.

44. For a discussion of the survival of class categories, see Seth Bernstein, "Class Dismissed? New Elites and Old Enemies among the 'Best' Socialist Youth in the Komsomol, 1939–1941," *Russian Review* 74 (2015): 97–116.

45. HPSSS, Schedule B, vol. 2, Case 1758 NY (interviewer M.F.), accessed August 14, 2018, 25, Widener Library, Harvard University, http://nrs.harvard.edu/urn-3:FHCL:939792?n=25.

46. HPSSS, Schedule B, vol. 2, Case 1758 NY, 25.

47. HPSSS, Schedule B, vol. 2, Case 1758 NY, 25.

48. *Fel'dsher*, no. 7 (1937): 11. By January 1940 there were 1,147 middle medical schools with 231,600 students in the USSR. N. A. Vinogradov, *Printsipy raboty s meditsinskimi kadrami* [Principles of work with medical cadres], (Moscow: Medgiz, 1955).

49. TsGAM, f. 552, op. 1, d. 36, l. 99 ob. Plans were afoot to drastically increase the numbers of medical workers with complete medical education for nurseries during the Third Five-Year Plan.

50. TsGAM, f. 552, op. 1, d. 36, l. 100.

51. TsGAM, f. 552, op. 1, d. 36, l. 100 ob.

52. GARF, f. 8009, op. 1, d. 67, l. 22 (Saminskii from Lenggorzdravotdel). The USSR figures for January 1, 1940, were 369,600 middle medical workers, 64.9 percent of

whom had legal middle medical education. Vinogradov, *Printsipy raboty s meditsinskimi kadrami*.

53. E. Thomas Ewing makes this point about mass education and modernization in relation to teachers and education more generally. See E. Thomas Ewing, *The Teachers of Stalinism: Policy, Practice, and Power in Soviet Schools of the 1930s* (New York: Peter Lang, 2002), 53–54; for wide scholarship, see 284n4. On other medical workers, see GARF, f. 9501, op. 3, d. 27, l. 46, 1936.

54. GARF, f. 5465, op. 17, d. 170, l. 21. Particular issues included no. 5–11 (1934).

55. GARF, f. 5465, op. 17, d. 170, l. 21.

56. GARF, f. 5465, op. 17, d. 168, l. 2 ob.

57. "Kak vypolniaetsia postanovlenie TsK VKP (b) i SNK ot 4/III 1935" [How to implement the resolution of the TsK VKP (b) from 4/III 1935], *Meditsinskii rabotnik*, no. 8 (1935): 12.

58. "Kak vypolniaetsia postanovlenie," 12.

59. "Kak vypolniaetsia postanovlenie," 13.

60. Basmannaia hospital, Novia Tasmania, 26. Number of beds: 470. Head doctor: Evg. Nik. Prozorovskii. *Vsia Moskva II chast'* [All Moscow: Part II] (Moscow, 1936), pt. 2, 303–304.

61. "Kak vypolniaetsia postanovlenie," 14–15.

62. "Kak vypolniaetsia postanovlenie," 14–15.

63. See B. Danilov, "Politicheskoe vospitanie mladshego meditsinskogo personala" [The political education of junior medical personnel], *Meditsinskii rabotnik*, no. 89 (1939): 3; M. Korman, "'Vrachebnye oshibki' ili vopiiushchie prestupleniia?" [Medical errors or egregious crimes?], *Meditsinskii rabotnik*, no. 17 (1938): 3.

64. N. N. Burdenko, "Rol' i zadachi meditsinskikh sester" [Role and tasks of the nurse], *Za sanitarnuiu oboronu*, no. 6 (1935): 9.

65. E. Gamarnikov, "Nurse or woman: Gender and professionalism in reformed nursing 1860–1923." In *Anthropology and Nursing*, eds P. Holden & J. Littlewood (London: Routledge, 1991), 123–126, cited in Rosemary Pringle, *Sex and Medicine: Gender, Power and Authority in the Medical Profession* (Cambridge: Cambridge University Press, 1998), 189.

66. If this person had not been an instructor, the monthly wage would have been 180–350 rubles. HPSSS, Schedule A, vol. 25, Case 490 (interviewer H.B., type A4), 13. Widener Library, Harvard University, accessed February 26, 2018, https://iiif.lib .harvard.edu/manifests/view/drs:5362752$13i. She received a decent monthly wage of 400 rubles owing to her length of service, her night-duty work, and the fact that she was an instructor.

67. HPSSS, Schedule A, vol. 25, Case 490, 10.

68. HPSSS, Schedule A, vol. 25, Case 490, 13.

69. HPSSS, Schedule A, vol. 25, Case 490, 15.

70. S. Rafal'kes (Moscow), "O kadrakh mladshego meditsinskogo personala" [About cadres of junior medical personnel], *Na fronte zdravookhraneniia*, no. 17–18 (1930): 52.

71. Grace Clement, *Care, Autonomy, and Justice: Feminism and the Ethic of Care* (Boulder, CO: Westview Press, 1991), 63.

72. V. Goriushkin, "Vnimanie k bol'nitsam dolzhno byt' usileno" [Attention to the hospitals should be strengthened], *Na fronte zdravookhraneniia*, no. 1 (1934): 25.

73. Rafal'kes, "O kadrakh," 52.

74. Goriushkin, "Vnimanie k bol'nitsam," 25.

75. Goriushkin, "Vnimanie k bol'nitsam," 25.

76. Michel Foucault, *The History of Sexuality*, vol. 1, *The Will to Knowledge*, trans. Robert Hurley (London: Penguin Books, 1998), 141. On states of exception, see Giorgio Agamben, *Homo Sacer: Sovereign Power and Bare Life*, trans. Daniel Heller-Roazen (Stanford, CA: Stanford University Press, 1995), 159.

77. Joseph Stalin, *Collected Works* (New York: Prism Key Press, 2013), 2:57. See also Kuromiya, *Stalin's Industrial Revolution*, 283.

78. "O povyshenii zarabotnoi platy meditsinskim rabotnikam i ob uvelichenii assignovanii na zdravookhranenie v 1935" [On increasing the wage of medical workers and on the increase in allocations in healthcare in 1935], *Meditsinskii rabotnik*, no. 2 (1935): 4–5. Sovnarkom also issued a decree on medical workers' salaries that would go into effect on January 1, 1936. GARF, f. 3316, op. 28, d. 560, Sovnarkom, December 26, 1935, Molotov. For a complete breakdown of all medical workers' wages, see also "O povyshenii zarabotnoi platy meditsinskim rabotnikam i ob uvelichenii assignovanii na zdravookhranenie v 1935" [On increasing the wage of medical workers and on the increase in allocations in healthcare in 1935], Na fronte zdravookhraneniia 3 (1935): 1–5.

79. Dr. Liubovskii, cited in "Ucheboi povysim kachestvo raboty" [We will increase the quality of work by studying], *Meditsinskii rabotnik*, no. 3 (1935): 18.

80. Liubovskii, cited in "Ucheboi povysim kachestvo raboty," 18.

81. "Ucheboi povysim kachestvo raboty," 18.

82. "Ucheboi povysim kachestvo raboty," 18.

83. "Ucheboi povysim kachestvo raboty," 19.

84. See also "Kak vypolniaetsia postanovlenie," 12–15.

85. GARF, f. 8009, op. 1, d. 95, l. 56, Obshche-gorodskoi aktiv medrabotnikov, November 30, 1937, Cheremushnikov, Leningrad. Orderlies earned 70–80 rubles a month and nurses working in a day nursery received 100 rubles.

86. GARF, f. 8009, op. 1, d. 95, l. 56.

87. GARF, f. 8009, op. 1, d. 95, l. 56 ob.

88. Susan M. Reverby, *Ordered to Care: The Dilemma of American Nursing, 1850–1945* (Cambridge: Cambridge University Press, 1987), 192.

89. GARF, f. 8009, op. 1, d. 95, l. 71, November 30, 1937. On labor turnover, see Donald Filtzer, *Soviet Workers and Stalinist Industrialization: The Formation of Modern Soviet Production Relations, 1928–1941* (London: Pluto Press, 1986), 49–63. On labor discipline during the Second Five-Year Plan, see Filtzer, *Soviet Workers and Stalinist Industrialization*, 134–144.

90. The Solovki islands were the site of a notorious labor camp.

91. GARF, f. 8009, op. 1, d. 95, l. 71.

92. "Vnimanie sanitarke" [Attention to the orderly], *Meditsinskii rabotnik*, no. 46 (1938): 3.

93. Nota-Bene, "V Botinskoi uravnilovka ne dobita" [In the Botkin equalization is not achieved], *Meditsinskii rabotnik*, no. 20–21 (1939): 9.

94. Nota-Bene, "V Botinskoi uravnilovka ne dobita," 9.

95. TsGAM, f. 552, op. 1, d. 46, l. 73 ob. On nurse achievements, see L. Lerov, "Meditsinskie sestry" [Nurses], *Meditsinskii rabotnik*, no. 46 (1939): 2.

96. "O 1-i obshchegorodskoi nauchno-prakticheskoi konferentsii akusherok i medit-sinskikh sester akushersko-ginekologicheskikh uchrezhdenii Leningrada 1939 g." [About the 1ˢᵗ general city scientific-practical conference of midwives and nurses of midwifery-gynecological institutions in Leningrad 1939], *Meditsinskaia sestra*, no. 5 (1980): 40–42.

97. TsGAM, f. 552, op. 1, d. 46, l. 73 ob.

98. TsGAM, f. 552, op. 1, d. 46, l. 80.

99. "Na Leningradskoi konferenstii akusherok i detskikh sester" [At the Leningrad conference of midwives and children's (pediatric) nurses] *Meditsinskii rabotnik*, no. 53 (1939): 1. For detailed discussion of the conference and published papers, see L. A. Emdin (head of Lengorzdravotdel), "Ocherednye zadachi zdravookhaneniia v Leningrade na 1939 g." [Outstanding tasks of healthcare in Leningrad in 1939] in *Trudy 1-i obshchegorodskoi konferentsii akusherok i sester akushersko-ginekologicheskikh uchrezhdenii gor. Leningrada* [Proceedings of the 1st general city conference of midwives and nurses of midwifery-gynecological institutions in Leningrad], (Leningrad: Izdanie Gosudarstvennogo tsentral'nogo nauchno-issledovatel'skogo akushersko-ginekologicheskogo instituta NKZ-SSSR, 1939), 9.

100. "Na Leningradskoi konferenstii akusherok i detskikh sester" [At the Leningrad conference of midwives and pediatric nurses], *Meditsinskii rabotnik*, no. 53 (1939): 1.

101. "Nauchnaia konferentsiia meditsinskikh sester v Leningrade" [Scientific conference of nurses in Leningrad], *Meditsinskii rabotnik*, no. 6 (1940): 3.

102. This group of hero workers was named for Aleksei Stakhanov, a miner who became famous for exceeding his work quota in 1935. Stakhanovite workers received a range of awards.

103. "Nauchnaia konferentsiia meditsinskikh sester v Leningrade," 3.

104. See P. A. Golonzko, ed., *Bol'nitsa imena Soiuza "Medsantrud," Moskva. Doklady I-i bol'nichnoi konferentsii meditsinskikh sester* [Hospital named for the union 'Medsantrud,' Moscow. Papers from the 1ˢᵗ hospital conference of nurses] (Moscow, 1939).

105. "SSSR. Sovet Narodnykh Komissarov. Postanovlenie Sovet Narodnykh Komissarov Soiuza SSSR (Moscow-Kremlin No. 637, 8 May 1939—O povyshenii zarabotnoi platy srednym i mladshim meditsinskim rabotnikam i rabotnikam aptechnykh uchrezhdenii i predpriiatii" [USSR. Council of Peoples' Commissars. Council of Peoples' Commissars resolution—On raising the wage of middle and junior medical workers and workers from pharmacy institutions and industries], (Chernigiv: Derzhdruk imena Kirova, 1939). This order was to take effect on June 1, 1939.

106. Ewing, *Teachers of Stalinism*, 115–116.

107. GARF, f. A-482, op. 52, d. 7, l. 87. Thanks to Donald Filtzer for pointing me in the direction of this collection.

108. GARF, f. A-482, op. 52, d. 7, l. 88.

109. GARF, f. A-482, op. 52, d. 7, l. 89.

110. GARF, f. A-482, op. 52, d. 7, l. 90.

111. Bol'nitsa imena Soiuza Medsantruda, formerly the Yauzkaia hospital, Internatsional'naia, 7. Number of beds: 550. Head doctor: Evg. Evg. Syroechkovskii; deputy head doctor El'sinovskii, Sol. Os. *Vsia Moskva* (Moscow, 1936), 305.

112. TsGAM, f. 2299, op. 1, d. 2, l. 1, January 17, 1934. The denunciation was communicated in a January 1934 letter from the head of the Medsantrud hospital, El'sinovskii, to the emergency room doctor. Shock workers were outstanding workers who often overfulfilled their work quotas.

113. TsGAM, f. 2299, op. 1, d. 2, l. 1.

114. TsGAM, f. 2299, op. 1, d. 2, l. 3.

115. TsGAM, f. 2299, op. 1, d. 2, l. 3.

116. HPSSS, Schedule B, vol. 22, Case 1158 (interviewer M.F.), accessed February 23, 2018, http://nrs.harvard.edu/urn-3:FHCL:981575?n=15.

117. RGASPI, f. 82, op. 2, f. 964, l. 64.

118. RGASPI, f. 82, op. 2, f. 964, l. 64.

119. RGASPI, f. 82, op. 2, f. 964, l. 65.

120. RGASPI, f. 82, op. 2, f. 964, l. 66.

121. RGASPI, f. 82, op. 2, f. 964, l. 70.

122. RGASPI, f. 82, op. 2, f. 964, l. 71.

123. Wendy Z. Goldman, *Inventing the Enemy: Denunciation and Terror in Stalin's Russia* (Cambridge: Cambridge University Press, 2011), 43.

124. TsGAM, f. 2299, op. 1, d. 5, l. 2, February 3, 1936.

125. TsGAM, f. 2299, op. 1, d. 5, 1. 2.

126. TsGAM, f. 2299, op. 1, d. 5, l. 55.

127. Goldman, *Inventing the Enemy*, 47.

128. TsGAM, f. 552, op. 1, d. 8, l. 78.

129. For more information on El'sinovskii, see the Sakharov Center, "Pamiat' o bespravii. Proekt muzeia i obshchestvennogo tsentra 'Mir, progress, prava cheloveka' imeni Andreia Sakharova," "El'sinovskii Solomon Osipovich," accessed February 24, 2018, http://www.sakharov-center.ru/asfcd/martirolog/?t=page&id=6751.

130. On the denouncement by the Basmannaia brigade, see TsGAM, f. 2299, op. 1, d. 4, ll. 6 ob–7. On the party committee secretary's accusation, see TsGAM, f. 2299, op. 1, d. 17, l. 1 ob, April 26–27, 1938. Present at the general meeting were 226 employees.

131. TsGAM, f. 2299, op. 1, d. 17, l. 1 ob, Prokhorova. In the claim, "isolated" seems to be a euphemism for arrest.

132. On compassion, see Nussbaum, *Upheavals of Thought*, 297–327; on disgust and the example of Nazi Germany, see 320, 348–350.

133. "Vnimanie sanitarke," 3. For a similar account, see L. Chemeris, "Akusherka sela Khrustal'nogo" [Midwife from the village of Khrustal'nii], *Meditsinskii rabotnik*, no. 34 (1939): 3; Lerov, "Meditsinskie sestry," 2. See also Grant, "Devotion and Revolution."

134. See David Priestland, *Stalinism and the Politics of Mobilization: Ideas, Power, and Terror in Inter-war Russia* (Oxford: Oxford University Press, 2007), 290–291.

135. Z. MED, "Slavnyi iubilei operatsionnoi sestry" [Renowned anniversary of a surgical nurse], *Meditsinskii rabotnik*, no. 24 (1938): 3.

136. K. Shil'dkret, *Znatnaia sestra: N. M. Anpilogova* [Noble sister: N. M. Anpilogova] (Moscow: Tsentr nauchno-metodicheskaia stanstiia Mosgorzdravotdela, 1939), 7.

137. Shil'dkret, *Znatnaia sestra*, 7.

138. Shil'dkret, *Znatnaia sestra*, 7.

139. Shil'dkret, *Znatnaia sestra*, 6, 22.

140. RGASPI, f. 82, op. 2, d. 965, l. 71.

141. RGASPI, f. 82, op. 2, d. 965, l. 71 For other cases of poor conditions in maternity wards, including the presence of rats, see Melanie Ilic, *Soviet Women—Everyday Lives* (London; New York: Routledge, 2020), 116–120.

142. RGASPI, f. 82, op. 2, d. 965, l. 71.

143. RGASPI, f. 82, op. 2, d. 965, ll. 71–72.

144. RGASPI, f. 82, op. 2, d. 965, l. 72.

145. GARF, f. A-482, op. 52, d. 7, l. 75, November 20, 1940.

146. GARF, f. A-482, op.52, d. 7, l. 82.

147. GARF, f. A-482, op.52, d. 7, l. 82.

148. GARF, f. A-482, op. 52, d. 7, ll. 83–84.

149. GARF, f. A-482, op. 52, d. 7, ll. 83–84. For a similar case of neglect, see Nina Markovna, *Nina's Journey. A Memoir of Stalin's Russia and the Second World War* (Washington D. C.: Regnery Gateway, 1989), 174–175. My thanks to Melanie Ilic for bringing this source to my attention.

150. Catriona Kelly, *Children's World: Growing up in Russia, 1890–1991* (New Haven, CT: Yale University Press, 2007), 321. Kelly uses the term "abjection displacement." For an example of an investigation of careless behavior, see GARF, f. A-482, op. 47, d. 26, l. 43, 1940.

151. Joan C. Tronto, "Beyond Gender Difference to a Theory of Care," in *An Ethic of Care: Feminist and Interdisciplinary Perspectives*, ed. Mary Jeanne Larrabee (New York: Routledge, 1993), 248.

152. On altruism, see Michaels, *Curative Powers*. On local officials on trial as "enemies of the people," see Sheila Fitzpatrick, "How the Mice Buried the Cat: Scenes from the Great Purges of 1937 in the Russian Provinces," *Russian Review* 52, no. 3 (1993): 299–320.

153. For a good historiographical discussion of state violence and terror, see Hoffmann, *Cultivating the Masses*, 279.

154. Kathleen Woodward, "Calculating Compassion," *Indiana Law Journal* 77, no. 2 (2002): 245. "Law, Morality, and Popular Culture in the Public Sphere" presented at a symposium, Indiana University School of Law, Bloomington, April 6, 2001.

155. There were 123,600 middle medical workers in 1930 and 276,800 in 1937. A. P. Zhuk, "Srednie meditsinskie kadry i ikh rol' v sovetskom zdravookhranenii" [Middle medical cadres and their role in Soviet healthcare], *Fel'dsher i akusherka*, no. 11 (1947): 5.

6. Fortresses of Sanitary Defense

1. See David L. Hoffmann, *Cultivating the Masses: Modern State Practices and Soviet Socialism, 1914–1939* (Ithaca, NY: Cornell University Press, 2011), especially chap. 2.

2. Aya Takahashi, *The Development of the Japanese Nursing Profession: Adopting and Adapting Western Influences* (London: Routledge, 2004), 95.

3. Anna Krylova, *Soviet Women in Combat: A History of Violence on the Eastern Front* (Cambridge: Cambridge University Press, 2010), 13.

4. Krylova, *Soviet Women in Combat*, 14.

5. Al'fa Del'ta, "Krasnokrestnyi urok" [Red cross lesson], *Zhenskii zhurnal*, no. 2 (1929): 4.

6. S.A., "Kakaia forma nam nuzhna [Which form do we need]," *Za sanitarnuiu oboronu*, no. 12 (1930): 5. The author argued that the crosses on the Red Cross nurse's uniform were different from the religious cross.

7. For more on *Za sanitarnuiu oboronu*, see Melanie Ilic, "Soviet Women and Civil Defense Training in the 1930s," *Minerva Journal of Women and War* 2, no. 1 (2008): 109. I am indebted to Melanie Ilic for bringing this publication to my attention. See also Susan Grant, "Nurses in the Soviet Union: Explorations of Gender in State and Society," in *The Palgrave Handbook of Women and Gender in Twentieth-Century Russia and the Soviet Union*, ed. Melanie Ilic (London: Palgrave Macmillan, 2018), 255–259.

8. R. Savel'eva, "Moskovskaia organizatsiia ROKK dolzhna stat' peredovoi" [The Moscow Red Cross organization should become advanced], *Za sanitarnuiu oboronu*, no. 7 (1933): 10.

9. Savel'eva, "Moskovskaia organizatsiia ROKK," 10.

10. See Sheila Fitzpatrick, *Tear off the Masks! Identity and Imposture in Twentieth-Century Russia* (Princeton, NJ: Princeton University Press, 2005), 15, 78–85. The state introduced passports to deal with peasant out-migration as a result of collectivization. Internal passports indicated social class and profession.

11. *Podrugi* [Girlfriends], directed by Lev Arnshtam (Leningrad: Lenfilm, 1936).

12. L. Bronshtein, "Delo chesti" [An honorable matter], *Za sanitarnuiu oboronu*, no. 3 (1936): 10–11. For more discussion of *Girlfriends*, see Alison Rowley, "Masha Grab Your Gun: 1930s Images of Soviet Women and the Defense of Their Country," *Minerva Journal of Women and War* 2, no. 1 (2008): 58–59.

13. See, for example, *Za sanitarnuiu oboronu*, no. 5, 6, 7, 9, and 11 (1939).

14. Bronshtein, "Delo chesti," 10–11.

15. Ia. I. Akodus and A. A. Skoriukova, *Meditsinskaia sestra Sovetskogo Krasnogo Kresta* [The Soviet Red Cross Nurse] (Moscow: Medgiz, 1955), 39.

16. Henry E. Sigerist, *Medicine and Health in the Soviet Union* (New York: Citadel Press, 1947), 83.

17. "Nagrada udarniki oborony" [Awards for Shock Workers of Defense], *Komsomol'skaia pravda*, February 20, 1935, 2, as cited in Seth Bernstein, "Communist Upbringing under Stalin: The Political Mobilization and Socialization of Soviet Youth, 1934–1941" (PhD diss., University of Toronto, 2013), 34.

18. *Frontovye podrugi* [Girlfriends at the front], directed by Viktor Eisymont (Leningrad: Lenfilm, 1941).

19. Seth Bernstein, *Raised under Stalin: Young Communists and the Defense of Socialism* (Ithaca, NY: Cornell University Press, 2018), 2.

20. The Communist Youth League was for young adults, usually between the ages of fourteen and twenty-three, and the Pioneers were for children. Anne E. Gorsuch, *Youth in Revolutionary Russia: Enthusiasts, Bohemians, Delinquents* (Bloomington: Indiana University Press, 2000), 15. For more on these organizations, see Bernstein, *Raised under Stalin*; and Matthias Neumann, *The Communist Youth League and the Transformation of the Soviet Union, 1917–1932* (London: Routledge, 2011).

21. GARF, f. 9501, op. 3, d. 1, l. 2, 1930.

22. Red Crescent organizations were established in the Uzbek SSR in 1925, in the Turkmen SSR in 1926, and in the Tajik SSR in 1929. While the international community recognized the Russian Red Cross in 1918, that did not extend to the Soviet Red Cross and Red Crescent until 1928. See L. A. Khodorkov, "Osnovnye etapy razvitiia sovetskogo obshchestva Krasnogo Kresta i Krasnogo Polumesiatsa" [The main stages of development

of the Soviet Society of the Red Cross and Red Crescent] in *Materialy nauchnoi konferentsii, posviashchennoi 100-letiiu Krasnogo Kresta v SSSR* [Scientific conference material dedicated to 100 years of the Red Cross in the USSR], (Moscow: Izdatel'stvo "Meditsina," 1968), 47–48.

23. TsDAVO, f. R-4616, op. 1, d. 109, l. 59.

24. Russian State Archive of Socio-Political History (Communist Youth League) (hereafter RGASPI-M), f. 1M, op. 23, d. 792, ll. 30, 32, 1927.

25. RGASPI-M, f. 1M, op. 23, d. 792, ll. 59, 68, 1927.

26. RGASPI-M, f. 1M, op. 23, d. 793, l. 55 ob, September 8, 1927.

27. RGASPI-M, f. 1M, op. 23, d. 793, l. 68.

28. RGASPI-M, f. 1M, op. 23, d. 792, l. 43.

29. RGASPI-M, f. 1M, op. 23, d. 792, l. 43.

30. RGASPI-M, f. 1M, op. 23, d. 792, l. 43.

31. Krylova, *Soviet Women in Combat*, 51.

32. Neumann, *Communist Youth League*, 45–52.

33. RGASPI-M, f. 1M, op. 23, d. 792, l. 65; Bernstein, *Raised under Stalin*, 64–65.

34. On the Communist Youth League and young women, see Bernstein, *Raised under Stalin*, 59–68.

35. Bernstein, *Raised under Stalin*, 42.

36. Roger D. Markwick and Euridice Charon Cardona, *Soviet Women on the Frontline in the Second World War* (London: Palgrave Macmillan, 2012), 8.

37. Sheila Fitzpatrick, *Education and Social Mobility in the Soviet Union, 1921–1934* (Cambridge: Cambridge University Press, 1979), 181. On the Communist Youth League as a "mass youth organization," see Seth Bernstein, *Raised under Stalin*, chapter 6.

38. GARF, f. 9501, op. 3, d. 20, l. 16.

39. GARF, f. 9501, op. 3, d. 20, l. 16.

40. GARF, f. 9501, op. 3, d. 20, l. 16.

41. Stone, *Hammer and Rifle*, 9.

42. GARF, f. 9501, op. 3, d. 20, l. 17.

43. GARF, f. 9501, op. 3, d. 27, l. 49.

44. Hoffmann, *Cultivating the Masses*, 228.

45. RGASPI-M, f. 1M, op. 23, d. 1362, l. 135, January 10, 1939.

46. RGASPI-M, f. 1M, op. 23, d. 1362, l. 135.

47. The Executive Committee of the Union of the Societies of the SOKK—one of the highest organs for administering SOKK societies—led ten central committees and oversaw four regional and forty-seven provincial committees. RGASPI-M, f. 1M, op. 23, d. 1362, l. 135.

48. RGASPI-M, f. 1M, op. 23, d. 1362, l. 148.

49. RGASPI-M, f. 1M, op. 23, d. 1362, l. 149.

50. Bernstein, *Raised under Stalin*, 177.

51. Bernstein, *Raised under Stalin*, 177.

52. RGASPI-M, f. 1M, op. 2, d. 170, l. 69. My thanks to Seth Bernstein for sharing this source.

53. Fitzpatrick, *Education and Social Mobility*, 238. The statistic on education did not include preschool-age children and older people. On the growth of trained cadres, see GARF, f. 9501, op. 3, d. 27, l. 46.

54. M. Kabe "Istoriia odnoi shkoly" [The history of one school], *Za sanitarnuiu oboronu*, no. 3 (1936): 13.

55. S. German, "Pered bol'shim prazdnikom" [Before the big holiday], *Za sanitarnuiu oboronu*, no. 3 (1934): 8.

56. E. Thomas Ewing, *The Teachers of Stalinism: Policy, Practice, and Power in Soviet Schools of the 1930s* (New York: Peter Lang, 2002), 169.

57. Ewing, *Teachers of Stalinism*, 169.

58. Ginzberg, "Kursam sester—postoiannoe pomeshchenie" (otvet na stat'iu v No. 10 zhurnala "Ne pora li pereiti k statsionarnym kursam") [Nurse/sister courses - permanent premises (response to article No. 10 of the journal "Is it not time to switch to hospital/statsionar courses")], *Za sanitarnuiu oboronu*, no. 3 (1935): 9.

59. Gartvig, "Vrachi plokho pomogaiut podgotovke medsester" [Doctors badly assist nurse training], *Za sanitarnuiu oboronu*, no. 4 (1935): 4; Ewing, *Teachers of Stalinism*, 169–171.

60. "Skryvaiut rabotu kursov sester (Ivanovskaia oblast')" [They hide the work of the nurses' courses (Ivanovo province)], *Za sanitarnuiu oboronu*, no. 4–5 (1930): 21.

61. Sigerist, *Medicine and Health*, 83.

62. Sigerist, *Medicine and Health*, 84.

63. Gr. Popovskii, "Berech' i leleiat' kadry" [Protect and cherish cadres], *Za sanitarnuiu oboronu*, no. 6 (1936): 4–5.

64. GARF, f. 9501, op. 3, d. 27, l. 48.

65. GARF, f. 9501, op. 3, d. 27, l. 48.

66. V. Smirnov, "Pod ogon' proletarskoi samokritiki" [Under the fire of proletarian self-criticism], *Za sanitarnuiu oboronu*, no. 1 (1931): 10.

67. HPSSS, Schedule B, vol. 22, Case 1158 (interviewer M.F.), accessed February 23, 2018, http://nrs.harvard.edu/urn-3:FHCL:981575?n=17.

68. HPSSS, Schedule B, vol. 2, Case 1758 NY (interviewer M.F.), accessed August 14, 2018, http://nrs.harvard.edu/urn-3:FHCL:939792?n=27.

69. HPSSS, Schedule B, vol. 2, Case 1758 NY.

70. G. M. Perfil'eva, "Sestrinskoe delo v Rossii (sotsial'no-gigienicheskii analiz i prognoz)" [Nursing in Russia (a social-hygiene analysis and forecast)] (PhD diss., Moscow Medical Academy named for I. M. Sechenov, 1995), 77–78.

71. See, for example, N. Sofina, "Voina s mikrobami" [The war with microbes], *Meditsinskii rabotnik*, no. 1 (1934): 36.

72. Sigerist, *Medicine and Health*, 84.

73. This was another badge of honor introduced in the early 1930s. This particular honor was for shooting and named after Kliment Voroshilov, Commissar of Defence at the time. For more on this and for wider context on these "badges," see Anna Krylova, *Soviet Women in Combat: A History of Violence on the Eastern Front* (Cambridge: Cambridge University Press, 2010), 52–53.

74. I Remember / Ia pomniu, accessed April 2, 2019, https://iremember.ru/memoirs/mediki/kravchenko-tsibrenko-mariya-pavlovna.

75. I Remember / Ia pomniu, accessed April 2, 2019, https://iremember.ru/memoirs/medik/chumachenko-valentina-anufrievna/.

76. I Remember / Ia pomniu, accessed April 2, 2019, https://iremember.ru/memoirs/medik/chumachenko-valentina-anufrievna/.

77. I Remember / Ia pomniu, accessed April 1, 2019, https://iremember.ru/memoirs/mediki/yureva-goryacheva-nadezhkda-stepanova/.

78. See Mikh. Tovbin, "V Odesskoi shkole medsester" [In the Odessa nursing school], *Za sanitarnuiu oboronu*, no. 12 (1938): 22.

79. See, for example, "Perepodgotovka srednego meditsinskogo personala" [Retraining middle medical personnel], *Meditsinskii rabotnik*, no. 51 (1939): 3.

80. K. Shashkova and N. Volkova, "Sanitarki" [Orderlies], *Meditsinskii rabotnik*, no. 92 (1939): 2.

81. Redaktsiia, "Zhenshchiny o sebe" [Women about themselves], *Meditsinskii rabotnik*, no. 2 (1935): 21–22. See also Susan Grant, "Creating Cadres of Soviet Nurses, 1936–1941," in *Russian and Soviet Health Care from an International Perspective: Comparing Professions, Practice and Gender, 1880–1960*, ed. Susan Grant (London: Palgrave Macmillan, 2017), 60–62.

82. Fitzpatrick, *Education and Social Mobility*, 205.

83. GARF, f. 8009, op. 14, d. 5, l. 134.

84. In the Soviet period, graduates were usually assigned work in provincial towns or in areas facing a shortage of medical workers. Eventually, these workers could apply to work elsewhere. A quota system determined certain employment needs. For example, in 1939 there were 250 positions for doctors in the Gulag system, with 247 filled. Or certain types of work, for example, prophylactic medicine, were oversubscribed. GARF, f. 8009, op. 14, d. 51, l. 23; GARF, f. 8009, op. 14, d. 55, l. 4. This system had its flaws, and the local authorities sometimes failed to provide an accurate picture. GARF, f. 8009, op. 14, d. 55, l. 8, Grashchenkov.

85. GARF, f. 8009, op. 14, d. 2, ll. 124–139, July 14, 1938.

86. GARF, f. 8009, op. 14, d. 5, l. 97, May 24–27, 1938. My thanks to Dan Healey for bringing this collection to my attention.

87. GARF, f. 8009, op. 14, d. 38, ll. 27–33.

88. HPSSS, Schedule B, vol. 22, Case 1158 (interviewer M.F.), Widener Library, Harvard University, accessed February 23, 2018, http://nrs.harvard.edu/urn-3:FHCL:981575?n=6. William A. Glaser confirms the trend. William A. Glaser, *Social Settings and Medical Organization: A Cross-National Study of the Hospital* (New York: Atherton Press, 1970), 101.

89. HPSSS, Schedule B, vol. 22, Case 1158.

90. The Lake Khasan affair was a conflict between the Soviet Union and Japan along the Manchurian border in 1938. See Paul W. Doerr, "The Changkufeng / Lake Khasan Incident of 1938: British Intelligence on Soviet and Japanese Military Performance," *Intelligence and National Security* 5, no. 3 (1990): 184–199.

91. Markwick and Cardona, *Soviet Women on the Frontline*, 59.

92. GARF, f. 8009, op. 5, d. 67, l. 46 (Prof. Landa, head doctor of the Second Odessa Clinical Hospital, October 21, 1939).

93. Olga Nikonova, "Soviet Amazons: Women Patriots during Prewar Stalinism," *Minerva Journal of Women and War* 2, no. 1 (2008): 88.

94. "Sestry (Okruzhim vnimaniem i zabotoi meditsinskuiu sestru)" [Nurses (We will surround the nurse with attention and care)] *Meditsinskii rabotnik*, no. 70 (1938): 3.

95. "Sestry (Okruzhim vnimaniem i zabotoi meditsinskuiu sestru)," 3.

96. Ellen D. Baer, "Women and the Politics of Career Development: The Case of Nursing," in *Nursing History and the Politics of Welfare*, ed. Anne Marie Rafferty, Jane Robinson, and Ruth Elkan (London: Routledge, 1997), 246.

97. Gordon Hyde, *The Soviet Health Service: A Historical and Comparative Study* (London: Lawrence and Wishart, 1974), cited in Elizabeth Murray, "Russian Nurses: From the Tsarist Sister of Mercy to the Soviet Comrade Nurse; A Case Study of Absence of Migration of Nursing Knowledge and Skills," *Nursing Inquiry* 11, no. 3 (2004): 137. Glaser describes this Soviet approach as combining medicine and nursing into "a single hierarchy characterized by degrees of education, skill and responsibility." Glaser, *Social Settings and Medical Organization*, 101.

98. Rosemary Pringle, *Sex and Medicine: Gender, Power and Authority in the Medical Profession* (Cambridge: Cambridge University Press, 1998), 201.

99. Pringle, *Sex and Medicine*, 201.

100. Pringle, *Sex and Medicine*, 201.

101. Baer, "Politics of Career Development," 247.

102. See Grant, "Creating Cadres of Soviet Nurses."

103. HPSSS, Schedule B, vol. 22, Case 490 (interviewer M.F.), accessed February 24, 2018, http://nrs.harvard.edu/urn-3:FHCL:981572?n=2.

104. HPSSS, Schedule B, vol. 22, Case 490. The training course was eighty hours.

105. HPSSS, Schedule B, vol. 22, Case 490.

106. K. Lugina, "Sestra Vtorova" [Nurse Vtorova], *Meditsinskii rabotnik*, no. 47 (1938): 3.

107. Lugina, "Sestra Vtorova," 3.

108. For the study program, see TsGAM, f. 552, op. 1, d. 15, ll. 1–3.

109. TsGAM, f. 552, op. 1, d. 31, ll. 29–31; TsGAM, f. 552, op. 1, d. 59, ll. 47–48 ob.

110. GARF, f. 9501, op. 3, d. 27, l. 73. For more on nurses and aviation, see Grant, "Nurses in the Soviet Union," 256–257.

111. GARF, f. 9501, op. 3, d. 27, l. 73. According to Sigerist, the Red Cross had 150 nurses trained in parachute jumping and 400 medical aviation personnel. Sigerist, *Medicine and Health*, 84.

112. Timothy Paynich, "Celebrities or Scapegoats? Women in Pre-war Soviet Aviation," *Minerva Journal of Women and War* 2, no. 1 (2008): 71.

113. Nikonova, "Soviet Amazons," 93.

114. Between 1934 and 1938, some 3 million passed the GSO norm (the badge for adults and high school students) and 250,000 were awarded the BGSO (Bud'gotov k sanitarnoi oborone) norm, the 'Be prepared for sanitary defense' badge for children in junior classes. *Materialy nauchnoi konferentsii* (Leningrad: Meditsina, 1968), 192.

115. Paynich, "Celebrities or Scapegoats?," 79–80.

116. TsGAIPD SPb, f. 24, op. 8, d. 578, ll. 64–65, 1939.

117. Natal'ia Aleksandrovna Ternova and Liudmilla Olegovna Chukhno, *Stranitsy istorii otechestvennogo Krasnogo Kresta* [Pages from the history of the national Red Cross] (Moscow: Meditsina, 1986), 25. The authors do not identify the original source.

118. Ternova and Chukhno, *Stranitsy istorii otechestvennogo Krasnogoi Kresta*, 26. Women tank drivers taking nursing courses held this opinion, as reported in *Red Star* (*Krasnaia zvezda*) on July 21, 1939.

119. GARF, f. 8009, op. 5, d. 63, ll. 14–15.

120. See Grant, "Creating Cadres of Soviet Nurses," 65–69.

121. GARF, f. 8009, op. 5, d. 63, l. 46. Some doctors took immense pride when noting that their nurses knew the blood groups. See also Grant, "Nurses in the Soviet Union," 256–257.

122. TsGAIPD SPb, f. K-598, op. 2, d. 832, l. 1.

123. GARF, f. 9501, op. 3, d. 82, l. 24, November 1939.

124. GARF, f. 9501, op. 3, d. 82, l. 24.

125. GARF, f. 9501, op. 3, d. 82, l. 24. The Sanitary Administration of the Red Army required 24,000 courses for women of war service, 16,000 courses for women workers without a break from work, and 10,000 courses for students. GARF, f. 9501, op. 3, d. 82, l. 26, August 22, 1939.

126. TsDAVO, f. R-4616, op. 1, d. 109, l. 59.

127. I Remember / Ia pomniu, accessed July 20, 2018, https://iremember.ru/memoirs/mediki/tarasova-kharchuk-evgeniya-filippovna/.

128. GARF, f. 9501, op. 3, d. 82, l. 27, October 15, 1939. The military–physical culture section of the Communist Youth League Central Committee organized nursing courses without a break from work. GARF, f. 9501, op. 3, d. 82, l. 31.

129. GARF, f. 9501, op. 3, d. 123, l. 7. After war broke out, the medical union wrote to the directors of universities and various institutes of higher education, as well as to representatives of the republic, regional, and provincial committees of the Red Cross. GARF, f. 9501, op. 3, d. 123, l. 86, July 8, 1941.

130. Barbara Brooks Tomblin, *G.I. Nightingales: The Army Nurse Corps in World War II* (Lexington: University Press of Kentucky Press, 1996), 8–9. In the United States, nurses qualified for military service only if they were "graduate nurses, unmarried, and under forty years of age." Tomblin, *G.I. Nightingales*, 9.

131. G. A. Miterev, ed., *Dvadtsat' piat' let sovetskogo zdravookhraneniia* (Moscow: NKZ SSSR, Gos. Izd. Meditsinskoi literatury, 1944), 241. At the time, there were an additional 49,784 kindergarten and school nurses.

132. GARF, f. 9501, op. 3, d. 130, l. 3, 1941.

133. GARF, f. 9501, op. 3, d. 130, l. 3.

134. I Remember / Ia pomniu, accessed July 20, 2018, https://iremember.ru/memoirs/mediki/tarasova-kharchuk-evgeniya-filippovna/.

135. A course of two and a half years' duration was organized for housewives and family members not working in industry, with courses also run in enterprises and institutes. Students at the Institute of Higher Education would undertake a period of five months' medical-sanitation study with no break from their primary course. GARF, f. 9501, op. 3, d. 130, l. 3, July 7, 1941, no. 317.

136. See *Pamiatka sestre-druzhinnitse partizanskogo otriada* [Memoir of a squad nurse in the partison brigade], (Moscow: Molodaia gvardiia, 1941).

137. M. K. Kuz'min, *Sovetskaia meditsina v gody Velikoi Otechestvennoi voiny* [Soviet medicine in the years of the Great Patriotic War], (Moscow: Meditsina, 1979), 18–19.

138. GARF, f. 9501, op. 3, d. 139, 1941, l. 3. For the years 1941–1942 the Red Cross trained 516,000 medical workers: 203,500 nurses, 285,000 sanitary brigade members, and 27,500 orderlies.

139. GARF, f. 9501, op. 3, d. 139, 1941, l. 3, l. 10.

140. TsGAM, f. 533, op. 1, d. 494, l. 18. Some put the number of Red Cross–trained personnel at 106,000 nurses and 100,000 members of sanitary brigades (*sandruzhinitsy*)

trained in the first six months of the war, with a total of 280,000 nurses, 500,000 *san-druzhinitsy*, and 36,000 orderlies trained over the course of the war. V. P. Romaniuk, V. A. Lapotnikov, and Ia. A. Nakatis, *Istoriia sestrinskogo dela v Rossii* [A History of nursing in Russia], (St. Petersburg: Sankt-Peterburgskaia gosudarstvennaia meditsinskaia akademiia, 1998), 83. The number of doctors at the start of the war has been cited elsewhere at 120,000. N. V. Kolesnikov, "Ocherednye zadachi srednei meditsinskoi shkoly" [Next tasks of the middle medical school], *Fel'dsher i akusherka*, no. 3 (1945): 5.

141. A. N. Shabanov, "Podgotovka srednikh meditsinskikh kadrov" [Training middle medical cadres], *Fel'dsher i akusherka*, no. 7 (1943): 6.

142. GARF, f. 9501, op. 3, d. 139, 1941, l. 11.

143. Markwick and Cardona, *Soviet Women on the Frontline*, 59.

144. GARF, f. A-482, op. 52, d. 9, l. 201; August 15, 1941, Tretiakov to Andreev and Miterev.

145. GARF, f. A-482, op. 52, d. 17, l. 41 ob, October 1941, Khabarovsk. See Grant, "Creating Cadres of Soviet Nurses," 65–69.

146. Geoffrey Roberts, *Stalin's Wars: From World War to Cold War, 1939–1953* (New Haven, CT: Yale University Press, 2006), 6.

7. A Decade of War and Reconstruction

1. V. P. Romaniuk, V. A. Lapotnikov, and Ia. A. Nakatis, *Istoriia sestrinskogo dela v Rossii* [A history of nursing in Russia] (St. Petersburg: Sankt-Peterburgskaia gosudarstvennaia meditsinskaia akademiia, 1998), 83.

2. Romaniuk, Lapotnikov, and Nakatis, *Istoriia sestrinskogo dela v Rossii*, 86. For more about the Florence Nightingale Medal, see the discussion in chapter 9.

3. For discussion of the complexities of Soviet patriotism during the war, see Roger R. Reese, *Why Stalin's Soldiers Fought: The Red Army's Military Effectiveness in World War II* (Lawrence: University Press of Kansas, 2011), 14–20. See also Oleg Budnitskii, "The Great Patriotic War and Soviet Society: Defeatism, 1941–42," trans. Jason Morton, *Kritika: Explorations in Russian and Eurasian History* 15, no. 4 (2014): 767–797; and Wendy Z. Goldman and Donald Filtzer, *Fortress Dark and Stern: The Soviet Home Front during World War II* (New York: Oxford University Press, 2021), chap. 9.

4. Roger D. Markwick and Euridice Charon Cardona, *Soviet Women on the Frontline in the Second World War* (London: Palgrave Macmillan, 2012), 56.

5. Markwick and Cardona, *Soviet Women on the Frontline*, 56.

6. TsGAM, f. 533, op. 1, d. 494, l. 18.

7. TsGAM, f. 533, op. 1, d. 494, l. 20.

8. RGASPI-M, f. 1M, op. 47, d. 106, l. 40.

9. RGASPI-M, f. 7M, op. 1, d. 6483, l. 1.

10. RGASPI-M, f. 7M, op. 1, d. 6744, l. 2.

11. RGASPI-M, f. 1M, op. 47, d. 106, l. 40.

12. TsGAIPD SPb, f. K-881, op. 10, d. 536, l. 5, July 22, 1940.

13. Ol'ga Ziv, *Meditsinskie sestry* [Nurses], (Moscow: Ogiz, Gospolitizdat, 1941), 5; TsGAIPD SPb, f. K-598, op. 2, d. 832, l. 11.

14. HPSSS, Schedule A, vol. 35, Case 386 / (NY)1495 (interviewer T.E., type A4), 78, Widener Library, Harvard University, accessed December 18, 2018, https://iiif.lib.harvard.edu/manifests/view/drs:5606072$78i.

15. HPSSS, Schedule A, vol. 35, Case 386 / (NY)1495, 78–79.

16. Svetlana Alexievich, *The Unwomanly Face of War: An Oral History of Women in World War II*, trans. Richard Pevear and Larissa Volokhonsky (New York: Random House, 2017), 62.

17. I Remember / Ia pomniu, accessed April 1, 2019, https://iremember.ru/memoirs/medik/kalinina-bormatova-nina-grigorevna/.

18. Alexievich, *Unwomanly Face of War*, 162.

19. RGASPI-M, f. 7M, op. 1, d. 6540, l. 1.

20. RGASPI-M, f. 7M, op. 1, d. 6540, l. 1.

21. Alexievich, *Unwomanly Face of War*, 34.

22. Elizabeth Scannell-Desch and Mary Ellen Doherty, *Nurses in War: Voices from Iraq and Afghanistan* (New York: Springer, 2010), 262.

23. June Wandrey, letter, cited in Barbara Brooks Tomblin, *G.I. Nightingales: The Army Nurse Corps in World War II* (Lexington: University Press of Kentucky Press, 1996), 147.

24. Mary Walker Randolph, "What Nurses Expect," *American Journal of Nursing* 45 (1945): 775–776, cited in Tomblin, *G.I. Nightingales*, 205.

25. Randolph, "What Nurses Expect," cited in Tomblin, *G.I. Nightingales*, 206.

26. Scannell-Desch and Doherty, *Nurses in War*, 163.

27. Alexievich, *Unwomanly Face of War*, 88. On the myth of the war, see Amir Weiner, *Making Sense of War: The Second World War and the Fate of the Bolshevik Revolution* (Princeton, NJ: Princeton University Press, 2001). Weiner argues that the war myth was represented as Russian rather than Soviet.

28. GARF, f. 9501, op. 3, d.188, l. 42, Rozhkova (Nach OPK Khar'kov). The file dates to 1944 and most likely refers to the second liberation of Kharkov (Kharkiv) in August 1943.

29. GARF, f. 9501, op. 3, d.188, l. 42.

30. I Remember / Ia pomniu, accessed April 3, 2019, https://iremember.ru/memoirs/mediki/koval-galina-petrovna/.

31. RGASPI-M, f. 1M, op. 47, d. 106, l. 40.

32. TsGAM, f. 533, op. 1, d. 494, l. 20.

33. I Remember / Ia pomniu, accessed 1 April 2019. https://iremember.ru/memoirs/medik/bogacheva-anna-vasilevna/.

34. I Remember / Ia pomniu, accessed April 2, 2019, https://iremember.ru/memoirs/mediki/chumachenko-valentina-anufrievna/.

35. Anna Krylova, *Soviet Women in Combat: A History of Violence on the Eastern Front* (Cambridge: Cambridge University Press, 2010), 101.

36. Alexievich, *Unwomanly Face of War*, 88.

37. Markwick and Cardona, *Soviet Women on the Frontline*, 78–80.

38. Markwick and Cardona, *Soviet Women on the Frontline*, 79.

39. *Letiat zhuravli* [The cranes are flying], directed by Mikhail Kalatozov (Moscow: Mosfilm, 1957).

40. Alexievich, *Unwomanly Face of War*, 235–236.

41. E. Fain, *Po dorogam, ne nami vybrannym* [On the roads not chosen by us], (London, 1990), 155–156, cited in Oleg Budnitskii, "Muzhchiny i zhenshchiny v Krasnoi armii (1941–1945)" [Men and women in the Red Army (1941–1945)], *Cahiers du Monde Russe* 52, no. 2–3 (2011): 413.

42. Budnitskii, "Muzhchiny i zhenshchiny," 412. Budnitskii adds that Zhukov later denied the "office romance" in a note to Stalin.

43. Budnitskii, "Muzhchiny i zhenshchiny," 420–421. Budnitskii notes that rumors included calling the medal for "wartime services" the medal for "sexual services."

44. Christine E. Hallett, *Containing Trauma: Nursing Work in the First World War* (Manchester: Manchester University Press, 2009), 194–195.

45. Hallett, *Containing Trauma*, 194.

46. Although considered a wartime measure, the labor law on shirking and quitting could also be viewed as "the culmination of a decade of conflict between the regime and its workforce." Peter H. Solomon, *Soviet Criminal Justice under Stalin* (Cambridge: Cambridge University Press, 1996), 300.

47. Goldman and Filtzer, *Fortress Dark and Stern*, 235; for detailed discussion of the labor laws, see chap. 7.

48. Goldman and Filtzer, *Fortress Dark and Stern*.

49. GARF, f. A-482, op. 52, d. 7, l. 86, November 20, 1940. The doctor was quoted in the report by the deputy head of state security for the Primorye Territory and the head of the NKVD department of state security.

50. GARF, f. A-482, op. 52, d. 7, l. 86. "Convictions" were frequently "meaningless." See Goldman and Filtzer, *Fortress Dark and Stern*, 237.

51. GARF, f. A-482, op. 52, d. 7, l. 86.

52. GARF, f. A-482, op. 52, d. 7, l. 87.

53. For further discussion of the challenges that medical workers in factories faced, see Donald Filtzer, "Factory Medicine in the Soviet Defense Industry during World War II," in *Russian and Soviet Health Care from an International Perspective: Comparing Professions, Practice and Gender, 1880–1960*, ed. Susan Grant (London: Palgrave Macmillan, 2017), 77–95.

54. For full discussion of starvation and other public health challenges on the home front, see Goldman and Filtzer, *Fortress Dark and Stern*, chap. 8.

55. I Remember / Ia pomniu, accessed April 2, 2019, https://iremember.ru/memoirs/mediki/vakhutina-serbienko-mariya-vasilevna/.

56. GARF, f. A-482, op. 52s, d. 16, l. 88, 1941. My thanks to Donald Filtzer for bringing this archive collection to my attention.

57. GARF, f. A-482, op. 52s, d. 16, l. 88.

58. I. K. Petrenko, "Kul'turnost' v rabote srednego meditsinskogo personala v evakogospitaliakh" [Level of culture in the work of middle medical personnel in evacuation hospitals], *Fel'dsher i akusherka*, no. 1 (1942): 41. Petrenko was deputy head of the Soviet Commissariat of Health's main administration for evacuation hospitals.

59. Goldman and Filtzer, *Fortress Dark and Stern*, 68–71; on evacuation and public health, see 68–82.

60. Petrenko, "Kul'turnost' v rabote," 42.

61. Petrenko, "Kul'turnost' v rabote," 42. Petrenko provides readers with examples of good nurses in an evacuation hospital and contrasts these with those of a less disciplined nurse.

62. G. A. Tukmanov, "Strana novykh popolnenii kvalifitsirovannymi srednimi meditsinskimi kadrami" [A country with new additions of qualified middle medical cadres], *Fel'dsher i akusherka*, no. 7 (1942): 48.

63. Tukmanov, "Strana novykh popolnenie," 48. Ironically, in 1947 Miterev was himself reprimanded for "anti-state and anti-patriotic actions" and removed from his

post. Viacheslav Rumiantsev (ed), Miterev Georgii Andreevich, *Khronos*, February 18, 2001: http://hrono.ru/biograf/miterev.html.

64. GARF, f. A-482, op. 52, d. 7, l. 81.

65. GARF, f. A-482, op. 52, d. 7, l. 81. Of these deaths in 1939, 396 were registered in Vladivostok.

66. GARF, f. A-482, op. 52, d. 7, l. 81. Of these deaths in 1940, 276 were again registered in Vladivostok.

67. For excellent and thorough discussion of public health during the Second World War, see Goldman and Filtzer, *Fortress Dark and Stern*, chap. 8.

68. Donald Filtzer, "Starvation Mortality in Soviet Home-Front Industrial Regions during World War II," in *Hunger and War: Food Provisioning in the Soviet Union during World War II*, ed. Wendy Z. Goldman and Donald Filtzer (Bloomington: Indiana University Press, 2015), 74, 268, 264.

69. On the response of authorities to disease, see John Barber and Mark Harrison, *The Soviet Home Front, 1941–1945: A Social and Economic History of the USSR in World War II* (London: Longman, 1991), 87. On local initiatives for disease control, see Goldman and Filtzer, *Fortress Dark and Stern*, 74, 264–266.

70. Barber and Harrison, *Soviet Home Front*, 87.

71. GARF, f. 8009, op. 5, d. 213, l. 246, June 2–4, 1942.

72. GARF, f. A-482, op. 52, d. 3, l. 27, June 14, 1940.

73. All medical personnel in the central health station from these two shops were to receive the salary outlined in 1935, along with a bonus of 30 percent for all medical workers in the first health center and 50 percent in the infirmary with the daytime shift work. GARF, f. A-482, op. 52, d. 3, l. 27.

74. Filtzer, "Factory Medicine," 79.

75. Filtzer, "Factory Medicine," 80–81; Goldman and Filtzer, *Fortress Dark and Stern*, chap. 8.

76. GARF, f. A-482, op. 52, d. 11, l. 78.

77. GARF, f. A-482, op. 52, d. 11, l. 79.

78. GARF, f. A-482, op. 52, d. 11.

79. GARF, f. A-482, op. 52, d. 11.

80. GARF, f. 8009, op. 5, d. 213, l. 246, June 2–4, 1942.

81. GARF, f. 8009, op. 5, d. 213, l. 246.

82. GARF, f. A-482, op. 52s, d. 16, l. 119.

83. GARF, f. A-482, op. 52s, d. 16, l. 119.

84. GARF, f. A-482, op. 52, d. 177, l. 308.

85. GARF, f. A-482, op. 52, d. 177, l. 314.

86. GARF, f. 8009, op. 5, d. 217, l. 117.

87. GARF, f. 8009, op. 5, d. 217, l. 117. Long stays were typical in Soviet hospitals.

88. See I Remember / Ia pomniu, accessed April 2, 2019, https://iremember.ru/memoirs/mediki/bykhovets-antonina-demyanovna/. This kind of nostalgia played out in other ways. Rebecca Manley argues that evacuees, especially some of the cultural elites who might not have ordinarily supported Soviet power, put the fight for their country ahead of politics during the war. Rebecca Manley, *To the Tashkent Station: Evacuation and Survival in the Soviet Union at War* (Ithaca, NY: Cornell University Press, 2009).

89. RGASPI, f. 603, op. 1, d. 19, l. 32. The hospital for the wounded was a community effort and could count up to fifteen hundred workers, employees, and students of several factories, plants, establishments, and educational institutions of the district.

90. RGASPI, f. 603, op. 1, d. 19, l. 38.

91. For examples of the work women took on, see Goldman and Filtzer, *Fortress Dark and Stern*, 48, 61, 87, 104.

92. RGASPI, f. 603, op. 1, d. 1, l. 24, November 28, 1941.

93. RGASPI, f. 603, op. 1, d. 1, l. 24.

94. RGASPI, f. 603, op. 1, d. 1, l. 52.

95. RGASPI, f. 603, op. 1, d. 2, l. 4.

96. RGASPI, f. 603, op. 1, d. 1, l. 24.

97. RGASPI, f. 603, op. 1, d. 2, ll. 1, 3.

98. RGASPI-M, f. 1M, op. 47, d. 119, 1943, l. 14.

99. RGASPI-M, f. 1M, op. 47, d. 119, 1943, l. 16. By 1943, raising qualifications was conducted internally, with young, inexperienced personnel shadowing their senior colleagues.

100. E. V. Murzanova, "Meditsinskie sestry—otlichnitsy zdravookhraneniia" [Nurses—excellent healthcare workers], *Meditsinskaia sestra*, no. 9–10 (1946): 21.

101. Murzanova, "Meditsinskie sestry," 20, 21. For further discussion of the narratives around nursing, see Susan Grant, "Devotion and Revolution: Nursing Values," in *Rethinking the Russian Revolution as Historical Divide*, ed. Matthias Neumann and Andy Willimott (London: Routledge, 2018), 171–185.

102. GARF, f. 9501, op. 3, d. 289, l. 18; GARF, f. 9501, op. 3, d. 193, l. 2 ob.

103. GARF, f. 9501, op. 3, d. 289, l. 15. The state position was outlined in relation to SOKK work.

104. GARF, f. 9501, op. 3, d. 289, l. 18.

105. GARF, f. 9501, op. 3, d. 289, ll. 19–20.

106. TsDAVO, f. R-4616, op. 1, d. 109, l. 60.

107. I Remember / Ia pomniu, accessed April 2, 2019, https://iremember.ru/memoirs/medik/kalinina-bormatova-nina-grigorevna/.

108. I Remember / Ia pomniu, accessed April 2, 2019, https://iremember.ru/memoirs/trishkina-lidiya-andreevna/.

109. See, for example, I Remember / Ia pomniu, accessed April 2, 2019, https://iremember.ru/memoirs/mediki/belskaya-tochilkina-lidiya-alekseevna/.

110. GARF, f. 9501, op. 3, d. 193, l. 2 ob.

111. GARF, f. 9501, op. 3, d. 193, l. 2 ob. The work in relation to SOKK courses went well in Leningrad, for example, but not in Ukraine.

112. TsDAVO, f. R-342, op. 14, d. 1912, l. 166, July 27, 1948.

113. TsDAVO, f. R-342, op. 14, d. 1912, l. 166.

114. I Remember / Ia pomniu, accessed April 1, 2019, https://iremember.ru/memoirs/medik/bogacheva-anna-vasilevna/.

115. I Remember / Ia pomniu, accessed April 2, 2019, https://iremember.ru/memoirs/mediki/onishchenko-kabalik-darya-aksentevna/. The railway medical system was superior to the Commissariat / Ministry of Health system (my thanks to Donald Filtzer for drawing my attention to this fact).

116. Michael Ryan, *The Organization of Soviet Medical Care* (New York: Professional Seminar Consultants, 1978), 63. For good discussion of postwar numbers of middle medical workers, see Ryan, *Organization of Soviet Medical Care*, 63–76. See also Mark G. Field, *Soviet Socialized Medicine: An Introduction* (New York: Free Press, 1967), 106–131. Field asserts that the number of nurses in Soviet Russia "increased about seven times" between 1910 and 1962. Field, *Soviet Socialized Medicine*, 126.

117. GARF, f. 9501, op. 3, d. 193, l. 6.

118. On the postwar number of nurses and middle medical personnel, see Ryan, *Organization of Soviet Medical Care*, 64, 71. On the number of war invalids, see Elena Zubkova, *Russia after the War: Hopes, Illusions, and Disappointments, 1945–1957*, trans. and ed. Hugh Ragsdale (Armonk, NY: M. E. Sharpe, 1998), 24. For further discussion of immediate postwar challenges, see Goldman and Filtzer, *Fortress Dark and Stern*, chap. 10.

119. Lavinia L. Dock to Secretary of State, General Marshall, May 31, 1947, MMC 2988, box 1, folder 2, Correspondence 1944–1949, Lavinia L. Dock Papers, Manuscript Division, Library of Congress, Washington, DC.

120. .A. Schwarzenberg to L. Dock, February 18, 1944, MMC 2988, box 1, folder 2 Correspondence 1944–1949, Lavinia L. Dock Papers, Manuscript Division, Library of Congress, Washington DC.

Lebedenko, according to Henry E. Sigerist, was a surgeon at a Moscow medical school and a representative of the Soviet Red Cross in the United States. Sigerist to Alan Gregg, 1943, in *Correspondence: Henry E. Sigerist–Alan Gregg, 1933–1955*, ed. and annotated by Marcel H. Bickel (Bern, 2012), an online publication of the Institute of the History of Medicine, University of Bern, Switzerland, accessed December 14, 2020, https://www.img.unibe.ch/unibe/portal/fak_medizin/ber_vkhum/inst_medhist /content/e40437/e40444/e153944/section154575/files154577/CorrespondenceHenry E.Sigerist-AlanGregg_ger.pdf.

121. LD to General Marshall, May 31, 1947, photocopy (emphasis in original), MMC 2988, box 1, folder 2, Correspondence 1944–1949, Lavinia L. Dock Papers, Manuscript Division, Library of Congress, Washington DC.

122. LD to General Marshall, May 31, 1947. Dock also wrote to the Soviet ambassador in Washington, DC.

123. Catherine Merridale, *Night of Stone: Death and Memory in Twentieth-Century Russia* (New York: Penguin Books, 2000), 268.

124. "Osnovye zadachi meditsinskikh sester v 1947 godu" [The main tasks of the nurse in 1947], *Meditsinskaia sestra*, no. 1 (1947): 2.

125. S. M. Raiskii, "O rabote palatnoi meditsinskoi sestry" [On the work of the ward nurse], *Meditsinskaia sestra*, no. 10 (1947): 24.

126. "Podnimem kul'turu ukhoda za bol'nym" [We will raise the culture of patient care], *Meditsinskaia sestra*, no. 2 (1948): 4.

127. S. I. Mokeev, "Oshibki i nedostatki v tekhnike raboty medistinskikh sester" [Mistakes and shortcomings in the technical work of the nurse], *Meditsinskaia sestra*, no. 1 (1947): 22–23, 24.

128. I. Trop, "Oshibka palatnoi sestry," *Meditsinskii rabotnik*, no. 8 (1948): 3.

129. Trop, "Oshibka palatnoi sestry," 3.

130. V. P. Yakovlev, "Uluchshim ukhod za bol'nymi v bol'nitse" [We will improve patient care in the hospital], *Meditsinskaia sestra*, no. 5 (1947): 1–3.

131. A. V. Ikonnikova (head doctor of the therapeutic department of the Fifth Soviet Hospital), "Opyt organizatsii sestrinskogo ukhoda v 5-i Sovetskoi bol'nitse" [The experience of organizing nursing care in the 5th Soviet hospital], *Meditsinskaia sestra*, no. 5 (1947): 11–14. For contrast, see A. Kurella, "O sestrinskom ukhode v bol'nitse" [On nursing care in the hospital], *Meditsinskii rabotnik*, no. 49 (1946): 3.

132. Christie Watson, *The Language of Kindness: A Nurse's Story* (London: Chatto & Windus, 2018), 249.

133. Watson, *Language of Kindness*, 283.

134. M. I. Reznikova (nurse), "Pis'mo v redaktsiiu" [Letter to the editor], *Meditsinskaia sestra*, no. 7 (1949): 32.

135. Reznikova, "Pis'mo v redaktsiiu," 32.

136. Juliane Fürst, ed., *Late Stalinist Russia: Society between Reconstruction and Reinvention* (London: Routledge, 2006), 5.

137. See Fürst, *Late Stalinist Russia*, 9.

138. "Podnimem kul'turu ukhoda za bol'nym," 2.

139. "Podnimem kul'turu ukhoda za bol'nym," 4.

140. GARF, f. 5451, op. 29, d. 161, l. 64, Babaev, Third Plenum of Medical Workers, Moscow, November 30, 1949.

141. Vladislav Zubok, *Zhivago's Children: The Last Russian Intelligentsia* (Cambridge, MA: Belknap Press of Harvard University Press, 2009), 34. Quotation by Leonid Gordon.

142. GARF, f. 5451, op. 29, d. 371, l. 140.

143. GARF, f. 5451, op. 29, d. 161, l. 42, Moscow, November 30, 1949.

144. TsDAVO, f. R-342, op. 14, d. 1912, l. 168, 1948.

145. TsDAVO, f. R-342, op. 14, d. 1912, l. 169.

146. For examples of "humane nurses," see V. V. Filippo, "Rol' Sovetskikh meditsinskikh sester i zadachi ikh ideino-politicheskogo vospitaniia" [The role of the Soviet nurse and the tasks of their ideological-political education], *Meditsinskaia sestra*, no. 8 (1948): 1–4; "Podnimem kul'turu ukhoda za bol'nym," 1–4.

147. TsDAVO, f. R-342, op. 14, d. 1912, l. 169.

148. TsDAVO, f. R-342, op. 14, d. 1912, l. 169.

149. Previously, all medical workers wore white gowns, but that changed in the late 1940s. From that time nurses working in wards wore gray dresses and white aprons, while orderlies wore dark navy dresses with black aprons. A. V. Ikonnikova, "Starshaia meditsinskaia sestra otdeleniia bol'nitsy" [Senior nurse of the hospital department], *Meditsinskaia sestra*, no. 3 (1948): 1–2. Further differentiation of medical worker uniforms happened ten years later. See "Forma odezhdy meditsinskikh rabotnikov" [Forms of clothing for medical workers], *Meditsinskii rabotnik*, no. 74 (1958): 4. For similar efforts in Moscow's Botkin hospital, see TsGAM, f. 1939, op. 1, d. 53, l. 1, 1948.

150. TsGAM, f. 1939, op. 1, d. 53, l. 1. For an emphasis on political education in medical institutes, see Chris Burton, "Medical Welfare During Late Stalinism. A Study of Doctors and the Soviet Health System, 1945–53," (PhD diss.: University of Chicago, 2000), 149–151.

151. TsGAM, f. 1939, op. 1, d. 53, l. 1, 1948.

152. GARF, f. 5451, op. 29, d. 371, l. 8, December 1, 1949.

153. GARF, f. 5451, op. 29, d. 371, l. 21, l. 26.

8. Caring for the Mind

1. See Irina Sirotkina, *Diagosing Literary Genius: A Cultural History of Psychiatry in Russia, 1880–1930* (Baltimore: Johns Hopkins University Press, 2002), 145–180.

2. Martin A. Miller, *Freud and the Bolsheviks: Psychoanalysis in Imperial Russia and the Soviet Union* (New Haven, CT: Yale University Press, 1998).

3. I. A. Berger, "Trud psikhiatricheskikh rabotnikov (Sanitarno-psikhopatolgicheskoe issledovanie)," *Psikhiatricheskie rabotniki. Trud i zdorov'e* [Pyschiatry workers. Work and health], no. 4 (1929): 6–8. *Collected Essays* (Moscow: TsK Medsantrud, 1929).

4. Berger, "Trud psikhiatricheskikh rabotnikov," 6–8.

5. For analysis, see Sidney Bloch and Peter Reddaway, *Soviet Psychiatric Abuse: The Shadow over World Psychiatry* (London: Victor Gollancz, 1984); Sidney Bloch and Peter Reddaway, *Russia's Political Hospitals: The Abuse of Psychiatry in the Soviet Union* (London: Victor Gollancz, 1977).

6. HPSSS, Schedule A, vol. 11, Case 139 (interviewer M.F.), accessed October 19, 2017, http://nrs.harvard.edu/urn-3:FHCL:948912?n=10.

7. Andrew Abbott, *The System of the Professions: An Essay on the Division of Expert Labor* (Chicago: University of Chicago Press, 1988), xi, 66.

8. Abbott, *The System of the Professions*, 66.

9. Benjamin Zajicek, "Scientific Psychiatry in Stalin's Soviet Union: The Politics of Modern Medicine and the Struggle to Define 'Pavlovian' Psychiatry, 1939–1953" (PhD diss., University of Chicago, 2009), 68–76.

10. Berger, "Trud psikhiatricheskikh rabotnikov," 7.

11. Berger, "Trud psikhiatricheskikh rabotnikov," 13.

12. Berger, "Trud psikhiatricheskikh rabotnikov," 15.

13. GARF, f. 8009, op. 5, d. 9, l. 2; "Rukovodstvo po ukhodu za dushevno-bol'nymi dlia mladshego meditsinskogo personala psikhiatricheskikh bol'nits" [Guidelines in caring for mentally ill patients for junior medical personnel in a psychiatric hospital] (unpublished manuscript, 1937). Doctors at the Odessa psychiatric hospital, named after P. Starostin, edited this volume.

14. GARF, f. 8009, op. 5, d. 9, l. 2; "Rukovodstvo po ukhodu."

15. GARF, f. 8009, op. 33, d. 618, ll. 197–217. My thanks to Ben Zajicek for sharing archive material about the Odessa clinic.

16. V. V. Mikheev and A. V. Neiman, eds., *Uchebnik nervnykh i psikhicheskikh boleznei dlia medsester* [Textbook for nurses on nervous and psychiatric illnesses], 2nd ed. (Moscow-Leningrad: Medgiz, 1939).

17. S. I. Konstorum, ed., *Uchebnik psikhiatrii dlia fel'dsherov. Rukovodstvo i posobie dlia srednei meditsinskoi shkoly* [Textbook on psychiatry for feldshers. Supervision and support for middle medical schools], 3rd ed. (Moscow-Leningrad, 1937). Konstorum published general textbooks on psychiatry too, the one first dating to 1935. The latest edition of his work dates to 2010.

18. Mikheev and Neiman, *Uchebnik nervnykh*, 149.

19. Mikheev and Neiman, *Uchebnik nervnykh*, 150–152.

20. Konstorum, *Uchebnik psikhiatrii*, 84.

21. V. V. Mikheev and A. V. Neiman, eds., *Uchebnik nervnykh i psikhicheskikh boleznei dlia srednikh meditsinskikh shkol* [Textbook of nervous and psychiatric illnesses for middle

medical schools], 3rd ed. (Moscow: Gosizdat meditsinskoi literatury, 1946); V. V. Mikheev, ed., *Uchebnik nervnikh boleznei*, 2nd ed. (Moscow: Gosizdat meditsinskoi literatury, 1962), with revisions and supplementary information. I am indebted to Ben Zajicek for sending me a copy of Mikheev's 1946 and 1962 editions of the publication.

22. TsGAM, f. 533, op. 1, d. 179, ll. 1–28 ob. Doctors at the Gannushkin hospital produced the following conference proceedings, and its head doctor was editor: O. V. Kondrashkova, ed., *Gorodskaia konferentsiia meditsinskikh sester psikhiatricheskikh bol'nits i psikhonevrologicheskikh dispanserov gor. Moskvy* [City conference of nurses of psychiatric hospitals and psychoneurological dispensaries in Moscow] (Moscow, 1966).

23. For an example of a "programme for advanced training for nurses working in psychiatric institutions compiled by M. S. Wol'f," see TsGAM, f. 533, op. 1, d. 405, ll. 1–15, 1972–1973.

24. "Meditsinskie sestry, nagrazhdennye Ministerstvom zdravookhraneniia SSSR znachkom, 'Otlichniku zdravookhraneniia'" [Nurses awarded the Ministry of Health USSR badge, 'Excellent healthcare worker'] *Meditsinskaia sestra*, no. 6 (1948): 31.

25. "Meditsinskie sestry," 31.

26. "Meditsinskie sestry," 31.

27. See Rosemary Pringle, *Sex and Medicine: Gender, Power and Authority in the Medical Profession* (Cambridge: Cambridge University Press, 1998), 189.

28. Mark G. Field tracks the feminization of the medical profession, noting that women accounted for 45 percent of those in medicine and stomatology by 1928, with the corresponding numbers at 62 percent by 1941 and 77 percent by 1950. These figures dipped slightly in the 1970s. Mark G. Field, "American and Soviet Medical Manpower: Growth and Evolution, 1910–1970," *International Journal of Health Services* 5, no. 3 (1975): 461; for the table with statistical comparisons, see 462. Field also adds some caveats about direct comparisons.

29. Pringle, *Sex and Medicine*, 189.

30. Chris Burton has made this point about a dearth of primary source literature. Christopher Burton "Gendered Healthcare and Postwar Stalinism: Soviet Women Practicing Medicine" (paper presented at the Workshop on Healthcare in History, University College Dublin, 2014).

31. Konstorum, *Uchebnik psikhiatrii*, 80.

32. Konstorum, *Uchebnik psikhiatrii*, 80.

33. Konstorum, *Uchebnik psikhiatrii*, 80–81.

34. L. Mackay, *Nursing a Problem* (Milton Keynes: Open University Press, 1989), 41, cited in Pringle, *Sex and Medicine*, 188.

35. Konstorum, *Uchebnik psikhiatrii*, 81.

36. TsGAM (formerly TsMAM), f. 533, op. 1, d. 55, l. 14, 1957–1962; TsMAM, f. 533, op. 1, d. 55, l. 74, 1957–1962. My thanks to Ben Zajicek for these references.

37. Hildegard Peplau, "Interpersonal Techniques: The Crux of Psychiatric Nursing," *American Journal of Nursing* 62, no. 6 (1962): 50–54, reprinted in Anita Werner O'Toole and Sheila Rouslin Welt (eds), *Hildegard E. Peplau, Selected Works. Interpersonal Theory in Nursing*, (New York: Macmillan, 1994), 177. See also Christie Watson, *The Language of Kindness: A Nurse's Story* (London: Chatto & Windus, 2018), 109.

38. Daniel M. Fox and Christopher Lawrence, *Photographing Medicine: Images and Power in Britain and America since 1840* (New York: Greenwood Press, 1988), 205.

I thank Christopher Burton for bringing this publication to my attention. I also thank Christopher Burton, Dan Healey, and Frances Bernstein for their detailed written comments on a version of this chapter presented at a workshop at St. Antony's College, Oxford University, in June 2014, as well as colleagues participating in the workshop.

39. Madeleine Elliott Ingram, *Principles and Techniques of Psychiatric Nursing*, 5th ed. (1939; Philadelphia: W. B. Saunders, 1960), 109–112.

40. John Foot, "Photography and Radical Psychiatry in Italy in the 1960s," *History of Psychiatry* 26, no. 1 (2015): 24.

41. Fox and Lawrence, *Photographing Medicine*, 6.

42. Raymond Williams, *Culture* (London: Fontana Paperbacks, 1981), 13, cited in Fox and Lawrence, *Photographing Medicine*, 6.

43. Michel Foucault, *Discipline and Punish: The Birth of the Prison*, trans. Alan Sheridan (1975; London: Penguin Books, 1991).

44. O'Toole and Welt, *Hildegard E. Peplau*, 177.

45. GARF, f. 8009, op. 5, d. 9, l. 142.

46. GARF, f. 8009, op. 5, d. 9, l. 28, l. 70.

47. TsGAM, f. 552, op. 1, d. 15, ll. 1–3.

48. GARF, f. 8009, op. 5, d. 209, l. 93 ob.

49. GARF, f. 8009, op. 5, d. 209, l. 93 ob.

50. GARF, f. 8009, op. 5, d. 212a, l. 64, l. 67, 1941.

51. GARF, f. 8009, op. 5, d. 212a, l. 68; on finance, see GARF, f. 8009, op. 5, d. 212a, l. 69. For discussion of curriculum development in medicine in late Stalinism, see Chris Burton, "Medical Welfare During Late Stalinism. A Study of Doctors and the Soviet Health System, 1945–53" (PhD diss.: University of Chicago, 2000), 158–160.

52. Watson, *Language of Kindness*, 143.

53. HPSSS, Schedule A, vol. 11, Case 139 (interviewer M.F., type A4), accessed October 19, 2015, https://nrs.harvard.edu/urn-3:FHCL:948912?n=10.

54. HPSSS, Schedule B, vol. 21, Case 139 (interviewer M.F.), last modified February 10, 2021, https://iiif.lib.harvard.edu/manifests/view/drs:5594824$5i.

55. Christopher Burton, "Soviet Medical Attestation and the Problem of Professionalisation under Late Stalinism, 1945–1953," *Europe-Asia Studies* 57, no. 8 (2005): 1211–1212.

56. Burton, "Soviet Medical Attestation," 1214.

57. Burton, "Soviet Medical Attestation," 1216.

58. Burton, "Soviet Medical Attestation," 1221–1222.

59. TsDAVO, f. R-342, op. 14, d. 1940, l. 23.

60. TsDAVO, f. R-342, op. 14, d. 1940, l. 62. The courses worked out to be two hours per day, one day a week, over a six-month period.

61. GARF, f. 8009, op. 33, d. 264, ll. 71–71 ob.

62. TsGAM, f. 533, op. 1, d. 28, ll. 38–45, especially l. 42, April 1954.

63. This career development path was also the case for Valentina Sarkisova, president of the Russian Nurses Association. Valentina Sarkisova, interview with the author, St. Petersburg, October 10, 2014.

64. Ingram, *Psychiatric Nursing*, 14–15. Their efforts resulted in the publication of *A Handbook for Psychiatric Aides* and in 1946 they founded the National Mental Hygiene Foundation.

65. Ingram, *Psychiatric Nursing*, 14–15.

66. L. I. Aikhenval'd and Ia. M. Kogan, eds., *Kratkoe rukovodstvo po psikhiatrii (dlia srednego medistinskogo personala psikhiatricheskikh uchrezhdenii)* [A brief guide to psychiatry for middle medical personnel of psychiatric institutions] (Kiev: Gosmedizdat UkSSR, 1947), 3.

67. Aikhenval'd and Kogan, *Kratkoe rukovodstvo*, 3–4.

68. Aikhenval'd and Kogan, *Kratkoe rukovodstvo*, inside cover "Tirazh" [circulation].

69. Aikhenval'd and Kogan, *Kratkoe rukovodstvo*, 90.

70. Aikhenval'd and Kogan, *Kratkoe rukovodstvo*, 138.

71. Aikhenval'd and Kogan, *Kratkoe rukovodstvo*, 138.

72. HPSSS, Schedule B, vol. 21, Case 139 (interviewer M.F.), 25, last modified February 10, 2021, https://iiif.lib.harvard.edu/manifests/view/drs:5594824$23i.

73. Aikhenval'd and Kogan, *Kratkoe rukovodstvo*, 246.

74. Aikhenval'd and Kogan, *Kratkoe rukovodstvo*, 246.

75. TsGAM, f. 533, op. 1, d. 143, l. 80, 1965.

76. For detailed discussion of science under Stalinism, see Ethan Pollock, *Stalin and the Soviet Science Wars* (Princeton, NJ: Princeton University Press, 2006).

77. Wage differentiation according to the nature of medical work was a feature of the Soviet system since the revolution. Nurses working with psychiatric patients fell into group 1 (the most difficult working conditions), and they received a higher rate of pay. GARF, f. 4094, op. 1, d. 3, l. 52, 1917–1919.

78. GARF, f. 8009, op. 5, d. 9, l. 157, 1917–1919.

79. GARF, f. 8009, op. 5, d. 9, l. 157.

80. GARF, f. 8009, op. 5, d. 9, l. 2. To improve workers' living and working conditions, longer holidays and resort passes were suggested.

81. See, for example, GARF, f. 8131, op. 31, dd. 84803, 36413, 17417, 18238, 23421, 26061.

82. GARF, f. 8131, op. 31, d. 27002, l. 5, l. 10 (citation).

83. GARF, f. 8009, op. 5, d. 209, l. 93, 1940.

84. GARF, f. 8009, op. 5, d. 209, l. 93.

85. GARF, f. 8009, op. 5, d. 209, l. 93.

86. TsDAVO, f. R-342, op. 14, d. 1940, l. 18.

87. TsDAVO, f. R-342, op. 14, d. 1940, l. 18.

88. GARF, f. A-482, op. 49, d. 1519, l. 28. Thanks to Ben Zajicek for bringing this file to my attention.

89. GARF, f. A-482, op. 49, d. 1519, l. 29.

90. GARF, f. A-482, op. 49, d. 1519, l. 32. On working two jobs, see also TsGAM, f. 533, op. 1, d. 143, l. 31, October 1, 1964.

91. GARF, f. A-482, op. 49, d. 6537, ll. 26–27, December 1953. The plans promised increased hospital construction and staffing. Thanks to Ben Zajicek for bringing this file to my attention. The corresponding pension conditions for middle medical workers more generally (based on the January 1, 1960, legislation) was a right to a pension after twenty-five years in rural areas and after thirty years in urban areas. L. I. Kaidashova, "O poriadke naznacheniia meditsinskim rabotnikam pensii za vyslugu let" [About the procedure of assigning medical workers a pension for long service] *Fel'dsher i akusherka*, no. 7 (1960): 57. GARF, f. A-482, op. 49, d. 6537, ll. 28–29. Benefits included increased salaries and longer holidays.

92. GARF, f. 9592, op. 1, d. 209, l. 7, 1955–1957. Letter from psychiatrists including V. A. Giliarovskii (representing the All-Union Society of Neuropathologists and Psychiatrists), V. M. Banshchikov (representing the Moscow Society of Neuropathologists and Psychiatrists) and I. A. Berger to Minister of Health M. D. Kovrigina. Thanks to Ben Zajicek for bringing this file to my attention. See also E. G. Genkin and E. A. Berger, "Travmatizm psikhiatricheskikh rabotnikov" [Traumatism of psychiatric workers], *Psikhiatricheskie rabotniki. Trud i zdorov'e*, no. 4 (1929): 79. Medical workers in dispensaries were also at risk. See TsGAM, f. 533, op. 1, d. 28, l. 89, 1954.

93. TsGAM, f. 533, op. 1, d. 28, l. 90, 1954.

94. Genkin and Berger, "Travmatizm psikhiatricheskikh rabotnikov," 80.

95. Denis Campbell, "Rise in Attacks on NHS Workers Blamed on Lack of Staff and Delays," *Guardian*, April 16, 2018, https://www.theguardian.com/society/2018/apr/17/rise-in-attacks-on-nhs-workers-blamed-on-lack-of-staff-money-and-delays.

96. Campbell, "Rise in Attacks."

97. Campbell, "Rise in Attacks."

98. TsGAM, f. 533, op. 1, d. 28, l. 90, 1954.

99. TsGAM, f. 533, op. 1, d. 28, l. 90, 1954.

100. TsGAM, f. 533, op. 1, d. 324, l. 2, 1970.

101. TsGAM, f. 533, op. 1, d. 324, l. 2.

102. TsGAM, f. 533, op. 1, d. 324, l. 3.

103. TsGAM, f. 533, op. 1, d. 324, l. 7. This was a response to the Ministry of Health resolution, No. 12–178, January 18, 1961, which outlined reforms relating to work and salary, specifically work trips (*komandirovki*) for middle medical workers and working two jobs. L. I. Tsareva, "O kompensatsiyakh, vyplachivaemykh srednim meditsinskim rabotnikam pri napravlenii v sluzhebnyiu komandirovku, na kursy usovershenstvovaniia i spetsializatsii i pri pereezde na druguiu rabotu" [On compensation paid to middle medical workers sent on work trips, advanced training courses and when moving to other work], *Fel'dsher i akusherka*, no. 7 (1961): 57; TsGAM, f. 533, op. 1, d. 324, l. 8.

104. TsGAM, f. 533, op. 1, d. 324, ll. 9–13.

105. GARF, f. 9592, op. 1, d. 73, l. 13.

106. See Benjamin Zajicek, "Banning the Soviet Lobotomy: Psychiatry, Ethics, and Professional Politics during Late Stalinism," *Bulletin of the History of Medicine* 91, no. 1 (2017): 33–61, and more specifically 56–61.

107. GARF, f. 9592, op. 1, d. 73, l. 14.

108. See Zajicek, "Banning the Soviet Lobotomy," 45–46.

109. Much has been written about Pavlov. For a good synopsis, see Zajicek, "Banning the Soviet Lobotomy," 47–48. For a more in-depth account, see Daniel P. Todes, *Ivan Pavlov: A Russian Life in Science* (Oxford: Oxford University Press, 2014).

110. TsGAM, f. 533, op. 1, d. 28, l. 17, April 1954.

111. TsGAM, f. 533, op. 1, d. 157, l. 1.

112. TsGAM, f. 533, op. 1, d. 157, l. 1.

113. TsGAM, f. 533, op. 1, d. 157, l. 1.

114. TsGAM, f. 533, op. 1, d. 157, l. 1.

115. TsGAM, f. 389, op. 1, d. 164; see nurse council meeting protocols, 1963–1968.

116. TsGAM, f. 533, op. 1, d. 157, l. 1.

117. TsGAM, f. 533, op. 1, d. 157, 3.

118. TsGAM, f. 533, op. 1, d. 157, l. 4.

119. Scholars working on the 1960s and 1970s have argued that the term "stagnation" is a misnomer and does not show the whole picture. See Dina Fainberg and Artemy M. Kalinovskii, eds., *Reconsidering Stagnation in the Brezhnev Era: Ideology and Exchange* (Lanham, MD: Lexington Books, 2016).

120. TsGAM, f. 533, op. 1, d. 257, l. 1.

121. TsGAM, f. 533, op. 1, d. 257, ll. 13–14.

122. TsGAM, f. 533, op. 1, d. 454, l. 5, July 28, 1974.

123. TsGAM, f. 533, op. 1, d. 454, l. 7, January 9, 1974.

124. TsGAM, f. 533, op. 1, d. 324, l. 1.

125. Michael Binyon, *Life in Russia* (London: Panther/Granada, 1983), 100–101.

126. Binyon, *Life in Russia*, 100–101.

127. See Maria Cristina Galmarini-Kabala, *The Right to Be Helped: Deviance, Entitlement, and the Soviet Moral Order* (DeKalb: Northern Illinois University Press, 2016), 117–133, especially 121–123, chapter five; Claire L. Shaw, *Deaf in the USSR: Marginality, Community and Soviet Identity, 1917–1991* (Ithaca, NY: Cornell University Press, 2017), 35–36.

128. Galmarini-Kabala, *Right to Be Helped*, 133.

129. Shaw, *Deaf in the USSR*, 36.

130. TsGAM, f. 533, op. 1, d. 615, l. 97.

131. TsGAM, f. 533, op. 1, d. 615, l. 97.

132. TsGAM, f. 533, op. 1, d. 615, l. 97, l. 98.

133. TsGAM, f. 533, op. 1, d. 615, l. 97.

134. Cited in Watson, *Language of Kindness*, 60.

135. Gaston Harnois and Phyllis Gabriel, *Mental Health and Work: Impact, Issues, and Good Practices* (Geneva: World Health Organization, 2000), 16, http://www.who.int/mental_health/media/en/712.pdf.

136. Harnois and Gabriel, *Mental Health and Work*, 16.

137. TsGAM, f. 533, op. 1, d. 690, l. 23. I have changed the original name and surname.

138. TsGAM, f. 533, op. 1, d. 690, l. 24.

139. TsGAM, f. 533, op. 1, d. 690, l. 24.

140. TsGAM, f. 533, op. 1, d. 690, l. 25.

141. TsGAM, f. 533, op. 1, d. 690, l. 25.

142. TsGAM, f. 533, op. 1, d. 690, l. 25.

143. TsGAM, f. 533, op. 1, d. 690, ll. 25–26.

144. TsGAM, f. 533, op. 1, d. 690, l. 27.

145. TsGAM, f. 533, op. 1, d. 690, ll. 27–28.

146. Harnois and Gabriel, *Mental Health and Work*, 21.

147. TsGAM, f. 533, op. 1, d. 690, ll. 27–28.

148. TsGAM, f. 533, op. 1, d. 643, ll. 32–33.

149. TsGAM, f. 533, op. 1, d. 643, l. 33.

150. TsGAM, f. 533, op. 1, d. 643, l. 34.

151. TsGAM, f. 533, op. 1, d. 643, l. 34.

152. For a good summary of the early literature on music therapy, see Rochelle P. Wortis, "Music Therapy for the Mentally Ill: II. The Effect of Music on Emotional

Activity and the Value of Music as a Resocializing Agent," *Journal of General Psychology* 62 (1960): 311–318.

153. Alexei Yurchak, *Everything Was Forever, Until It Was No More: The Last Soviet Generation* (Princeton, NJ: Princeton University Press, 2006), 2.

154. Yurchak, *Everything Was Forever*, 2.

155. Kate Sara Schecter, "Professionals in Post-Revolutionary Regimes: A Case Study of Soviet Doctors" (PhD diss., Columbia University, 1992), 182.

156. TsGAM, f. 533, op. 1, d. 690, l. 13. I have changed the original name and surname.

157. TsGAM, f. 533, op. 1, d. 690, l. 14.

158. TsGAM, f. 533, op. 1, d. 690, l. 14.

159. TsGAM, f. 533, op. 1, d. 690, l. 14. For Vinokourov's analysis of Chulak's characters and plot, see TsGAM, f. 533, op. 1, d. 690, l. 16.

160. TsGAM, f. 533, op. 1, d. 690, l. 15.

161. TsGAM, f. 533, op. 1, d. 690, l. 16.

162. TsGAM, f. 533, op. 1, d. 690, l. 17.

163. TsGAM, f. 533, op. 1, d. 690, l. 18.

164. TsGAM, f. 533, op. 1, d. 690, l. 21.

165. TsGAM, f. 533, op. 1, d. 690, l. 21. Here Vinokourov referenced the professor S. Fedorov's *Pravda* article "Warriors with Arrows" ("Voinstvo so strelami"), from September 28, 1987.

166. TsGAM, f. 533, op. 1, d. 690, l. 22.

167. TsGAM, f. 533, op. 1, d. 690, l. 22.

9. Communist Morality, Activism, and Ethics

1. Susan M. Reverby, "The Duty or Right to Care? Nursing and Womanhood in Historical Perspective," in *Circles of Care: Work and Identity in Women's Lives*, ed. Emily K. Abel and Margaret K. Nelson (Albany: State University of New York Press, 1990), 132–149.

2. When I use the term "emotional labor" I draw on Arlie Russell Hochschild's conceptualization, in her book *The Managed Heart: Commercialization of Human Feeling* (Berkeley: University of California Press, 1983).

3. Many nurse councils were set up after the war, but they were first established in 1938/1939. Nurse council structures depended on the institution. For example, in one Leningrad institute's clinic the nurse council included the head doctor as the council's representative; two senior nurses and a nurse from the institute's hospital as deputy representatives; twenty senior nurses, of whom two were secretaries and two were nurse bureau members. In the Leningrad clinic, power lay with the bureau, with the head doctor subordinate to it. This structure changed and expanded over time, with various subcommittees and sections established, a pattern evident in many institutions. N. L. Bedeker, "Opyt raboty pervogo soveta meditsinskikh sester v Leningrade" [The experience of work of the first council of nurses in Leningrad], *Meditsinskaia sestra*, no. 1 (1951): 29–31; on council structure, see 29. See also M. S. Kalmykova, "O rabote soveta sester klinicheskoi Ordena Lenina bol'nitsy imeni S. P. Botkina v 1951 g." [On the work of the council of nurses of the clinical Order of Lenin hospital named after S. P. Botkin in 1951], *Meditsinskaia sestra*, no. 3 (1952): 26–27. Smaller medical institu-

tions had fewer nurses on the council; for instance, an institution with up to seventy-five nurses would have seven to fifteen on the council. T. L. Neupokoeva, "O soveta meditsinskikh sester pri lechebno-profilakticheskom uchrezhdenii" [On the council of nurses under the medical-prophylactic institution], *Meditsinskaia sestra*, no. 1 (1956): 7. The Soviet Ministry of Health officially recognized the councils in 1955, and the network expanded from 1959 on. See "Sovety meditsinskikh sester" [Councils of nurses], *Meditsinskaia sestra*, no. 2 (1960): 44–47. One can read reports from the nurse councils in the archives, and in this chapter some of the examples specific to hospitals come from nurse council reports. One can find many articles about nurse councils and their activities in *Meditsinskaia sestra*.

4. TsGAM, f. 1939, op. 1, d. 133, l. 1, February 29, 1952.

5. The growing involvement of nurses in their profession reflects Stephen V. Bittner's argument that some reform was under way before 1953. Stephen V. Bittner, *The Many Lives of Khrushchev's Thaw: Experience and Memory in Moscow's Arbat* (Ithaca, NY: Cornell University Press, 2008), 216.

6. TsGAM, f. 1939, op. 1, d. 133, l. 1.

7. TsGAM, f. 1939, op. 1, d. 133, l. 5.

8. TsGAM, f. 1939, op. 1, d. 133, l. 1.

9. TsGAM, f. 1939, op. 1, d. 133, l. 1.

10. Vladislav Zubok, *Zhivago's Children: The Last Russian Intelligentsia* (Cambridge, MA: Belknap Press of Harvard University Press, 2009), 52.

11. State Archive of the City of Sochi (hereafter GAGS), f. 175, op. 1, d. 73, ll. 9–10, 1959–1960.

12. GAGS, f. 175, op. 1, d. 95, l. 19. My thanks to Johanna Conterio for pointing me in the direction of this archive.

13. GAGS, f. 175, op. 1, d. 95, l. 31.

14. Valentina Sarkisova, interview with the author, St. Petersburg, October 10, 2014. Sarkisova qualified as a nurse in 1964.

15. I. Zhordania and L. Novikova, "Pervyi aziatskii congress akusherov i ginekologov" [First Asian Congress of Midwives and Gynecologists]. *Meditsinskii rabotnik*, no. 62 (1957): 4. The congress focused on toxicosis of pregnancy, poor-quality chorionepithelioma, and uterine cancer.

16. M. Pokhvalova, "Pod emblemoi Sovetskogo Krasnogo Kresta" [Under the emblem of the Soviet Red Cross], *Meditsinskii rabotnik*, no. 20 (1960): 4.

17. TsGAM, f. 1939, op. 1, d. 133, l. 12.

18. TsGAM, f. 1939, op. 1, d. 133, l. 12.

19. TsGAM, f. 1939, op. 1, d. 133, l. 12.

20. This figure was for 1963. There were 364,100 feldshers, 154,300 midwives, and 443,300 physicians. Mark G. Field, *Soviet Socialized Medicine: An Introduction* (New York: Free Press, 1967), 109, 108.

21. TsDAVO, f. R-4616, op. 1, d. 97, l. 27.

22. N. G. Lin'kova, "Moral'nyi oblik meditsinskoi sestry" [Moral character of the nurse], *Meditsinskaia sestra*, no. 1 (1951): 23–24. Chief nurses were also the heads of the nurse councils. Valentina Sarkisova, interview, October 10, 2014. Nursing has three main levels: nurse, head nurse (department), and chief nurse (hospital nursing director), followed by chief nurse at the regional and national level. Many thanks to Natalia Serebrennikova and Valentina Sarkisova for this succinct explanation. For a review

of the first conference of the heads of nursing schools, held on April 19–21, 1950, see "Vsesoiuznoe soveshchanie shkol meditsinskikh sester" [All-Union conference of nursing schools], *Meditsinskaia sestra*, no. 8 (1950): 30–31. Lin'kova, in her role as representative of the Moscow Council of Nurses, was quite active. See TsGAM, f. 533, op. 1, d. 19, l. 1. See also Susan Grant, "Devotion and Revolution: Nursing Values," in *Rethinking the Russian Revolution as Historical Divide*, ed. Matthias Neumann and Andy Willimott (London: Routledge, 2018), 173.

23. Lin'kova, "Moral'nyi oblik meditsinskoi sestry," 23–24. Some of the language here is similar to that in Pavel Beilin's 1949 work, as discussed by Burton. Pavel Beilin, "Chustvo dolga," *Chuvstvo dolga* (Kiev: Gosmedizdat, 1949), 222, in Chris Burton, "Medical Welfare During Late Stalinism. A Study of Doctors and the Soviet Health System, 1945–53," (PhD diss.: University of Chicago, 2000), 254. Burton argues that "in many ways, his writings resemble nineteenth century duties literature."

24. Lin'kova, "Moral'nyi oblik meditsinskoi sestry," 23–24.

25. E. A. Vsiukova, "Sanitarki" [Orderlies], *Meditsinskii rabotnik*, no. 46 (1957): 4.

26. Vsiukova, "Sanitarki," 4.

27. TsDAVO, f. R-4616, op. 1, d. 97, l. 3, 1956.

28. TsDAVO, f. R-4616, op. 1, d. 97, l. 4.

29. TsDAVO, f. R-4616, op. 1, d. 97, l. 9.

30. TsDAVO, f. R-4616, op. 1, d. 109, l. 48, 1957. Films and documentaries were also used as a teaching device in other medical institutes such as the Russian Academy of Medical Sciences, although there was a "complete absence of cinematic films on the academic program." See S. M. Reznikov, "Podgotovka meditsinskikh sester v meditsinskom uchilishche AMN SSSR" [Training nurses in medical colleges of the Soviet Academy of Medical Sciences], *Meditsinskaia sestra*, no. 2 (1961): 18 (citation), 19.

31. TsDAVO, f. R-4616, op. 1, d. 109, l. 52.

32. TsDAVO, f. R-4616, op. 1, d. 109, l. 53.

33. For more on Khrushchev's "crackdown" on young intellectuals after the Hungarian intervention, see Zubok, *Zhivago's Children*, 79–84. On the sense of confusion caused by de-Stalinization, see Cynthia Hooper, "What Can and Cannot Be Said: Between the Stalinist Past and New Soviet Future," *Slavonic and East European Review* 86, no. 2 (2008): 306–327.

34. Zubok, *Zhivago's Children*, 160.

35. TsDAVO, f. R-4616, op. 1, d. 97, ll. 27–28.

36. Marianne Liljestrom notes with regard to autobiographical texts that "idealised womanhood (and femininity) [was made] an effective tool of collectivist policies." Marianne Liljestrom, "Monitoring Selves: Soviet Women's Autobiographical Texts in the Khrushchev Era," in *Women in the Khrushchev Era*, ed. Melanie Ilic, Susan E. Reid, and Lynne Attwood (Basingstoke: Palgrave Macmillan, 2004), 141. See also Susan Grant, "Nurses in the Soviet Union: Explorations of Gender in State and Society," in *The Palgrave Handbook of Women and Gender in Twentieth-Century Russia and the Soviet Union*, ed. Melanie Ilic (London: Palgrave Macmillan, 2018), 259–261.

37. On the 1950s: Philip A. Kalisch and Beatrice J. Kalisch, "Nurses on Prime-Time Television," *American Journal of Nursing* 82, no. 2 (1982): 265; on the 1960s and 1970s: Philip A. Kalisch and Beatrice J. Kalisch, "The Image of the Nurse in Motion Pictures," *American Journal of Nursing* 82, no. 4 (1982): 610.

38. Christine Varga-Harris, *Stories of House and Home: Soviet Apartment Life during the Khrushchev Years* (Ithaca, NY: Cornell University Press, 2016), 135.

39. TsGAM, f. 1939, op. 1, d. 459, l. 1, February 14, 1962.

40. TsGAM, f. 1939, op. 1, d. 459, l. 2. See also Grant, "Nurses in the Soviet Union," 261.

41. TsGAM, f. 1939, op. 1, d. 459, l. 2.

42. TsGAM, f. 1939, op. 1, d. 459, l. 3.

43. TsGAM, f. 1939, op. 1, d. 459, l. 5.

44. Liljestrom avers that "ideologically and discursively women were expected to follow and internalise a certain set of gendered characteristics of 'emancipated womanhood.'" Liljestrom, "Monitoring Selves," 141.

45. "Vrach i bol'noi" [Doctor and patient], *Meditsinskii rabotnik*, no. 53 (1962): 13.

46. Victoria Smolkin, *A Sacred Space Is Never Empty: A History of Soviet Atheism* (Princeton, NJ: Princeton University Press, 2018), 141.

47. Tat'iana Tess, "Prizvanie k dobrotu" [Calling to kindness], *Izvestiia*, no. 272 (1964): 3.

48. "O medsestre, o niane" [On the nurse, on the nanny], *Meditsinskaia gazeta*, no. 80 (1971): 4.

49. Tess, "Prizvanie k dobrotu," 3.

50. V. Kalin', "Sestra miloserdiia" [Sister of mercy], *Izvestiia*, no. 65 (1975): 6.

51. Kalin', "Sestra miloserdiia," 6.

52. TsDAVO, f. R-4616, op. 1, d. 97, l. 29.

53. *Vracha vyzyvali?* [Did You Call for a Doctor?], directed by Vadim Gauzner (Leningrad: Lenfilm, 1974).

54. TsDAVO, f. R-4616, op. 1, d. 97, l. 28.

55. TsDAVO, f. R-4616, op. 1, d. 97, l. 28. The Soviet approach to diagnosis was based on the premise that too much information would inhibit recovery. See William A. Knaus, *Inside Russian Medicine: An American Doctor's First-Hand Report* (New York: Everest House, 1981), 126–127.

56. "Biuro meditsinskikh sester" [Nurse bureau], *Izvestiia*, no. 4 (1961): 4.

57. Tess, "Prizvanie k dobrotu," 3.

58. "Imeni Florens Naitingeil" [Named after Florence Nightingale], *Meditsinskaia sestra*, no. 1 (1975): 52. A maximum of thirty-six medals were awarded every two years. Here the author argued that Soviet success was recognition of the Soviet contribution to the Second World War.

59. TsDAVO, f. R-4616, op. 1, d. 198, l. 1. Here Z. Maiorova, deputy representative of the Executive Committee of the Soviet Red Cross and Red Crescent, wrote to her Ukrainian counterpart to forward three candidates, December 14, 1962. Also on expanding contacts, see TsDAVO, f. R-4616, op. 1, d. 198, l. 43. There is also material on Soviet contact with the International Committee of the Red Cross as well as the Nightingale Medal in GARF, from 1961 through to the 1980s (for example, GARF, f. 9501, op. 5, d. 634).

60. International Committee of the Red Cross, "Eighteenth Award of the Florence Nightingale Medal," 1961, accessed January 25, 2021, https://international-review.icrc.org/sites/default/files/S0020860400010366a.pdf.

61. V. Zaitseva, "Odna is 36," *Meditsinskii rabotnik* 8 (1966): 4. For information on and photographs of the five winners and the local award ceremonies, see International

Committee of the Red Cross, "Twentieth Award of the Florence Nightingale Award," 1965, accessed January 25, 2021, https://international-review.icrc.org/sites/default/files/S0020860400090318a.pdf.

62. "Na perednem krae sovetskogo zdravookhraneniia," *Meditsinskaia sestra*, no. 8 (1965): 44. In 1966 middle medical personnel numbered 1,777,500 and doctors 577,700. A. A. Romenskii, "Sovetskoe zdravookhraneniia za 10 let v tsifrakh" [Soviet health-care over 10 years in figures], *Meditsinskaia sestra*, no. 11 (1967): 12.

63. The number of beds and medical workers increased. There were about 300,000 doctors and 900,000 middle medical workers in 1955, compared to 130,400 doctors in 1940 and 421,200 middle medical workers by January 1, 1941. I. B. Rostotskii, "Istoricheskoe reshenie" [Historical decision], *Meditsinskaia sestra*, no. 8 (1955): 4, 5.

64. In the Ukrainian SSR, Red Cross nurses were not paid to study after 1950 (they had previously been paid owing to nursing shortages), and that year 27 nursing courses were organized on a voluntary basis (*na obshchestvennykh nachalakh*). By 1951 the number had increased to 180 courses with 5,069 students. TsDAVO, f. R-4616, op. 1, d. 109, l. 60. The Red Cross trained two types of nurse at that time: "nurses with complete middle medical education and reserve nurses with 8 months study on a paid basis."

65. GARF, f. 9501, op. 3, d. 289, l. 1, 1954–1956. The number graduating from SOKK courses was to increase further, with a target of 200,000 nurses set for 1955–1957; 50,000 of these would be in two-year courses and 150,000 in short-term courses.

66. Zubok, *Zhivago's Children*, 161–162.

67. GARF, f. 9501, op. 3, d. 509, l. 1, July 1, 1960–January 1, 1961; "Biuro meditsinskikh sester," 4.

68. "Biuro meditsinskikh sester," 4.

69. Alison Bashford, "Domestic Scientists: Modernity, Gender, and the Negotiation of Science in Australian Nursing, 1880–1910," *Journal of Women's History* 12, no. 2 (2000): 128.

70. "Biuro meditsinskikh sester," 4.

71. GARF, f. 9501, op. 3, d. 509, l. 2. Over the course of two months in 1960, SOKK nurses served over 8,000 people in Leningrad. See "Biuro meditsinskikh sester," 4.

72. GARF, f. 9501, op. 3, d. 509, l. 2. Some of the nurses were awarded monetary prizes.

73. See Melanie Ilic, "What Did Women Want? Khrushchev and the Revival of the *Zhensovety*," in *Soviet State and Society under Nikita Khrushchev*, ed. Melanie Ilic and Jeremy Smith (London: Routledge, 2009), 104–121.

74. A. I. Rogov, "O rabote Moskovskogo gorodskogo soveta meditsinskikh sester" [On the work of the Moscow city council of nurses], *Meditsinskaia sestra*, no. 10 (1962): 62.

75. Rogov, "O rabote Moskovskogo gorodskogo soveta," 62.

76. Oleg Kharkhordin, *The Collective and the Individual in Russia: A Study of Practices* (Berkeley: University of California Press, 1999), 280.

77. Donald Filtzer, *Soviet Workers and De-Stalinization* (Cambridge: Cambridge University Press, 1992), 42–43.

78. GARF, f. 9501, op. 3, d. 509, l. 3.

79. GARF, f. 9501, op. 3, d. 509, l. 4.

80. GARF, f. 9501, op. 3, d. 509, l. 7.

81. GARF, f. 9501, op. 3, d. 509, l. 7.

82. GARF, f. 9501, op. 3, d. 509, l. 7.

83. GARF, f. 9501, op. 3, d. 538, l. 1, 1974.

84. GARF, f. 9501, op. 3, d. 538, l. 3. The Soviet Union had three categories of disability and corresponding social welfare benefits. Those in the first category, known as Group I, were "severely disabled and unable to work," Group II "had loss of more than one organ" but could "work only in special conditions," while Group III "had loss or impairment of one limb or organ" and could work. See Shaw, *Deaf in the USSR*, 95; Burton, "Medical Welfare During Late Stalinism," 268.

85. GARF, f. 9501, op. 3, d. 538, l. 4.

86. GARF, f. 9501, op. 3, d. 538, l. 7.

87. "Zabotlivo okhranit' zdorov'e i trud medikov" [Carefully protecting the health and work of medics], *Meditsinskii rabotnik*, no. 82 (1956): 4.

88. "Zabotlivo okhranit' zdorov'e i trud medikov," 4.

89. "Zabotlivo okhranit' zdorov'e i trud medikov," 4.

90. "Uluchshat' usloviia truda meditsinskikh rabotnikov" [Improving working conditions for medical workers], *Meditsinskii rabotnik*, no. 41 (1957): 1.

91. "Zabotlivo okhranit' zdorov'e i trud medikov," 4.

92. "Uluchshat' usloviia truda," 1.

93. "Uluchshat' usloviia truda," 1.

94. See, for example, the Ministry of Health decree on patient and medical workers' safety with regard to radioactivity. The Library of normative-legal acts of the Union of the Soviet Socialist Republic (Biblioteka normativno-pravovykh aktov Soiuza Sovetskikh Sotsialisticheskikh Respublik), LibUSSR.RU, May 25, 1977, accessed June 12, 2019, http://www.libussr.ru/doc_ussr/usr_9314.htm.

95. A. Tentsova, "Aktual'nye voprosy srednego meditsinskogo obrazovaniia" [Actual Questions of middle medical education], *Meditsinskii rabotnik*, no. 72 (1955): 2. Tentsova was the deputy head of the Ministry of Health USSR's main administration for medical institutes.

96. "Luchshe gotovit' srednie meditsinskie kadry" [It is better to train middle medical workers], *Meditsinskii rabotnik*, no. 100 (1961): 1.

97. "Luchshe gotovit' srednie meditsinskie kadry," 1.

98. E. A. Kolesnikova, "Oshibki i nedostatki v tekhnike raboty meditsinskikh sester i ikh preduprezhdenie" [Errors and shortcomings in the technical work of nurses and their prevention], *Meditsinskaia sestra*, no. 4 (1956): 14.

99. TsGAM, f. 498, op. 1, d. 246, l. 3.

100. V. Poltoranov and L. Gol'dfail', "N. A. Semashko i kurorti" [N. A. Semashko and resorts], *Meditsinskaia gazeta*, no. 75 (1974): 4.

101. GAGS, f. 180, op. 1, d. 18, l. 86, 1950.

102. Statistics from the first half of 1950 showed that southern Crimea had the most patient complaints (fifty-two in 1949, or 25 percent of all Union complaints). Complaints touched on, for example, medical service, diet, and cultural service. The republic with the most complaints was Georgia, where patient service was "particularly bad." GARF, f. 9228, op. 1, d. 645, l. 298.

103. GAGS, f. 180, op. 1, d. 18, l. 87.

104. GAGS, f. 180, op. 1, d. 18, l. 60.

105. GAGS, f. 180, op. 1, d. 18, l. 60.

106. GAGS, f. 180, op. 1, d. 18, l. 87.

107. "Nurses at the Moscow Exhibition," *American Journal of Nursing* 59, no. 11 (1959): 1594–1595.

108. TsGAM, f. 1939, op. 1, d. 439, ll. 12–13, August 11, 1961.

109. TsGAM, f. 1939, op. 1, d. 439, l. 14.

110. TsGAM, f. 1939, op. 1, d. 439, l. 14.

111. TsGAM, f. 1939, op. 1, d. 439, l. 15.

112. TsGAM, f. 1939, op. 1, d. 439, l. 19.

113. Catriona Kelly, *Refining Russia: Advice Literature, Polite Culture, and Gender from Catherine to Yeltsin* (Oxford: Oxford University Press: 2001), 331.

114. Marina Balina and Evgeny Dobrenko, eds., *Petrified Utopia: Happiness Soviet Style* (London: Anthem Press, 2009), xvi.

115. Vladimir A. Tsesis, *Communist Daze: The Many Misadventures of a Soviet Doctor* (Bloomington: Indiana University Press, 2017), 22.

116. Tsesis, *Communist Daze*, 22.

117. Tsesis, *Communist Daze*, 31.

118. Kate Sara Schecter, "Professionals in Post-Revolutionary Regimes: A Case Study of Soviet Doctors" (PhD diss., Columbia University, 1992), 192.

119. GAGS, f. 175, op. 1, d. 79, ll. 24–24 ob, April 13, 1961. On the patient experience of sanatoria, see Johanna Conterio, "Places of Plenty: Patient Perspectives on Nutrition and Health in the Health Resorts of the USSR, 1917–1953," *Food and History* 14, no. 1 (2016): 135–169.

120. GAGS, f. 120, op. 1, d. 40, ll. 53–53, April 12, 1960; GAGS, f. 120, op. 1, d. 62, l. 53, March 23, 1963 (Metallurg).

121. GAGS, f. 120, op. 1, d. 63, June 8, 1963.

122. M. Kaziev, "Povyshat' kachestvo raboty kurortov" [Raising the quality of work of resorts], *Meditsinskii rabotnik*, no. 27 (1960): 2.

123. Varga-Harris, *Stories of House and Home*, 222.

124. TsGAM, f. 498, op. 1, d. 500, l. 19, 1976. The Ostroumova hospital received thirteen complaints in 1976.

125. GAGS, f. 120, op. 1, d. 17, l, 5, *kniga otzyvov* (comment book); GAGS, f. 120, op. 1, d. 193, January 24, 1974–December 8, 1976.

126. GAGS, f. 21, op. 1, d. 284, ll. 28–29, November 18, 1976.

127. GAGS, f. 21, op. 1, d. 284, l. 30.

128. GAGS, f. 21, op. 1, d. 92, l. 6, June 10, 1970.

129. D. A. Vershadskii, *Nekotorye osobennosti raboty sotrudnikov sanatorno-kurortnykh uchrezhdenii v svete trebovanii deontologii i maloi psikhoterapii* [A few particularities in the work of employees of sanitorium-resorts institutions in light of the demands of deontology and minor psychotherapy], (Sochi: VTsSPS, 1971), 4–8.

130. GAGS, f. 21, op. 1, d. 196, l. 10 ob, 11. 15, 17. See also, for example, GAGS, f. 21, op. 1, d. 209, ll. 13–14, 52; GAGS, f. 21, op. 1, d. 227, ll. 78–79.

131. GAGS, f. 21, op. 1, d. 209, ll. 2, 3.

132. Diane P. Koenker mentions this kind of template in *Club Red: Vacation Travel and the Soviet Dream* (Ithaca, NY: Cornell University Press, 2013), 179.

133. Varga-Harris, *Stories of House and Home*, 203.

134. Alexei Yurchak, *Everything Was Forever, Until It Was No More: The Last Soviet Generation* (Princeton, NJ: Princeton University Press, 2006), 8.

135. Vladimir E. Shlapentokh, "Two Levels of Public Opinion: The Soviet Case," *Public Opinion Quarterly* 49 (2001): 448.

136. Shlapentokh, "Two Levels of Public Opinion," 449–450.

137. "Doklad Tovarishch N. S. Khrushcheva" [Address by Comrade N. S. Khrushchev], *Izvestiia*, no. 166 (1964): 4; Field, *Soviet Socialized Medicine*, 128–130.

138. Field, *Soviet Socialized Medicine*, 131.

139. Linda J. Cook, *The Soviet Social Contract and Why It Failed: Welfare Policy and Workers' Politics from Brezhnev to Yeltsin* (Cambridge, MA; Harvard University Press, 1993), 20, 23.

140. Smolkin, *Sacred Space*, 197.

141. Smolkin, *Sacred Space*, 197.

142. "Edinstvo i sotrudnichestvo—vo imia gumanizma," [Unity and solidarity—in the name of humanism], *Meditsinskaia gazeta*, no. 86 (1975): 1–2.

143. "Edinstvo i sotrudnichestvo," 1–2. See also M. Ogurtsova, A. Popov, and M. Pokhvalova, "V dukhe solidarnosti i edinstva deistvii" [In the spirit of solidarity and united action], *Meditsinskaia gazeta*, no. 87 (1975): 2.

144. "Pod znamenem edinstva i gumanizma" [Under the banner of unity and humanism], *Meditsinskaia gazeta*, no. 5 (1975): 1.

145. V. Pravilova and A. Mamosueva, "Meditsinskaia sestra, ee spetsializatsiia" [The nurse, her specialization], *Meditsinskaia gazeta*, no. 96 (1967): 2. For similar accounts of nurses seeking improvement and professional development, see E. Korovina, "Sovet sester" [The council of nurses], *Meditsinskii rabotnik*, no. 79 (1968): 2; S. A. Beliaev, "Voprosy attestatsii srednikh meditsinskikh rabotnikov" [Questions of attestation for middle medical workers], *Fel'dsher i akusherka*, no. 12 (1966): 3–7.

146. There was an order on attestation for nurses in certain institutions in Moscow issued in 1973 and updated in 1977. The Library of normative-legal acts of the Union of the Soviet Socialist Republic (Biblioteka normativno-pravovykh aktov Soiuza Sovetskikh Sotsialisticheskikh Respublik), LibUSSR.RU, accessed June 12, 2019, http://www.libussr.ru/doc_ussr/usr_14330.htm. See also G. M. Perfil'eva, "Sestrinskoe delo v Rossii (sotsial'no-gigienicheskii analiz i prognoz)" Nursing in Russia (a socio-hygienic analysis and forecast)], (PhD diss., Moscow Medical Academy named for I. M. Sechenov, 1995), 82.

147. G. Ustinov, "Zdorov'e—tsennost' gosudarstvennaia," *Izvestiia*, no. 196 (1971): 3.

148. "Uchatsia meditsinskie sestry" [Nurses are studying] *Meditsinskaia gazeta*, no. 81 (1974): 1.

149. "Uchatsia meditsinskie sestry," 1.

150. *Oi, spasibo doktor* [Oh, Thank You Doctor], directed by A. Andreev (Moscow: TsSDF. RTsSDF, 1990). Available at Net-Film, http://net-film.ru/film-9818/?searchqой%20спасибо%20доктор.

151. Statistic for 1979. There were 960,500 doctors and 3 million junior medical personnel working in Soviet medical institutions (including educational institutes). *Bol'shaia meditsinskaia Entsiklopedia*, accessed November 27, 2020. https://бмэ.орг/index.php/МЕДИЦИНСКИЕ_КАДРЫ. At the end of 1974 there were 1,185,500 nurses, 525,100 feldshers, and 78,500 feldsher midwives and 244,100 midwives. Michael

Ryan, *The Organization of Soviet Medical Care* (New York: Professional Seminar Consultants, 1978), 71. Original source cited: *Narodnoe khoziaistvo SSSR* [National Economy of the USSR], 730 (for 1974).

152. "Meditsinskaia sestra" [Nurse], *Pravda*, no. 280 (1973): 1.

153. "Meditsinskaia sestra," 1.

154. L. Dvoinin, "Sestra miloserdiia—ne atlet" [The Sister of mercy—is not an athlete], *Izvestiia*, no. 78 (1974): 3. Problems in the healthcare service were also blamed on poor organization. See "Na prieme polyklinika" [In the polyclinic reception], *Izvestiia*, no. 68 (1975): 1; and the interview by S. Tutorskaia with Alexei G. Safonov, deputy minister for health, "Prakticheskaia meditsina: Problem i puti razvitiia" [Practical medicine: Problems and the paths to development], *Izvestiia*, no. 75 (1976): 5.

155. G. Gukasov, V. Komov, P. Novokshonov, and S. Tutorskaia (*Izvestiia*'s editorial brigade), "Tekhnika miloserdiia" [The technique of mercy], *Izvestiia*, no. 252 (1974): 2.

156. Gukasov et. al, "Tekhnika miloserdiia," 2.

157. E. Rapaport, "Medsestra u pribora . . ." [Nurse at the device . . .], *Meditsinskaia gazeta*, no. 41 (1973): 2.

158. P. Novokshonov, "Sestra miloserdiia" [Sister of mercy] *Izvestiia*, no. 259 (1971): 5.

159. I. Borich, ed., "Tvoi zaboty, medsestra" [Your concern, nurse], *Meditsinskaia gazeta*, no. 11 (1974): 2.

160. Tsesis, *Communist Daze*, 33.

161. Ogurtsova, Popov, and Pokhvalova, "V dukhe solidarnosti i edinstva deistvii," 2.

162. TsGAM, f. 498, op. 1, d. 462, l .3.

163. *Vracha vyzyvali?*

164. Filtzer, *Soviet Workers and De-Stalinization*, 53.

165. Filtzer, *Soviet Workers and De-Stalinization*, 53–54.

166. See Elena Zdravomyslova and Anna Temkina, "The Crisis of Masculinity in Late Soviet Discourse," *Russian Studies in History* 51, no. 2 (2012): 21.

167. Donald Filtzer, "Women Workers in the Khrushchev Era," in *Women in the Khrushchev Era*, ed. Melanie Ilic, Susan E. Reid, and Lynne Attwood (Basingstoke: Palgrave Macmillan, 2004), 47.

168. Natalia Baranskaia's "A Week Like any Other" was published in *Novyi mir* in 1969 and first published in English in 1974.

169. TsGAM, f. 498, op. 1, d. 526, l. 1.

170. TsGAM, f. 498, op. 1, d. 526, l. 1.

171. TsGAM, f. 498, op. 1, d. 526, l. 1.

172. TsGAM, f. 498, op. 1, d. 526, l. 1.

173. TsGAM, f. 498, op. 1, d. 526, l. 1.

174. TsGAM, f. 498, op. 1, d. 526, l. 3.

175. For more on Znanie, see Smolkin, *Sacred Space*, 61, 140.

176. TsGAM, f. 498, op. 1, d. 526, l. 3.

177. *Oi, spasibo doktor.*

178. V. S. Grazhul', "Etika meditsinskogo rabotnika" [Ethics of the medical worker], *Fel'dsher i akusherka*, no. 11 (1966): 24–29. Medical workers were told not to conceal the mistakes of colleagues, but not to identify any perceived mistakes in the patient's company. See also A. L. Ostapenko, "Etiket srednego meditsinskogo rabotnika" [Etiquette of the middle medical worker], *Fel'dsher i akusherka*, no. 1 (1985): 7–8.

179. R. M. Sokirianskaia, "Ateisticheskoe vospitanie uchashchikhsia meditsinskikh uchilishch" [Atheist education of students in medical college], *Fel'dsher i akusherka*, no. 11 (1971): 44, 48. The author encouraged more widespread propaganda work, including talks on the topics of "medicine and religion" and "women and religion."

180. Michael Binyon, *Life in Russia* (London: Panther/Granada, 1983), 83. Many of the articles on ethics and moral character in *Meditsinskaia sestra* also referred to a lack of care or negative attitudes.

181. A. Terekhov, "Vera Bezukh, Sestra miloserdiia" [Vera Bezukh, Sister of mercy], *Meditsinskaia gazeta*, no. 56 (1974): 4.

182. Knaus, *Inside Russian Medicine*, 130.

183. Knaus, *Inside Russian Medicine*, 131.

184. L. Cherpakova, "Oshibka medsestry . . . tol'ko li?," *Meditsinskaia gazeta*, no. 67 (1974): 2.

185. TsAGM f. 1939, op. 1, d. 723, l. 89, March 5, 1976; report, 1975–1976. I have changed the nurse's name and surname.

186. TsGAM, f. 1939, op. 1, d. 723, l. 89.

187. Knaus, *Inside Russian Medicine*, 111.

188. R. Nazarov, in "Dlia medsester i sanitarok" [For nurses and orderlies], *Meditsinskaia gazeta*, no. 103 (1976): 2.

189. See the Ministry of Health USSR, decree issued on May 25, 1977, accessed June 12, 2019, http://www.libussr.ru/doc_ussr/usr_9314.htm.

190. Binyon, *Life in Russia*, 83.

191. Schecter, "Professionals in Post-Revolutionary Regimes," 107.

192. Sarah Helmstadter, "Splitting Headache," *New Republic* (1990), cited in Schechter, "Professionals in Post-Revolutionary Regimes," 107.

193. Schechter, "Professionals in Post-Revolutionary Regimes," 176–177.

194. James R. Millar, "The Little Deal: Brezhnev's Contribution to Acquisitive Socialism," *Slavic Review* 44, no. 4 (1985): 696.

195. Cook, *Soviet Social Contract*, 52.

196. "Blago naroda—vysshaia tsel'" [The welfare of the people—is the highest goal], *Izvestiia*, no. 63 (1981): 2.

197. L. Ivchenko, "Poluchite niania, progressivku . . ." [Get a nanny, a progressive], *Izvestiia*, no. 193 (1984): 3. The statistic on nurses is for 1982. S. I. Korovina, "Rol' medsestry v sokhranenii meditsinskii tainy" [The role of the nurse and preserving medical confidentiality], *Meditsinskaia sestra*, no. 5 (1983): 50.

198. Ivchenko, "Poluchite niania, progressivku," 3. Ibid.

199. S. Gladysh, "Medsestra" [Nurse], *Izvestiia* (1984): 3.

200. Gladysh, "Medsestra," 3.

201. Gladysh, "Medsestra," 3.

202. TsGAM, f. 498, op. 1, d. 631, ll. 32–34, Moscow, April 12, 1982; TsGAM, f. 1939, op. 1, d. 665, l. 17 ob.

203. G. V. Dvorkin, "Liudi dumaiut o liudiakh" [People are thinking about people], *Meditsinskaia sestra*, no. 6 (1982): 3.

204. Dvorkin, "Liudi dumaiut o liudiakh," 4.

205. A. Serdiuk, "Belyi khalat i chistaia sovest'" [A white gown and a clean conscience], *Izvestiia*, no. 38 (1982): 2. Serdiuk was speaking about Ukraine.

206. Serdiuk, "Belyi khalat i chistaia sovest'," 2.

207. The code included attentiveness, confidentiality, humanity, and conscientiousness. For a full list, see A. L. Ostapenko, "Obshchie pravovye i deontologicheskie normy vzaimootnoshenii meditsinskoi sestry i bol'nogo" [General legal and deontological norms between a nurse and a patient], *Meditsinskaia sestra*, no. 2 (1985): 61–63.

208. A. L. Ostapenko, "Miloserdie sestry v sovremennykh usloviiakh" [Sisters of mercy in modern conditions], *Meditsinskaia sestra*, no. 2 (1986): 63.

209. Ostapenko, "Obshchie pravovye," 61–63.

210. A. L. Ostapenko, "Professional'naia etika i moral' srednego meditsinskogo rabotnika" [The professional ethics and morality of the middle medical worker], *Fel'dsher i akusherka*, no. 10 (1983): 9. The Engels quotation is from Karl Marx and Friedrich Engels, *Sochineniia* [*Essays*] (Second edition: volume 21), 298–299.

211. Andropov, Iu. *Izbrannyie Rechi i Stati* [Selected speeches and articles], (Moscow: Politizdat, 1983), cited in Shlapentokh, "Two Levels of Public Opinion," 447.

212. N. V. Erenkova, "O nravstvennom oblike i delovykh kachestvakh srednego meditsinskogo rabotnika" [On the moral character and business qualities of the middle medical worker], *Meditsinskaia sestra*, no. 3 (1985): 62.

213. Erenkova, "O nravstvennom oblike," 62.

214. Mark G. Field, "Soviet Health Problems and the Convergence Hypothesis," in Anthony Jones (ed.), *Soviet Social Problems* (Boulder: Westview Press, 1991), 79–80 cited in Schecter, "Professionals in Post-Revolutionary Regimes," 193.

215. TsGAM, f. 1939, op. 1, d. 875, l. 8, 1986.

216. TsGAM, f. 1939, op. 1, d. 875, l. 8.

217. TsGAM, f. 1939, op. 1, d. 875, l. 9.

218. TsGAM, f. 1939, op. 1, d. 875, l. 9.

219. TsGAM, f. 1939, op. 1, d. 665, l. 26.

220. TsGAM, f. 1939, op. 1, d. 665, l. 29.

221. See Prikaz, October 9, 1987, accessed June 12, 2019, The Library of normative-legal acts of the Union of the Soviet Socialist Republic (Biblioteka normativno-pravovykh aktov Soiuza Sovetskikh Sotsialisticheskikh Respublik), LibUSSR.RU, http://www.libussr.ru/doc_ussr/usr_14330.htm. This source also references the Ministry of Health 1986 decree, issued on October 24, 1986. Attestation for these categories was due to begin in 1988. These are all outlined in the decree on the LibUSSR.RU website with Soviet laws.

222. R. Talyshinskii and T. Khudiakova, "Nado li platit' za lechenie?" [Is it necessary to pay for treatment?], *Izvestiia*, no. 267 (1987): 3. The article covered the views of specialists and patients.

223. Talyshinskii and Khudiakova, "Nado li platit' za lechenie?," 3.

224. Talyshinskii and Khudiakova, "Nado li platit' za lechenie?," 3.

225. Talyshinskii and Khudiakova, "Nado li platit' za lechenie?," 3.

226. *Chetvertyi son Anny Andreevny* [The fourth sleep of Anna Andreevna], directed by N. Obukhovich (Leningrad: Leningradskii studiia dokumental'nykh filmov, 1988), accessed April 4, 2019, https://www.net-film.ru/film. N. G. Chernyshevsky was a Russian writer and theoretician who was influential in the revolutionary thought of V. I. Lenin.

227. Cook, *Soviet Social Contract*, 129.

228. Cook, *Soviet Social Contract*, 129.

229. *Oi, spasibo doktor*. See also the film's notes identifying those interviewed.

230. Vera Dunham, *In Stalin's Time: Middleclass Values in Soviet Fiction*, enlarged and updated ed. (Durham, NC: Duke University Press, 1990). First published 1976 by Cambridge University Press.

231. Smolkin, *Sacred Space*.

Epilogue

1. N. A. Beliakova, *Sestry miloserdiia Rossii* (St. Petersburg: Liki-Rossii, 2005), 313.

2. Beliakova, *Sestry miloserdiia Rossii*, 313.

3. For more on study plans and resolutions, see G. M. Perfil'eva, "Sestrinskoe delo v Rossii (sotsial'no-gigienicheskii analiz i prognoz)" (PhD diss., Moscow Medical Academy named for I. M. Sechenov, 1995), 82.

4. The Soviet Interview Project was conducted in the early 1980s. Similar to the HPSSS project before it, respondents were recent Soviet emigrants to the United States. For full discussion of the origins and development of the Soviet Interview Project, see the foreword and chapter 1 in Alex Inkeles and Raymond A. Bauer, *The Soviet Citizen: Daily Life in a Totalitarian Society* (New York: Atheneum, 1968), vii–30.

5. Inkeles and Bauer, *The Soviet Citizen: Daily Life in a Totalitarian Society*, 236–237.

6. For more, see James R. Millar and Elizabeth Clayton, "Quality of Life: Subjective Measures of Relative Satisfaction," in *Politics, Work, and Daily Life in the USSR: A Survey of Former Soviet Citizens*, ed. James R. Miller (Cambridge: Cambridge University Press, 1987), 50–51.

7. Perfil'eva, *Sestrinskoe delo v Rossii*, 82.

8. *ILO Nursing Personnel Convention No. 149* (Geneva: International Labor Organization, 1977), 1, accessed December 4, 2018, http://www.who.int/hrh/nursing_midwifery/nursing_convention_C149.pdf. This publication was updated in 2002. The 1979 ratification refers to the Russian Federation, Belarus, and Ukraine (4).

9. *ILO Nursing Personnel Convention No. 149*, 2.

10. Perfil'eva, *Sestrinskoe delo v Rossii*, 83.

11. Perfil'eva, *Sestrinskoe delo v Rossii*, 82.

12. For more on the Russian Nurses Association, see "Obshcherossiiskaia obshchestvennaia organizatsiia 'Assotsiatsiia meditsinskikh sester Rossii'" [The general Russian social organization 'The Association of Nurses of Russia'], https://medsestre.ru/istorija/, accessed July 14, 2021.

13. Valentina Sarkisova, interview with the author, St. Petersburg, October 10, 2014.

14. Sarkisova, interview.

15. Sarkisova, interview.

16. Nurses in St. Petersburg, interview with author, March 2015. The nurses in these cases are anonymous.

17. Sarkisova, interview.

18. Nurses in St. Petersburg, interview.

19. "What Do Nurses in Russia Really Earn?," Woman.ru forum, accessed December 12, 2018, http://www.woman.ru/health/medley7/thread/4082492/2/.

20. Again, this is an international problem. See Howard Catton, *International Council of Nurses Workforce Forums* (International Center on Nurse Migration: Philadelphia,

PA, May 2018), 14, accessed December 12, 2018, https://www.icn.ch/sites/default/files/inline-files/2018_Pay%20data%20analysis.pdf.

21. Catton, *International Council of Nurses Workforce Forums*, 14.

Coda

1. Karin Hedlund Morris, "Profile of a Russian Nurse," *American Journal of Nursing* 66, no. 3: (1966): 550.

Archives and Libraries Consulted

Archives

Moscow, Russian Federation

Gosudarstvennyi arkhiv Rossiiskoi Federatsii [State Archive of the Russian Federation] (GARF)

Reading Room 1: USSR

f. 3316	Tsentral'nyi Ispolnitel'nyi Komitet SSSR (TsIK SSSR)
f. 3341	Tsentral'nyi Komitet Rossiiskogo Obshchestva Krasnogo Kresta (Tsentrokrest, TsK ROKK)
f. 4094	Upravleniia predstavitelei Rossiiskogo Obshchestva Krasnogo Kresta pri Armiiakh zapadnogo fronta i 6-i armii
f. 5451	Vsesoiuznyi Tsentral'nyi Sovet Professional'nykh Soiuzov (VTsSPS)
f. 5515	Narodnyi Komissariat Truda SSSR (Narkomtrud, NKT SSSR)
f. 5532	Tsentral'noe pravlenie Vserossiiskogo Soiuza Sester Miloserdiia
f. 5465	Tsentral'nye Komitety Professional'nykh Soiuzov Meditsinskikh Rabotnikov
f. 8009	Ministerstvo Zdravookhraneniia SSSR
f. 8131	Prokuratura SSSR
f. 9501	Soiuz Obshchestv Krasnogo Kresta i Krasnogo Polumesiatsa SSSR (SOKK i KP SSSR)
f. 9228	Glavnoe Upravlenie Kurortov i Sanatoriev (Glavkursanupr) Ministerstva Zdravookhraneniia SSSR
f. 9592	Gilyarovskii Vasili Alekseevich, chlen-korrespondent Akademii Meditsinskikh Nauk SSR, Obshchestvennyi deiatel', zasluzhennyi deiatel' nauki RSFSR

Reading Room 2: RSFSR

f. A-482   Ministerstvo Zdravookhraneniia RSFSR (Minzdrav RSFSR)

f. A-1565   Glavnoe Upravlenie Professional'nogo Obrazovaniia (Glavpro-fobr) Narkomata Prosveshcheniia RSFSR

ROSSIISKOGO GOSUDARSTVENNYI ARKHIV SOTSIAL'NO-POLITICHESKOI ISTORII [RUSSIAN STATE ARCHIVE OF SOCIO-POLITICAL HISTORY] (RGASPI)

f. 17   Tsentral'nyi komitet KPSS (1898, 1903–1991)

f. 82   Molotov Viacheslav Mikhailovich

f. 603   Vsesoiuznyi komitet pomoshchi po obsluzhivaniiu bol'nykh i ranenykh boitsov i komandirov Krasnoi Armii

ARCHIVE REPOSITORY NO. 2: COMMUNIST YOUTH LEAGUE (RGASPI-M)

f. 1M   Central Committee of the VLKSM

f. 7M   Vystavka TsK VLKSM "Leninsko-Stalinskii Komsomol"

ROSSIISKII GOSUDARSTVENNYI VOENNYI ARKHIV [RUSSIAN STATE MILITARY ARCHIVE] (RGVA)

f. 19032   Kommunisticheskaia krasnoarmeiskii gospital' Moskvy

TSENTRAL'NYI GOSUDARSTVENNYI ARKHIV GORODA MOSKVY [CENTRAL STATE ARCHIVE OF THE CITY OF MOSCOW] (TsGA MOSKVY)

Otdel khraneniia dokumentov posle 1917 goda (OKhD posle 1917 g.)—Fondy byvshego Tsentral'nogo arkhiva goroda Moskvy (TsAGM) from 2005 to 2013, and TsMAM from 1993–2013

f. 389   Psikhonevrologicheskaia gorodskaia klinicheskaia bol'nitsa No. 1 im. P. P. Kashchenko Mosgorzdravotdela

f. 498   Gorodskaia klinicheskaia bol'nitsa No. 33 im. A. A. Ostroumova

f. 533   Psikhonevrologicheskaia gorodskaia bol'nitsa No. 4 im. Gan-nushkina. Mosgorzdravotdela

f. 552   Moskovskii gorodskoi otdel zdravookhraneniia Mosgorispolkoma

f. 1939   Moskovskaia gorodskaia klinicheskaia bol'nitsa imena S. P. Botkina

f. 2299   Moskovskaia gorodskaia klinicheskaia bol'nitsa imena soiuza Medsantrud

TSENTRAL'NYI GOSUDARSTVENNYI ARKHIV MOSKOVSKOI OBLASTI [CENTRAL STATE ARCHIVE OF MOSCOW OBLAST] (TsGAMO)

f. 975   Moskovskii uezdnyi zdravotdel

St. Petersburg, Russian Federation

Tsentral'nyi gosudarstvennyi arkhiv istoriko-politicheskikh dokumentov Sankt-Peterburga [Central State Archive of Historico-Political Records of St. Petersburg] (TsGAIPD SPb)

f. 1	Petrogradskii Komitet RKP (B). Petrograd. 1917–1920.
f. 24	Leningradskii oblastnoi komitet KPSS. Smol'ninskii raion, Leningrad. 1927–1991.
f. 235	Fraktsiia VKP (B) Leningradskogo oblastnogo otdela professional'nogo soiuza rabotnikov lechebno-sanitarnogo dela "Medsantrud" (1919–1930). Tsentral'no-gorodskoi raion, Leningrad.
f. K-598	Leningradskii oblastnoi komitet VLKSM. Smol'ninskii raion, Leningrad. 1925–1996.
f. K-881	Leningradskii gorkom VLKSM. Leningrad. 1931–1990.

Tsentral'nyi gosudarstvennyi arkhiv Sankt-Peterburga [Central State Archive of St. Petersburg] (TsGASPb)

f. 2738	Bol'nitsa "V Pamiat' 5-letiia Oktiabr'skoi revoliutsii" otdela zdravookhraneniia Petrogradskogo soveta rabochikh, krest'ianskikh i krasnoarmeiskikh deputatov. Petrograd. 1918–1939.
f. 2745	Gavanskaia bol'nitsa otdela zdravookhraneniia Petrogradskogo gubernskogo ispolnitel'nogo komiteta soveta rabochikh, krest'ianskikh i krasnoarmeiskikh deputatov. Petrograd. 1918–1922.
f. 2916	Bol'nitsa imeni Karla Marksa Petrogradskogo gubernskogo otdela zdravookhraneniia. Petrograd. 1919–1923.

Sochi, Russian Federation

Gosudarstvennyi Arkhiv Goroda Sochi [State Archive of Sochi] (GAGS)

f. 21	Sanatarii "Kavkazskaia Riv'era"
f. 120	Sanatarii "Metallurg"
f. 175	Sochinskii sanatoria "Primor'e"
f. 180	Sochinskii sanatorii "Dendrarii"

Tambov, Russian Federation

Gosudarstvennyi arkhiv Tambovskoi oblasti [State Archive of Tambov Oblast] (GATO)

f. 1512	Otdel zdravookhraneniia ispolnitel'nogo komiteta Tambovskogo gubernskogo Soveta rabochikh, krest'ianskikh i krasnoarmeiskikh deputatov (gubzdravotdel)

Kyiv, Ukraine

Tsentral'nyi derzhavnyi arkhiv vishchikh organiv vladi ta upravleniia Ukrainy [Central State Archive of the Supreme Organs of Government and Administration of Ukraine] (TsDAVO)

f. R-342   Ministerstvo okhorony zdorov'ia Ukrainy, m. Kyiv / Ministerstvo Zdravookhraneniia USSR, g. Kiev

f. R-4616   Tsentral'nyi Komitet Tovarystva Chernogo Khresta, URSR, m. Kyiv / Tsentral'nyi Komitet Obshchestva Krasnogo Kresta USSR g. Kiev

London, United Kingdom

Imperial War Museum

Florence Farmborough, Oral History, 000312/17/06

Library of the Society of Friends (LSF), Quakers in Britain, Friends House

FSC/RU/PO/2 Russia and Poland Committee: Folders 2, 3, 4
FWR/RU/1/5 From Moscow No. 2 October 1926–December 1927
GQM Europe

Philadelphia, United States

American Friends Service Committee (AFSC) Archive

AFSC Committee Minutes
AFSC Minutes
Foreign Service (FS), Russia General
Foreign Service Section (FSS), Russia
General Administration
General Files: Foreign Service

Barbara Bates Center for the Study of the History of Nursing, University of Pennsylvania School of Nursing

International Council of Nurses (ICN) Refugee Nurses Series, MC112, box 16

New York City, United States

Columbia University Rare Book and Manuscript Library

Andrea Aleksandra Stegman Memoirs, 1954–1968 (Bakhmeteff Archive)
Lillian Wald Papers

Rockefeller Archive Center (RAC), Sleepy Hollow

Collection: Rockefeller Foundation Records (RF); record group (RG) 1.1 Projects; Series: 785 USSR; Sub-Series: A Medical Sciences; box 2; folders 15, 16, 17
Collection: RF; RG 1.1 Projects; Series: 785 USSR; Subseries: C Nursing; box 1; folders 2, 4
Collection: RF; RG 1.1 Projects; Series: 785 USSR; Subseries: C Nursing; box 3; folders 28, 29

Collection: RF; RG 1.1 Projects; Series: 100 c International; Subseries: C Nursing; box 37; folder 314

Collection: RF; RG 1.1 Projects; Series: 100 c International; Subseries: C Nursing; box 38; folder 341

Collection: RF; RG 1.1 Projects; Series: 100 c Progress Report; Subseries: C Nursing; box 38; folder 332

Collection: RF; RG 1.1 Projects; Series: 100 c Original Box 38; Subseries: C Nursing; box 38; folder 332

Collection: RF; RG 1.1 Projects; Series: 100 c Original Box 37; Subseries: C Nursing; box 4; folders 302, 341, 342

Collection: RF; RG 1.1 Projects; Officer Diaries RG 12, A-E. Disc 2 Mary Beard, 1911–1992

Collection: RF; RG 1.1 Projects; Officer Diaries RG 12, A-E. Disc 1 Alan Gregg

Washington DC, United States

Library of Congress

Lavinia L. Dock Papers

Libraries

Aldham Library, Liverpool John Moores University
Brotherton Library, University of Leeds
Moscow State Library
National Library of Russia, St. Petersburg
Robarts Library and Gerstein Library, University of Toronto
Sechenov Central Scientific Medical Library, Moscow

Periodicals

Biulleten' Narodnogo Kommissariata zdravookhraneniia / Biulleten' Narkomzdrava
Bol'nichnoe delo
Damskii mir
Fel'dsher
Fel'dsher i akusherka
Fe'ldsherskii mysl'
Gigiena i sotsialisticheskoe zdravookhranenie
Istoricheskii vestnik
Istoriia zdravookhraneniia i meditsina
Izvestiia
Krest'ianka
Meditsina
Meditsinskaia sestra
Meditsinskii rabotnik / Meditsinskaia gazeta
Na fronte zdravookhraneniia / Voprosy zdravookhraneniia
Pervyi vestnik sestry miloserdiia
Pravda

Rabotnitsa
Sestrinskoe delo
Sovetskaia meditsina
Vestnik Krasnogo Kresta
Vestnik sovremennoi meditsiny
Voenno-meditsinskii zhurnal
Voprosy zdravookhraneniia
Za kadry srednego meditsinskogo personala
Za sanitarnuiu oboronu
Zhenskii mir
Zhenskii vestnik
Zhenskii zhurnal
Zhenskoe delo

Index

Ingram Content Group UK Ltd.
Milton Keynes UK
UKHW040314240323
419035UK00019B/422